S0-BQY-737

Endoscopic Surgery of the Paranasal Sinuses and Anterior Skull Base

Malte Erik Wigand

with the collaboration of W. Hosemann
and contributions
by M. Brandl and M. Weidenbecher

Translated by P. M. Stell

Foreword by David W. Kennedy

183 color plates, 14 tables

1990
Georg Thieme Verlag Stuttgart · New York
Thieme Medical Publishers, Inc., New York

Prof. Dr. med. M. E. Wigand, Direktor der Klinik und Poliklinik für Hals-Nasen-Ohrenkranke der Universität Erlangen-Nürnberg, Waldstraße 1, 8520 Erlangen, West Germany

Dr. med. W. Hosemann, Oberarzt der Klinik und Poliklinik für Hals-Nasen-Ohrenkranke, Universität Erlangen-Nürnberg, Waldstraße 1, 8520 Erlangen, West Germany

Translator:
Prof. P. M. Stell, Ch. M., F. R. C. S., University of Liverpool, Royal Liverpool Hospital, Prescot St. P.O. Box 147, Liverpool L69 3BX, United Kingdom

Prof. Dr. med. M. Brandl, Institut für Anaesthesiologie der Universität Erlangen-Nürnberg, Krankenhausstraße 12, 8520 Erlangen, West Germany

Prof. Dr. med. M. Weidenbecher, Leitender Oberarzt der Klinik und Poliklinik für Hals-Nasen-Ohrenkranke der Universität Erlangen-Nürnberg, Waldstraße 1, 8520 Erlangen, West Germany

ESKIND BIOMEDICAL LIBRARY

DEC 0 6 1996

VANDERBILT UNIVERSITY
NASHVILLE, TN 37232-8340

Important Note: Medicine is an ever-changing science. Research and clinical experience are continually broadening our knowledge, in particular our knowledge of proper treatment and drug therapy. Insofar as this book mentions any dosage or application, readers may rest assured that the authors, editors and publishers have made every effort to ensure that such references are strictly in accordance with the **state of knowledge at the time of production of the book.** Nevertheless, every user is requested to examine carefully the manufacturer's leaflets accompanying each drug to check on his own responsibility whether the dosage schedules recommended therein or the contraindications stated by the manufacturers differ from the statements made in the present book. Such examination is particularly important with drugs that are either rarely used or have been newly released on the market.

Library of Congress Cataloging-in-Publication Data

Wigand, M. E.
[Endoskopische Chirurgie der Nasennebenhöhlen und der vorderen Schädelbasis. English]
Endoscopic surgery of the paranasal sinuses and anterior skull base / Malte Erik Wigand: with the collaboration of W. Hosemann and contributions by M. Brandl and M. Weidenbecher.
p. cm.
Translation of: Endoskopische Chirurgie der Nasennebenhöhlen und der vorderen Schädelbasis.
Includes bibliographical references.
1. Paranasal sinuses – Endoscopic surgery. 2. Skull base – Surgery, I. Title.
[DNLM: 1. Endoscopy. 2. Paranasal Sinuses – surgery, 3. Skull – surgery. WV 340 W654e]
RF 421.W5413 1990
617.5'1 – dc20
DNLM/DLC
for Library of Congress 90–10814

This book is an authorized and revised translation from the 1st German edition, published and copyrighted 1989 by Georg Thieme Verlag, Stuttgart, Germany. Title of the German edition: Endoskopische Chirurgie der Nasennebenhöhlen und der vorderen Schädelbasis.

Some of the product names, patents and registered designs referred to in this book are in fact registered trademarks or proprietary names even though specific reference to this fact is not always made in the text. Therefore, the appearance of a name without designation as proprietary is not to be construed as a representation by the publisher that it is in the public domain.

This book, including all parts thereof, is legally protected by copyright. Any use, exploitation or commercialization outside the narrow limits set by copyright legislation, without the publisher's consent, is illegal and liable to prosecution. This applies in particular to photostat reproduction, copying, mimeographing or duplication of any kind, translating, preparation of microfilms, and electronic data processing and storage.

© 1990 Georg Thieme Verlag, Rüdigerstraße 14, D-7000 Stuttgart 30, Germany
Thieme Medical Publishers, Inc., 381 Park Avenue South, New York, N.Y. 10016

Typesetting by Ludwig Auer GmbH, D-8850 Donauwörth (Linotype System 4/202)
Printed in Germany by Karl Grammlich, D-7401 Pliezhausen

ISBN 3-13-749401-X (Georg Thieme Verlag, Stuttgart)
ISBN 0-86577-369-6 (Thieme Medical Publishers, Inc., New York)

3 4 5 6

Foreword

This is a book that has been eagerly awaited by many otolaryngologists. It is a comprehensive and beautifully illustrated work by one of the recognized pioneers and leading experts in this field. Professor Wigand carefully documents the changes which have occurred in our concepts regarding the pathogenic mechanisms and treatment of chronic sinusitis. The difficult regional anatomy is presented in an organized fashion with sections on endoscopic, radiologic and cadaver anatomy. Each section is meticulously illustrated.

In addition to presenting both the anteroposterior and posteroanterior surgical approaches, Professor Wigand discusses endoscopic surgery for lesions of the anterior skull base, tumors, and dacryocystorhinostomy. He highlights the importance of careful endoscopic follow-up and postoperative care when surgery is performed for chronic inflammatory disease. He also details the results obtained in over 10 years' experience at the Erlangen University Clinic.

Some years ago I had the opportunity to visit Professor Wigand and to scrub with him in the operating room. As soon as he began the first case, it was obvious that I was in the presence of a master. As I have gotten to know him better, my initial observation has been reinforced. He approached that first case with meticulous atraumatic technique and clear knowledge of the anatomy, and maintained excellent hemostasis throughout. He has written this book with the same attention to detail. However, perhaps more importantly, he brings to his book a wealth of personal experience, the salient points of which are carefully elucidated in his writing. The advent of this book is a significant milestone in the field of sinus surgery.

David W. Kennedy, M.D., F.R.C.S.
Associate Professor
Departments of Otolaryngology –
Head and Neck Surgery and Neurosurgery
The Johns Hopkins Medical Institutions
Baltimore, Maryland

Preface

"To be successful, intranasal operations must be so designed as to restore the normal physiologic function of the nose. It is impossible with impunity to operate upon the interior of the nose as though it were simply an air flue and on the sinuses as though they were boxes."

Anderson C. Hilding, 1950

Eleven years ago we gave our first report of the advantages of endoscopy in intranasal surgery (Wigand and Steiner 1977). Now we feel able to produce a comprehensive account of this theme. This technique was originally thought to be merely a modification of the long-established procedures for the treatment of inflammations of the paranasal sinuses, but this view had to be rapidly adapted to changing views of the pathological and regenerative processes of the respiratory mucosa. The established surgical principle "where there is pus let it out" is inadequate for this complex system of rigid epithelial surfaces with a highly organized self-cleansing system. Understanding of this system, of the importance of the mucociliary transport system discovered in the 1930s by Anderson C. Hilding and so beautifully illustrated in recent years with endoscopic films by Messerklinger and his colleagues, and adaptation to the many new concepts demanded time and scientific proof.

Experience has justified our initial optimism that even the most severely inflamed hyperplastic mucosa could recover after restoration of ventilation and drainage, and this has led to a general decline in radical surgery. Hosemann has shown that the concept of complete elimination of mucosa thought to be irreversibly damaged is no longer tenable. Furthermore, the good results of tympanoplasty for infections of the middle ear have supported our confidence in a similar resolution of the chronically inflamed air cells of the anterior skull, and have shown that the concept of a constitutionally determined biological mucosal inferiority (Wittmaack) is no longer valid. Nonetheless many interactions between micro-anatomy and the local immune reponses and healing processes of the mucosa remain unexplained. It is difficult in the midst of continuing research to declare a technique "ready" for a book. It is clear, however, that this new method must now be propagated and taught, and we as authors must accept the fact that criticisms, corrections and further developments will be made by others.

We have deliberately avoided writing a surgical atlas. Good surgical results demand an understanding of pathophysiology and surgical anatomy, experience in diagnosis and surgical skill. Therefore the chapter on operative technique is only a limited part of the book, and perhaps not the most essential. Neither is this book intended as a compendium of all known operations on the nasal and paranasal sinuses, but is restricted to those procedures which have become established and taught at the Erlangen Clinic. Concentration on personally proven methods imposes some limitations, but also guarantees wide application and reliability. A good example of this is the personal modification of septal correction. This monograph is not intended as a didactic operative atlas, but rather a handbook based on the personal views and experiences of the author. For this reason the very extensive literature on intranasal surgery of the paranasal sinuses is only referred to sporadically, and many techniques are not mentioned.

Despite numerous publications from many centers, intranasal endoscopy in the surgical management of chronic sinusitis remains widely unknown and neglected, probably because the nasal surgeon does not feel at ease working in a delicate anatomical region through narrow access. Even until recent times intranasal ethmoidal surgery has been regarded as being fraught with complications, including severe hemorrhage, blindness and intracranial infection. It must be emphasized that these fears are much less with experienced endoscopic nasal surgeons. If the jaws of the instrument can no longer be seen by the naked eye, and working distances and the direction of dissection are difficult to estimate, then naturally the procedure is unsafe. Safe dissection demands thorough study of endoscopic anatomy, and practice of endoscopic manipulations with both hands. It is hoped that the results given in Chapter 7 will be proof of this. The last section of the chapter on operative techniques shows that the range of indications has been extended to include surgery of the anterior base of the skull, and of obstructed lacrimal ducts, as described by Professor Dr. M. Weidenbecher.

A wide range of illustrations is necessary to demonstrate all these procedures. Dr. Hosemann has been particularly helpful with the organization of the material and recording of the operative steps on practice models. I am also very grateful to my colleagues Dr. Burlein, Dr. Kachlik, Dr. Riemann and Herr Gerard for taking the endoscopic pictures, and for other photographs. I am very grateful to Herr M. Jauch of Richard Wolf (Kittlingen) for a series of diagrams to illustrate the use of the instruments.

Not all the operative steps could be illustrated on one specimen, so the figures had to be taken from various dissections. Since only one side of the nose is presented to give a better insight into endoscopic anatomy, many original figures had to be transposed.

I am particularly grateful to Professor Dr. Brandl, and his many colleagues of the Institute of Anesthesiology (Director, Professor Dr. E. Ruegheimer) of the University of Erlangen-Nuremberg for their contributions to general anesthesia for this form of surgery, for their patience and understanding and for providing a bloodless field.

I wish to thank my former colleague Professor Dr. W. Steiner, now Director of the Department of ORL at the University in Goettingen, for his thoughtful and practical support in the early phase of our joint venture into this previously unknown field of endoscopy. I am also indebted to Professor Dr. J. Lang, Director of the Anatomical Institute of the University of Wuerzburg, and to Dr. M. P. Jaumann of Goeppingen for the loan of anatomical and endoscopic illustrations.

I would like to record my thanks to my secretary Karin Sippel for skilled assistance in the revision of the manuscript under difficult circumstances; sadly she died in July 1988.

Our librarian Beate Broghammer has worked tirelessly and carefully in accumulating the references, and on the input of data for the index as outlined by Dr. Hosemann. I wish to express my sincere gratitude to her, both for the present work and for help with papers and courses over many years.

I am very grateful to my wife Monika Christina whose careful reading has eliminated many unclear points from the text, and who has compiled the index.

Finally I wish to express my thanks to Dr. med. L. C. G. Hauff of Georg Thieme for his untiring encouragement to write this monograph, and to Herr W. Tannert for the high quality which is characteristic of this publishing house.

Erlangen, Spring 1988 *Malte Erik Wigand*

Acknowledgment

It is my privilege to express both my gratitude and appreciation to Prof. Philip M. Stell, Liverpool, who kindly took on the task of translating this book into current medical English. The text was reread by Prof. Stanley E. Thawley, who added special terms used in the United States, where endoscopic sinus surgery has become very popular during recent years. I am very grateful to both Prof. Stell and Dr. Thawley for their careful work.

February 1990 *Malte Erik Wigand*

Contents

Abbreviations used in the Figures

A. car. i.	Internal carotid artery
A. eth. A.	Anterior ethmoid artery
Ag. n.	Agger nasi
Bu	Ethmoid bulla
C. e. a.	Anterior ethmoid cells
C. e. p.	Posterior ethmoid cells
Ch.	Choana
Cl.	Clivus
Co. i.	Concha inferior, inferior turbinate
Co. m.	Concha media, middle turbinate
Co. s.	Concha superior, superior turbinate
D. nf.	Frontonasal duct
D. nl.	Nasolacrimal duct
H. sl.	Semilunar hiatus
Hyp.	Pituitary gland
I. e.	Ethmoid infundibulum
Lam. p.	Lamina papyracea
M. r. m.	Medial rectus muscle
N. max.	Maxillary nerve
N. o.	Optic nerve
N. pet. m.	Greater petrosal nerve
O. m.	Maxillary ostium
O. s.	Secondary ostium
P.	Pons
Pr. un.	Uncinate process
Re. zy.	Zygomatic recess
S.	Nasal septum
Sin. cav.	Cavernous sinus
Sin. f.	Frontal sinus
Sin. m.	Maxillary sinus
Sin. s.	Sphenoid sinus

1. Concepts of Intranasal Surgery of the Paranasal Sinuses

Intranasal endoscopic surgery of the paranasal sinuses is mainly indicated in the management of chronic sinusitis. It is based on entirely different concepts from those of radical surgery, and several prerequisites must be fulfilled if this alternative to the classical operations is to succeed. Intranasal procedures on the paranasal sinuses were first developed about 100 years ago, but were quickly abandoned because of uncertain results and frequent complications. Intranasal surgery of the paranasal sinuses has undergone a renaissance in the last decade, due to many technical advances and improved understanding of the biology and clinical behavior of sinusitis.

This change is based on the following:

- modification of long-standing concepts of mucosal pathophysiology,
- a more thorough knowledge of topographic anatomy,
- adaptation to endoscopic operative techniques using special angled telescopes and instruments through a narrow access,
- abandoning cherished principles of *en-bloc* clearance via wide access,
- a long-term treatment plan that includes supplementary procedures and time-consuming endoscopic aftercare, which the patient must accept as an important part of the treatment

Attention to the details of this complex treatment strategy is needed to reap the full benefit of intranasal surgery, to avoid complications and disappointing results, and to recognize the unsolved problems obstructing the development of ideal treatment.

The local patho-histomorphological appearance of the mucosa in one sinus does not reflect the actual stage of the disease in other compartments.

Surgical Pathology of the Sinus Mucosa

The respiratory mucosa of the nose and paranasal sinuses does not present a homogenous histological structure throughout its extent. Its texture depends on site, age and physical/biological responses to metabolic, endocrine and other factors.

In the nasal cavity, secretory elements (goblet cells and mucosal glands) are abundant where the mucosa carries a dense ciliary layer. In the more remote niches of the large sinuses these typical characteristics are sparser, and the histological picture more nearly resembles that of a mucoperiosteum with, at times, a thin serosal layer resembling the pattern of the middle ear and mastoid. Tos et al. (1978) have measured accurately the normal variation in density of the mucosal glands in the sinuses: under pathological conditions this pattern of distribution can change radically. The frequent macroscopical variants of the mucosa, even in the absence of inflammation, are already familiar to the rhinologist: dry, thickened regions at the nasal valve, atrophic areas over bony ridges, succulent velvety ends of the turbinates with arterial, or venous coloration, and finally the swollen, pale mulberry-like, bluish-red colored mucosa on the posterior end of the turbinates.

The local appearances of the mucosa show even more marked variations in sinusitis. The endoscopist is familiar with the various swellings, edematous areas, papillary hyperplasia and polyps that differ between the two sides and even within one nasal cavity. Using standardized mucosal biopsies Hosemann (1985) has demonstrated the wide variation in histopathology of sinus mucosa in diffuse polypoid hyperplastic sinusitis (Figures 1.**1**–1.**4**). A diagnosis of sinusitis by the histopathologist does not apply to the entire mucosa but only to that part which is sampled. This conclusion is self-evident, but conflicts with the concept of radical surgery that demands complete mucosal clearance.

In our experience temporal factors are as important as local factors because histomorphological findings change enormously over time. After a successful tympanoplasty even the most severe mucosal lesions have often regressed when the ear is later re-opened after aeration and internal drainage have been restored. A previously very hyperplastic layer will be found to have been replaced by non-inflamed, soft mucosa. The same results have now been found many times after surgery for severe sinusitis with

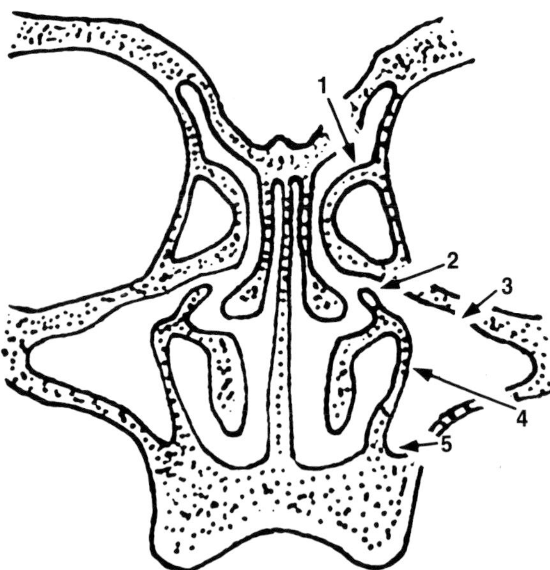

Figure 1.1 Local variation in chronic sinusitis. Five standard areas for the removal of tissue (Hosemann):
1. Anterosuperior ethmoid cells.
2. Maxilloethmoid junctional region.
3. Roof of the antral cavity.
4. Medial antral wall.
5. Floor of the antrum.

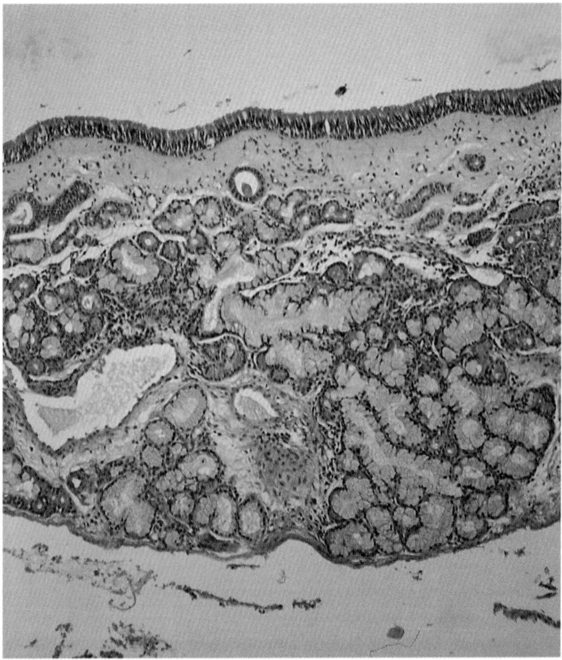

Figure 1.2 Relatively thin mucosa of the maxillo-ethmoid junctional zone in chronic sinusitis, showing numerous glands, but little cellular infiltrate (H and E 20×).

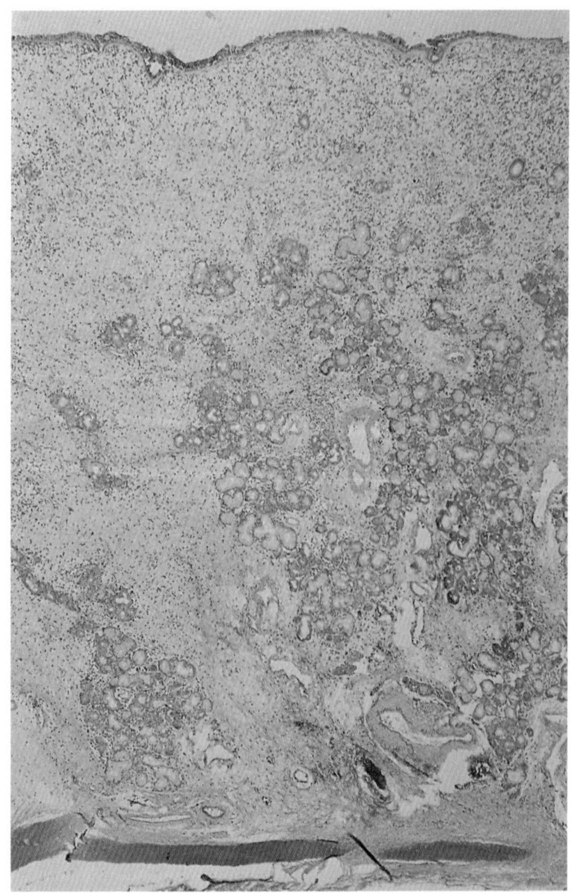

Figure 1.3 Relatively thick mucosa in the upper ethmoid cells in chronic sinusitis showing loose edematous connective tissue, many glands and dilated submucosal vessels (elastic-van Gieson, 8×).

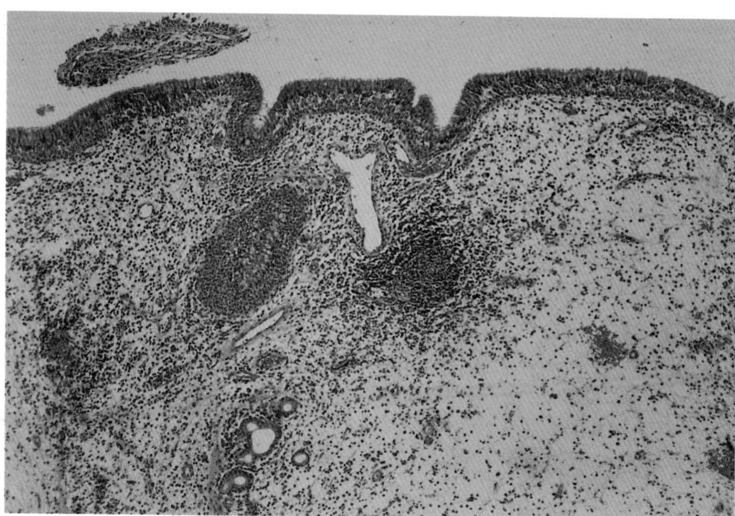

Figure 1.4 Ethmoid mucosa in chronic sinusitis showing loose stroma with disseminated clumps of cells but no glands (Goldner, 7×).

mucosal preservation: even previously thick, spongy, injected and indurated mucosa presents a completely healthy appearance after conservative sinus operations that restore drainage and aeration. Thus neither the surgeon's eye nor the results of a frozen tissue section can predict whether inflamed mucosa is capable of resolution.

At the time of a first operation the surgeon can by no means predict whether the chronically diseased mucosa will recover or not.

Mucositis

Little is known of the morphological and functional changes in acute and chronic inflammation of the respiratory mucosa or of the healing processes, either with or without surgery. Numerous histomorphological and structural investigations have been done of the mucosal response pattern, the lymphatic system and the pathological ciliary activity of the mucosa of men and animals (e.g. Naumann 1961, Jahnke 1972 and Terrahe 1970), but an overall view of nonspecific mucosal inflammation is not available. The temporal course of the phenomena associated with spread of inflammation from the nasal cavity into the sinuses is not known.

We suspect that an intermediate stage of hyperemia, lymphatic swelling, stasis in the blood and lymphatic pathways, and increased secretion of mucus succeeds an initial stage of hyperemia with reduced mucociliary transport. This is followed either by resolution or by progression to a chronic stage with pathological increase in the elements of the lamina propria such as cells, fibers and ground substance, and resultant permanent disruption of the mucociliary transport and lymphatic drainage. The resulting obstruction of the narrow ducts between the paranasal sinuses and the nasal cavity leads to a vicious circle of retention of secretions, obstruction of lymphatic drainage, edema, and finally organized connective tissue and mucosal hyperplasia. The causes of local and temporal variations of pathology probably depend on anatomy, the local mucosal response, the influence of other body systems, pathogens and on external noxious agents. The factors which influence spontaneous recovery of the inflamed mucosa and determine its remarkable regenerative capacity even though it has been diseased for many years, remain unknown.

Polyps, retention cysts and fistulae do not have a high potential for recovery, so that removal of mucosa should be restricted to these lesions, whereas smooth swellings, cushions of edema and areas of papillary mucosa can be preserved and given the chance to recover. It is uncertain whether polyps and retention cysts in children heal spontaneously.

In sinusitis, the removal of mucosal lesions which appear to be incapable of resolution is limited to polyps and (pseudo) cysts. Flat edematous swellings and broad-based mucosal cushions can be preserved. The treatment of granulations follows the principles of the treatment of ulcers (see below).

Doctors and patients often ask whether the chance of healing is reduced by allergy, particularly of the respiratory, immediate type. Basically, it is not: data in the literature about this question are scarce, and the conclusion is based on only a proportion of patients because it is impossible to subject a large number of subjects to complete allergy tests including all possible provocation tests before and after operation.

About 10% of the population including those with chronic polypoid sinusitis demonstrate an allergic response, and eosinophilia is often found in polyps. These two facts have led to overestimation of the importance of Type I allergy in the genesis and prognosis of nasal polyps. However, tissue eosinophilia is also found in primary non-allergic rhinitis, a disease which is often combined with endogenous asthma and sensitivity to analgesics. Furthermore, the typical immune reactive elements, such as eosinophils, plasma cells and immunoglobulin deposits, are so varied (Figures 1.**5**–1.**6**) that local mucosal individual responses must be recognized. *In-vitro* experiments after a challenge with allergens showed no difference in the basic histamine release of polyps from allergic and non-allergic subjects (Baenkler et al. 1983, 1987).

There is no correlation between the histological and immunohistochemical findings and the clinical and immunological response of patients with severe polypoid sinusitis (Waller et al. 1976). This fact is borne out by the smooth healing independent of proven allergy.

Whereas antiallergic conservative treatment of patients with nasal polyps can obviously lead to some reduction in size of the polyps, on account of reduction of the edema it is not adequate long-term therapy. In the author's own follow-up investigations after intranasal ethmoid operations the results of the operation did not depend on respiratory allergy or on treatment by desensitization. Surgery influences the allergic mucosal response favorably by controlling the inflammation, and often leads to complete or at least considerable relief of symptoms. Supplementary measures, for example septal correction, also play a role in this process.

Surgical Principles

The main goal of intranasal endoscopic surgery for chronic sinusitis is the maximal preservation of mucosa achieved by restoration of drainage and ventilation. This principle stands in marked contrast with radical surgery in which mucosa regarded as irreversibly damaged or as "biologically inferior" is completely removed and the bony framework is also widely sacrificed. In this surgery, for instance, the maxillary sinus is deprived of its rigid anterior wall so that the facial soft tissues can prolapse, and the upper jaw may later shorten due to scar tissue contracture (Figure 1.**7**). Also much of its medial wall is lost if a large window is created into the inferior meatus through which a flap of nasal mucosa is turned. The external frontal and ethmoid operations also change the bony structures of the frontal infundibulum and anterior ethmoid decisively. Mucosal flaps are often turned in to prevent the penetration of scar tissue into this sensitive area, but they do not always ensure aeration, and mucoceles can arise later.

Intranasal endoscopic surgery has two goals: maximal preservation of all living mucosa, and a secure communication between the nasal cavity and the paranasal sinuses via the natural channels. In the maxillary sinus the latter is achieved by creation of a new window in the middle nasal meatus, complemented if necessary by an inferior meatal antrostomy, without reflection of a flap of nasal mucosa whose direction of ciliary stream is unknown, and without distortion of the bony anterior wall. In the frontal sinus the aim is to restore ventilation and drainage into the nose via the original frontonasal duct or a channel of maximal width but not by weakening of the bone around the infundibulum.

The same concept also applies to the ethmoid and sphenoid sinuses: of necessity many cells must be removed, but not every cell must be denuded or drilled out into every last corner. Only the narrow points are opened up in "isthmus surgery" (Figure 1.**8 a** and **b**). The improved aeration and drainage and supplementary procedures (see below) can be confidently expected to achieve permanent resolution of the chronically inflamed mucosa (Figure 1.**9**). The entire circumference of ducts and antrostomies must not be completely denuded of mucosa as this leads to stenosis.

Mucosal continuity of the sinus cavities with each other and the nose is important, to restore mucociliary transport, to prevent granulations arising form denuded bone, and, more importantly, to supplement the abnormal or absent lymphatic drainage. Although this matter has received little attention, the author's own endoscopic dissections show that the diversion or abnormal function of the lymphatic network can cause serious problems. Even minor manipulations at the ostium or in a duct can lead to long-standing mucosal edema within the sinus

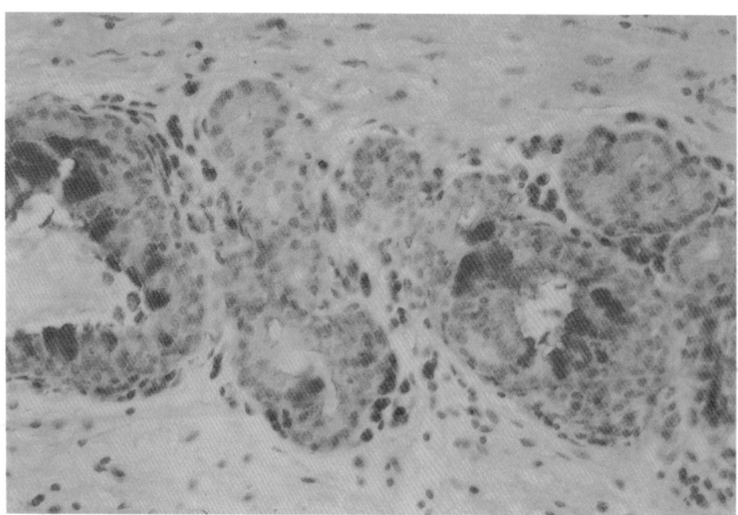

Figure 1.**5** Ethmoid mucosa in chronic sinusitis showing cells heavily laden with IgA (brown granules) lying close to the gland (immunoperoxidase, 80×).

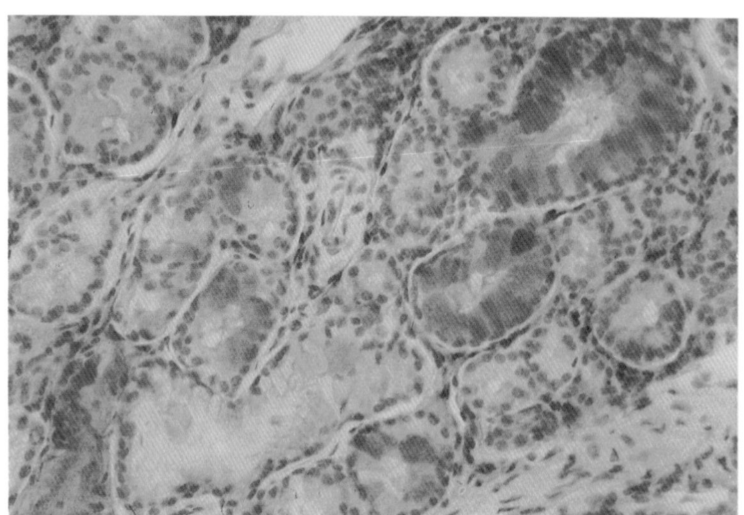

Figure 1.**6** Ethmoid mucosa in chronic sinusitis showing no underlying IgA laden cells around the glands (immunoperoxidase, 250×) (same ethmoid as in Figure 1.**5**).

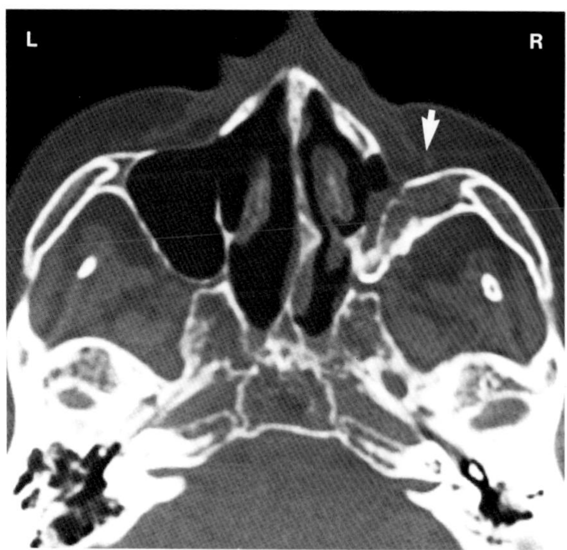

Figure 1.**7** Scar tissue deformity of the right maxilla after a Caldwell-Luc radical antrostomy. The medial and posterior walls are drawn together, and the anterior wall (marked by an arrow) has collapsed. Axial CT scan.

a

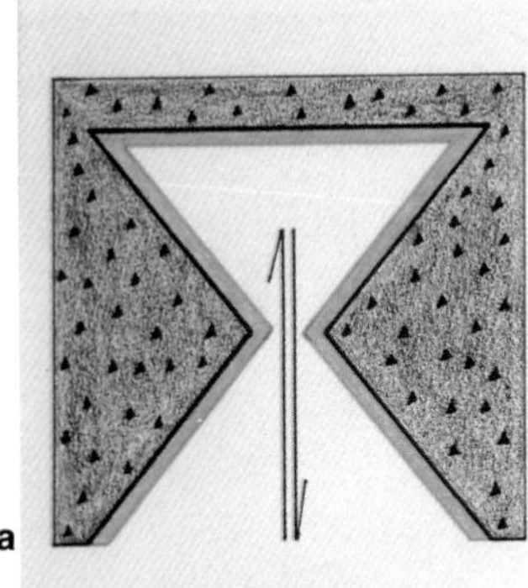

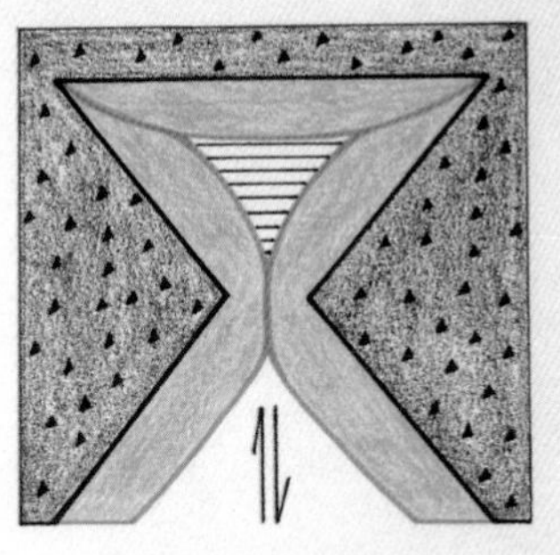

b

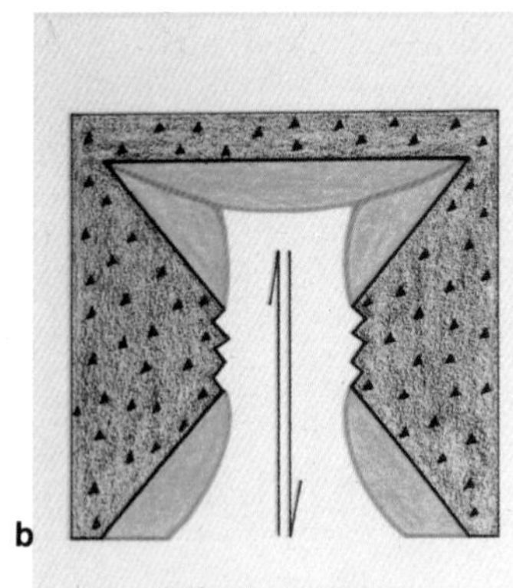

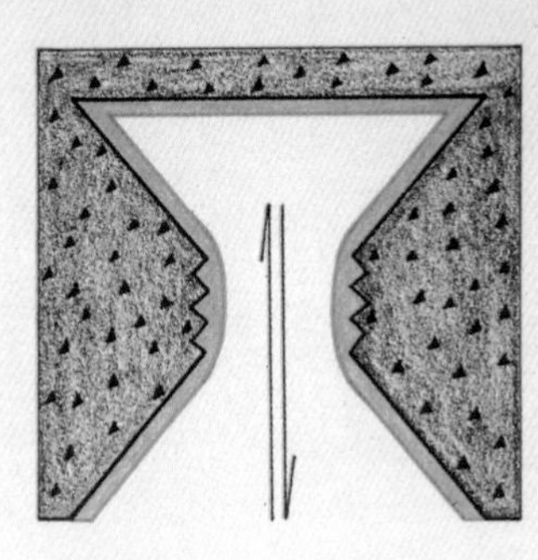

Figure 1.**8** Diagram of the principle of isthmus surgery.
a Vicious circle due to mucosal edema of the antrostomy. The stasis facilitates inflammation and hyperplasia.
b Reventilation and drainage are encouraged by widening of the functionally closed window.

interfering with healing as much as disordered mucociliary transport.

> Intranasal endoscopic operations on the paranasal sinuses for chronic sinusitis are mainly limited to opening the narrow bony points to restore ventilation and internal drainage.

The recommendation to open narrow areas should not be interpreted as an invitation to create large cavities: respect for natural sinus physiology is the guideline running through this type of surgery. On the other hand, the long-held view that wide nasal cavities automatically carry the danger of drying and atrophy of the mucosa, and even of ozena, must be challenged. Despite relatively generous septal correction, partial resection of the middle turbinate with complete ethmoidectomy (see below) and limited inferior turbinectomy, we have so far seen not one single case of true ozena after intranasal ethmoidectomy. Although poor aftercare can cause crusting in the ethmoid sinuses, careful removal of the crusts reveals that the underlying mucosa is not dry and atrophic but oversecreting with resultant granulations.

> Enlargement of the nasal cavity by ethmoidectomy, partial turbinectomy, and septum correction does not provoke atrophic rhinitis (ozena).

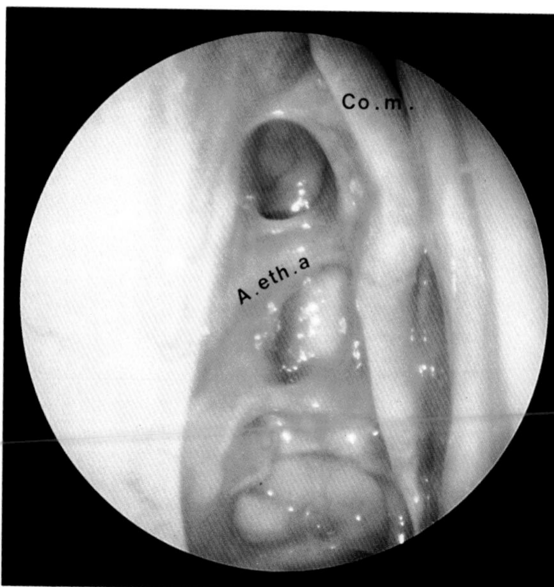

Figure 1.**9** Regeneration of previously polypoid-hyperplastic ethmoid mucosa after endoscopic ethmoidectomy with preservation of the sinus mucosa. The surgically opened areas are healed. The medial lamella (or wall) of the middle turbinate is still present, and the olfactory cleft is normal. Right ethmoid (70° telescope).

Textbooks of general pathology and general surgery fail to mention the spontaneous healing of defects of the respiratory mucosa. Little is known of the inflammatory reaction, the speed of formation of replacement tissue in mucosal ulcers, the proliferative power of the underlying bone and its periosteum or of the edges of a mucosal defect, and whether metaplasia is to be expected as an intermediate stage (Lenz and Preussler 1986). Few histological investigations have been performed which evaluate the influence of medical treatment on the local healing of defects of the respiratory mucosa.

The physiological transport pathways can be seen by applying particles to the mucosa of live or dead animals and observing the particle movement (Hilding 1932, Proetz 1941, Messerklinger 1960). However, it is not known whether the pathways regenerate following inflammation and/or surgery, or whether regenerated mucosa incorporates mucociliary action. The importance of replacement mechanisms, such as expulsion of secretion by pressure changes during breathing is also unknown. Hosemann (1985) used photography to show that carbon particles placed on the floor of the maxillary antrum are transported upwards over the maxillary walls and through the antrostomy into the nasal cavity after either an inferior or middle meatal antrostomy (Figure 1.**10**). Also, he showed by endoscopy that secretions drain continuously through a newly created antrostomy, and that the edges of the antrostomy are covered by ciliated respiratory epithelium (Figure 1.**11 a, b**). It is uncertain how this phenomenon is restored in the frontal infundibulum, the ethmoid niches and the sphenoid sinus, and how mucus, bacteria, etc., are transported. The basic studies of mucociliary transport carried out by Hilding (1932, 1941) were the first to show that mucus and particles were moved along preordained corkscrew pathways to the ostia by the coordinated ciliary beat of the respiratory epithelium. New windows in the wall of the maxilla are bypassed, and the transport pathway can even carry the particle out of the cavity and then back in again at the opposite edge of the antrostomy. Hilding showed that ridges of scar tissue can easily arise in a hollow organ forming an insurmountable barrier even if their height is minimal. He showed also that collections of mucus can be carried along by neighboring mucociliary epithelial activity, so that cleansing of mucosal surfaces with no ciliary activity can still be achieved. The concept of minimal injury to the mucosa during endoscopic surgery developed from this insight. In particular the formation of a ridge of scar tissue is to be avoided.

Data in the literature about reversal of the direction of the ciliary beat after transplantation of the mucosa are contradictory. The possible serious disadvantages following the rotation of mucosal flaps (Uffenorde or Boenninghaus) or free transplants of mucosal islands (Wigand) is ignored in practice.

Healing Problems

The preceding goals are often not achieved: exact resection of bone, and precise removal of mucosal lesions are often not accomplished for the lack of suitable instruments, leading to the creation of unnecessarily large mucosal defects that heal by scar tissue. Remote ethmoidal cells may be hidden from inspection and remain unopened, and they can stimulate recurrent ethmoiditis. Also, some obstructions to drainage can be overlooked. However, at every point where bone has been denuded new mucosa must grow over a granulating intermediate layer before healing can be expected. The outcome is jeopardized by three factors: failure of reorganization of mucociliary transport, excessive granulations and abnormal lymphatic drainage.

From every mucosal defect can arise granulation tissue preventing mucosal regeneration. The resulting scar tissue distorts mucociliary transport and lymphatic drainage which can produce retained secretions even in an open sinus cavity.

Excessive granulation tissue in surgically created mucosal defects is even more important because of the resultant obstruction of narrow ducts, outflow tracts or neighboring mucosal niches. The race between formation of new granulation tissue in a vertical direction, and re-epithelialization in a horizontal plane is a wellknown phenomenon in cutaneous wound healing. Slowly-healing ulcers can usually be controlled by superficial cautery with a silver nitrate stick because the squamous epithelium can grow more readily over the flat fresh wound. This healing process has not been investigated satisfactorily in the respiratory mucosa.

Endoscopic study of healing shows that the shape of the wound surface influences the healing of the ulcer. The concave gutters in the anterior ethmoid, the antrostomies and ducts are ideal sites for the formation of granulation tissue which is converted to scar tissue by the normal contraction of collagen fibers, leading to restenosis and polyp formation. This epithelialized granulation tissue, like the middle-ear polyp, must be distinguished from the true edematous mucosal polyp. Obstruction of the anterior ethmoid and the frontal duct by scar tissue or by a granular polyp is a common cause of recurrent sinusitis after ethmoid operations. To what extent the shape of the "concave ulcer", and obstruction to aeration by the agger nasi, the nasal septum or other factors such as disorganized mucociliary transport are responsible for this common cause of failure is unknown. Systemic factors such as allergy, immune deficiencies, exogenous toxins, etc., must be taken into account, but local biomechanical causes also need attention during the postoperative phase.

If a surgeon finds that the polyps often arise in the anterior ethmoid area after sphenoethmoidectomy, whereas the posterior ethmoidal walls and the sphenoidal cavity heal, then he should ask the following questions:

- have the anterior ethmoid cells been completely exposed?
- has unsatisfactory resection of the agger nasi created a narrow pit which is inefficiently aerated?
- is the anterior ethmoid gutter narrow due to an uncorrected upper nasal septum?
- are all cells and niches open and draining properly; this can be assessed reliably by high resolution CT scan (Figure 1.**12**).

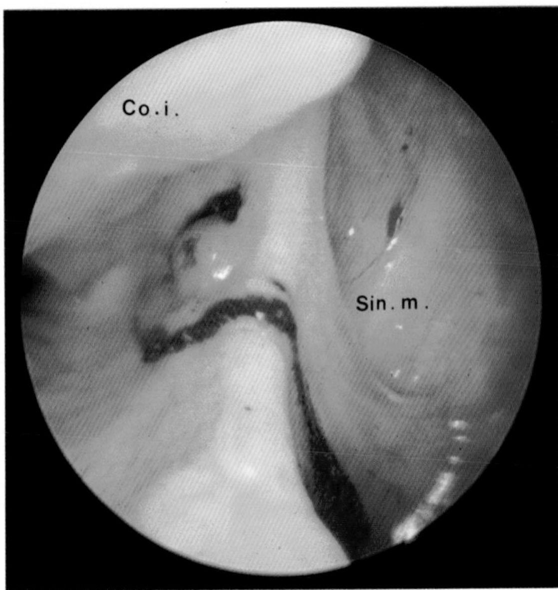

Figure 1.**10** Mucociliary transport pathways of carbon particles from the left antral cavity over the threshold of an inferior meatal antrostomy into the floor of the nose (from Hosemann) (25° telescope).

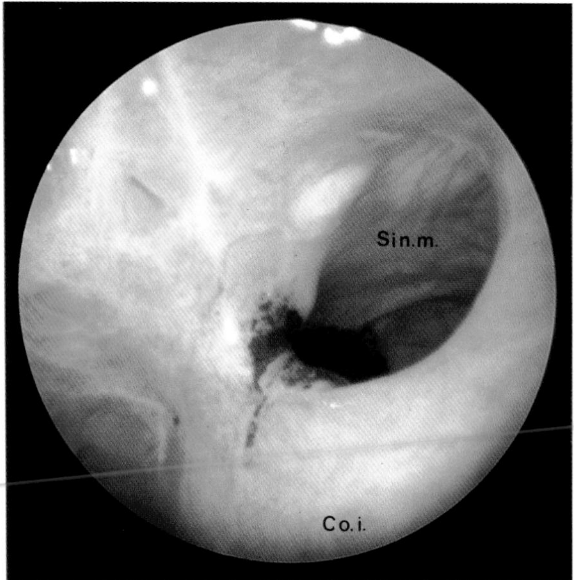

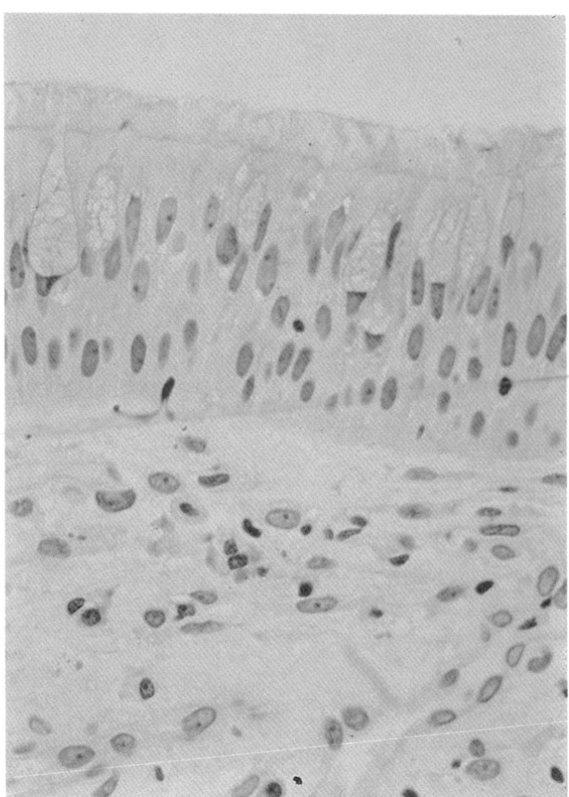

Figure 1.**11** **a** Mucociliary transport pathways of carbon particles over the inferior edge of a middle meatal antrostomy into the left antral cavity (photographed by Hosemann) (70° telescope).
b Regenerated ciliated epithelium of the inferior edge of the middle meatal antrostomy of Figure 1.**11 a**) (Semi-thin section, H and E 130×).

Supplementary Procedures

Healing of chronic sinusitis is not ensured by an endonasal procedure: all factors contributing to the pathogenesis demand attention. The history, examination and investigation should reveal the severity and extent of the mucosal disease, and explain its cause (see Chapter 3). Operative clearance of the affected sinus should be paralleled by treatment of the suspected causal factors (Table 1.**1**). These factors may be neglected because the surgeon concentrates on the visible disease, and underestimates the influence of neighboring tissue and of systemic factors.

Table 1.1 Accesory procedures for operative treatment of sinusitis.
Normalization of ventilation of the nose and sinuses (correction of septal deviation or cleft palate, turbinectomy, adenoidectomy, tonsillectomy)
Elimination of septic foci (dental attention, tonsillectomy, elimination of exogenous toxins)
Treatment of systemic disorders (such as allergy, immune deficits, hormonal disorders, mucoviscidosis, etc.)

A common cause of chronic sinusitis is abnormal ventilation of the nasal cavity and the ostia of the sinuses. Whether abnormal ventilation and obstruction to drainage play an equal part, or whether the disorder of drainage is due to the deficient aeration is unknown. Endoscopic findings, and possibly rhinomanometry, indicate whether a *septal correction or reduction of the turbinates* is indicated. The decision to carry out septoplasty cannot always be based on the patient's symptoms, such as nasal obstruction, or on objective data provided by rhinomanometry. It is frequently based on consideration of the pathogenesis of the sinusitis, such as pronounced narrowing of the middle meatus by a septal spur (Figure 1.**13**). Also a free exposure for the operating instruments and for the postoperative manipulation has to be calculated. A septum which has previously been operated on, a perforated septum, narrow nostrils due to a wide *columella*, or *nasal alae* which are too lax and prolapse on inspiration may need to be corrected. In children, enlarged tonsils or adenoids are potential causes of obstruction to breathing or drainage and their removal often cures chronic or recurrent sinusitis in children, without any further procedure being necessary.

The effects of *congenital clefts* and their surgical repair are difficult to evaluate. Chronic sinusitis is

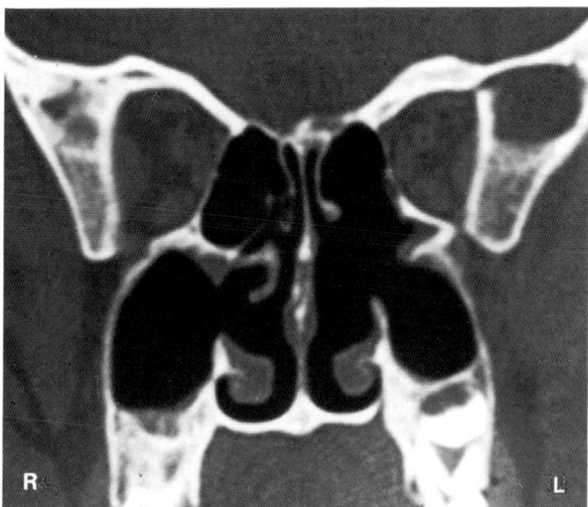

Figure 1.**12** Follow-up CT scan showing healing of polypoid-hyperplastic sinusitis after endoscopic ethmoidectomy (left side) and middle meatal antrostomy on both sides.

Surgical treatment of chronic sinusitis must include the diagnosis and elimination of co-factors by flanking measures.

encouraged by displacement or widening of the septum, an elevated floor of the nose, and anomalies of the soft palate. Thus reconstruction of the floor of the nose or the soft palate may be needed for functional reasons. It is more important to look for a dental cause of inflammation of the sinus mucosa such as *a root abscess* and a dental consultation is often advisable. Reports of the frequency of dental disease vary widely. Since the dentist is often unable to find a focus in the dental roots to explain mucosal proliferations on the floor of the antrum, it may be possible that periodontal mucosal disease alone can lead to circumscribed areas of osteitis with resultant sinusitis. Polyps on the floor of the antrum often lie very close to a conserved molar or premolar even if their roots do not appear to be diseased or visible within the antral lumen.

A proven dental cause for the sinusitis does not demand transoral opening of the sinus. Dental treatment combined with endoscopic management of the sinuses fulfills the same purpose, and avoids the well known disadvantages of the Caldwell-Luc operation.

Other *exogenous agents* which should be eliminated include:

- inhaled industrial irritants,
- cigarettes and snuff,
- side effects of drugs.

The treatment of *allergy* before and after operation should also be mentioned. However, operative correction of narrow areas of the nose and/or the sinuses cannot be replaced by treatment of the allergy. Surgery should be carried out if indicated on its own merits, even in patients with sensitivity to aspirin, or in those with *endocrine diseases*.

Surgery may also be useful for *systemic diseases* in childhood such as mucoviscidosis. Previously, surgery to the sinuses in these cases was thought to be useless or even harmful, but pediatricians now find increasingly that surgery to the sinuses improves the course of asthma, bronchitis and mucoviscidosis. The main contraindication to surgery is not the difficulty of the operative technique in the small sinus system, or reduced healing ability, but the inability of children to tolerate the essential endoscopic aftercare. Close cooperation with neighboring disciplines such as pediatrics, pulmonology and immunology is important in achieving a good result from intranasal sinus surgery in children.

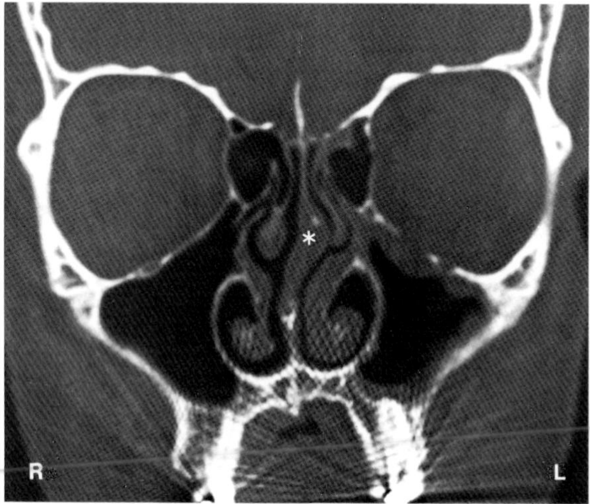

Figure 1.**13** Development of chronic sinusitis due to narrowing of the middle meatus by a projecting septal spur (*). High-resolution coronal CT scan.

Endoscopic Aftercare

Endoscopic postoperative care is important for the success of endoscopic sinus surgery. Even patients who have undergone a minor procedure such as antrostomy, removal of a cyst, etc., benefit from follow-up for a few weeks to allow the sinuses to be irrigated, secretions to be removed by suction, adhesions within the antrostomy and nasal ducts or between the turbinate and the ethmoid wall to be divided and granulations at the wound edge to be cauterized. These steps are even more necessary after ethmoidectomy for profuse polyposis or other diseases. It can never be assumed that recovery and regrowth of the mucosa will proceed smoothly and spontaneously. The guidelines (Table 1.**2**) for aftercare described below rely more on intuition and experience than on a scientific basis, and need basic investigation. Follow-up may be needed for up to 2 years.

Table 1.**2** Methods for endoscopic aftercare following surgery for chronic sinusitis.

Removal of crusts and clots
Cautery and removal of granulations
Division of synechiae
Treatment of infection by antibiotics
Treatment of edema with inhalations and steroids
Elimination of causative factors such as allergy, immune deficits, etc.

Acute Postoperative Phase

Clots and crusts often cause renewed obstruction of the nasal passages after the nasal packing is removed on the second day after operation, and require careful suction once a day to guarantee nasal patency. In this phase the inhalation of a saline solution increases the fluidity of fibrin clots and crusts. Prophylactic antibiotics are usually given, preferably a broad-spectrum agent such as doxycycline which penetrates the mucosa well. Swelling of the septal and turbinate mucosa should be treated by nonsteroidal anti-inflammatory agents. Allergic and asthmatic subjects may need temporary treatment with systemic corticosteroids, because of their superior effect in comparison to sprays and nasal drops.

After a few days when the acute danger of reactionary hemorrhage has passed, the all important narrow areas – the frontal duct, the superior ethmoid gutter, the sphenoid cavity and the antrostomy – are cleaned by daily endoscopy. The middle turbinate should be replaced in its correct position using a slightly curved suction tube or a curved elevator to prevent it swinging laterally and adhering to the lateral nasal wall in the absence of the supporting ethmoid cells. Mechanical trauma to the mucosa must be avoided. Irrigation with saline solution or installation of gel solutions mixed with antibiotics and steroids into the frontal and antral cavities are useful.

The patient is soon able to dissolve the crusts for himself with saline irrigation several times a day, and by repeated inhalation of antibiotic solutions. A double inhalation supplemented by Tacholiquin (Tyloxapol) and Nebacetin (neomycin plus bacitracin) solution has proved useful for persisting suppuration.

Massive edema of the remaining antral or ethmoid mucosa is found in many cases a few days after the operation, particularly at the edges of the wound or the antrostomy (Figures 1.**14**–1.**17**). It is not clear whether this is due to inflammation or to lymphatic stasis. *Cushions of edema* can be very persistent and lead to recurrence of edematous pseudocysts and polyps. At the same time *granulations* often spring from the bony wall which has been denuded of mucosa. Endoscopic incision or cauterization with 10–20% silver nitrate is used in an attempt to suppress these swellings which can obstruct the narrow areas and lead to a vicious circle. Short courses of systemic steroids are often helpful. Occasionally the initial tendency to crusting can be suppressed by loose daily packing of the ethmoid cavity with gauze strips soaked in aureomycin. Crusting should never be interpreted as indicating mucosal atrophy: it is caused by secretions drying out on ulcerated or overreactive mucosa. The old dermatological principle of "treat moisture with moisture" is also valid in this situation.

Late Postoperative Phase

If excess, possibly purulent, secretion is a prominent feature in the early healing phase, the wound will form profuse granulation tissue 3–4 weeks later (Figure 1.**18**), demanding even more careful endoscopic control and energetic countermeasures. The sites of predilection for granulation tissue are the edges of an antrostomy, a sphenoidectomy, or the edge of the frontal duct. Often in this stage the middle turbinate tends to abut against the lateral ethmoidal wall because it has lost its support, and the anterior ethmoid gutter is obstructed if the turbinate is not replaced in its correct position. Endoscopic attention to this site of obstruction ensures freedom from crusts under which fibrin adhesions can develop to be followed rapidly by synechiae. Small granulation tissue polyps (Figure 1.**19**) must be distinguished from edema of the mucosal edges; they may be cauterized with 10–20% silver nitrate. Adhesions (Figure 1.**20**) can be divided easily with the scissors, the cutting diathermy or the laser, but sheets of scar tissue require revision surgery. Revision surgery is particularly valuable if the sense of smell can be restored by reopening of the olfactory cleft, or if inflammation of the mucosa of the frontal sinuses resolves after a second-stage, wider opening of the frontal duct.

This phase of reparative granulations and scar tissue formation can last for several months. Healing is complete and the danger of scar formation obstruction is past only when complete re-epithelialization by respiratory mucosa or by metaplastic stratified epithelium is complete. However, if wound healing is

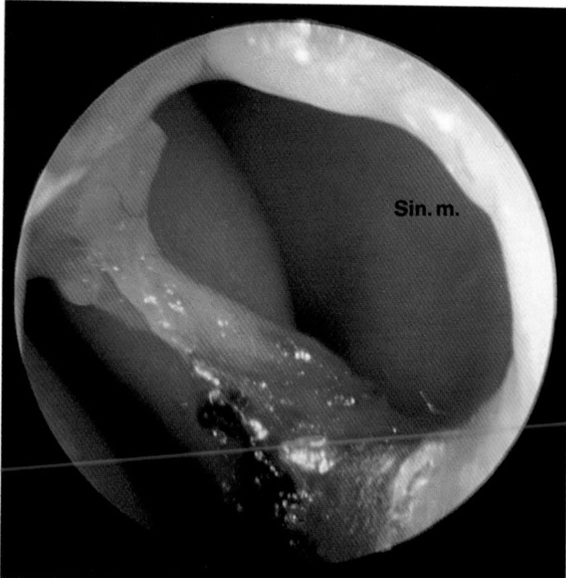

Figure 1.**14** Deposits of secretion and fibrinous inflammation on the edges of a middle meatal antrostomy 9 days after the operation.

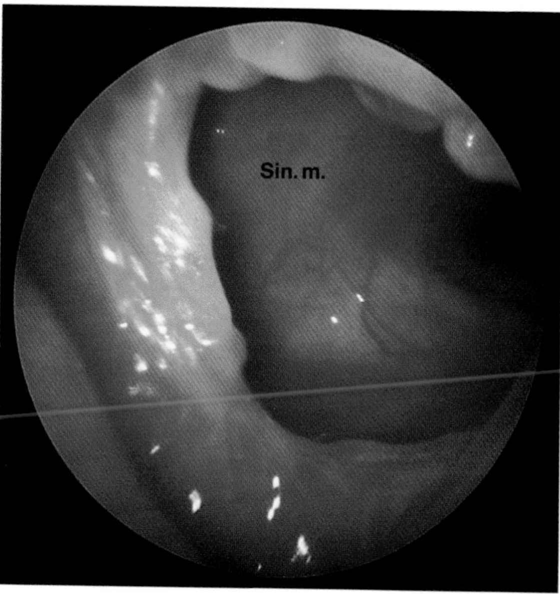

Figure 1.**15** Subsiding crusting and granulation of a middle meatal antrostomy 4 weeks after operation.

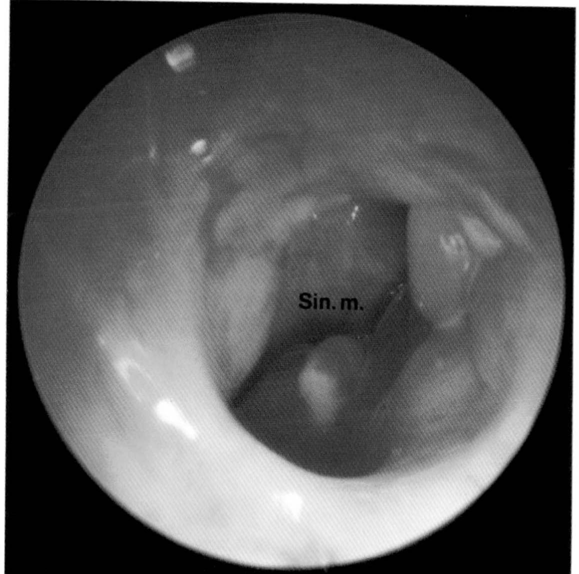

Figure 1.**16** Persisting edema of the neighboring mucosa and excessive formation of scar tissue in a middle meatal antrostomy.

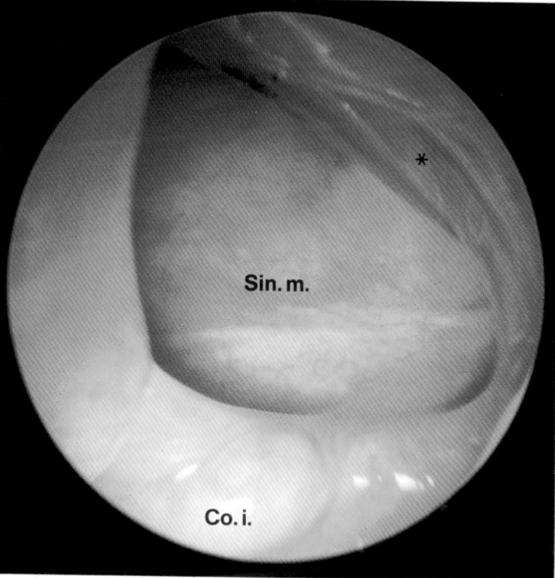

Figure 1.**17** Transport of mucus (*) over the upper edge of the middle meatal antrostomy. Despite the recent scar tissue healing the self-cleaning function has been reorganized within months of the operation.

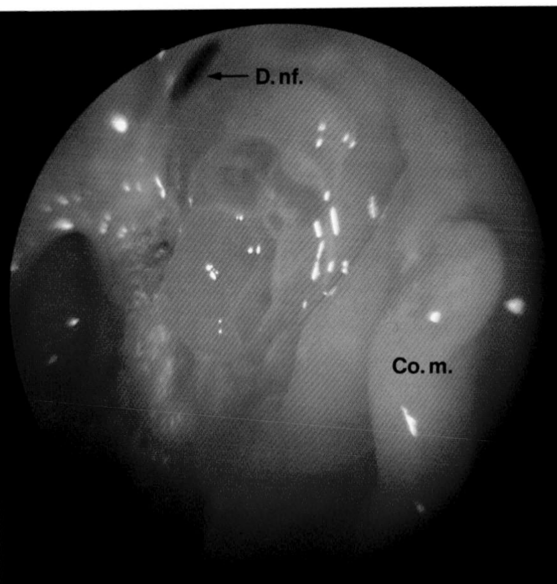

Figure 1.**18** Excessive mucosal granulation on the roof of the right ethmoid several weeks after the operation due to damage at ethmoidectomy (70° telescope).

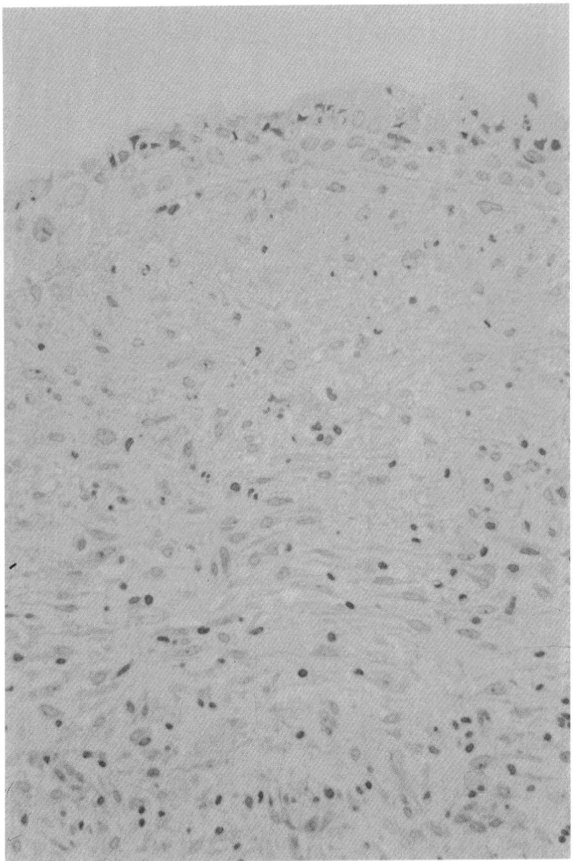

Figure 1.**19** Typical granulation tissue polyp 8 days after ethmoidectomy. It has a loose edematous stroma and is largely covered by a single layer of cubical epithelium (semi-thin section, H and E, 66×).

left to its own devices there is a danger of stenosis of the antrostomy or closure of the narrow outflow tract of the frontal sinus and the upper ethmoid gutter (Figure 1.**21**).

This period is often also marked by recurrence of the symptoms of asthma or bronchitis. It is suspected that breakdown products of bacteria and secretions become noxious due to renewed stasis in the cell recesses and hollow niches. A pre-existing hypersensitivity of the bronchial mucosa may worsen, precipitating an attack of asthma, by neural reflexes, or by intraluminal or hematogenous spread of toxins or allergens. Recovery can be achieved in these cases by reopening the narrow areas, either by cautery of the bands of scar tissue as an outpatient, or by curettage under surgical conditions.

Before the first operation the patient with severe polyposis must be warned of the difficulties of the postoperative phase, and be prepared for the program of aftercare during which further surgery may be necessary. This applies particularly to children who need a general anesthetic for effective endoscopic procedures. The surgery should be supplemented by conservative methods such as drugs, sprays, nasal emulsions, etc., dictated by the surgeon's personal experience.

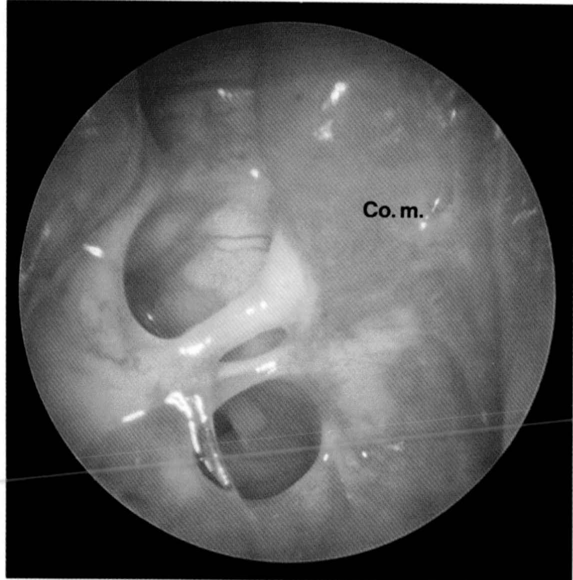

Figure 1.**20** Bands of scar tissue arising from granulation tissue, and bridging the ethmoid gutter between the middle turbinate and the lateral wall of the right ethmoid (70° telescope).

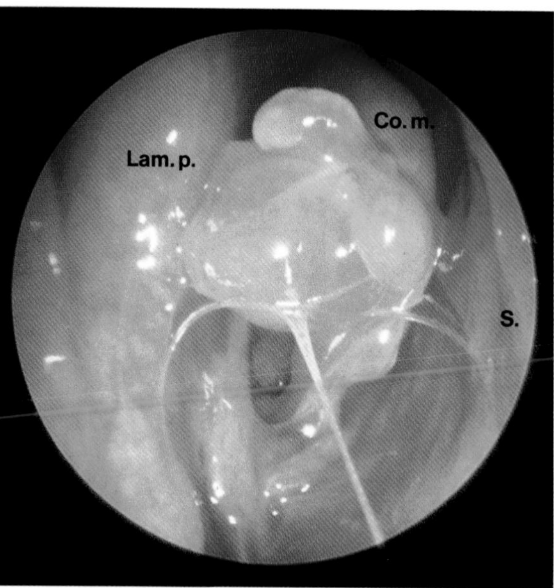

Figure 1.**21** Obliteration of the frontal duct by a mass of scar tissue lying between the middle turbinate and the lateral wall of the right ethmoid.

Maintenance of the Olfactory Cleft

Chronic rhinosinusitis extends to much of the mucosa of the olfactory area. Superficial swelling of this area causes intermittent or permanent dysosmia. Polyps seldom form in the superior and supreme nasal meatus: they consist of granulation tissue and sometimes of edematous mucosa, and are caused solely by injury to the mucosa of this region. This fact should be remembered in surgery of the nose and ethmoid sinuses, even simple polypectomy, but particularly during ethmoidectomy. The mucosa should be preserved very carefully to prevent later closure of the olfactory cleft by granulations or scar tissue.

Sheets of silicone or similar material placed in the olfactory cleft, fixed to the septum by interrupted sutures are often useful, but cautery, curettage removal of tissue with the punch and the use of pressure should be avoided (see also reconstruction of the olfactory cleft during ethmoidal operations).

Informed Consent

Operations on the nose and sinuses require careful explanation to the patient. The legal system expects the surgeon to discuss typical dangers and rarer complications before the operation. In the author's experience the rhinologist can find himself in a dilemma: a too-wide ranging explanation can lead to unnecessary anxiety, and many patients are frightened off a necessary procedure.

It is advisable to record in the case sheet the dangers and results of the operation which have been discussed with the patient. When drawing up the operation notes it should be remembered that judges, administrators and the general public now expect that the case sheet be made available. This process may lead to an overly pessimistic description of the likely outcome of the operation. One can imagine that the scientific value of such reports may be reduced in the future.

The complications are determined by the neighboring structures which are in danger. After *endoscopy or operations on the antrum* these include:

- spread of inflammation to the mouth, jaw and cheek,
- disturbances of vision and lacrimal function,
- loss of sensation and neuralgia in the face and anterior scalp.

The complications of procedures on the ethmoid, sphenoid and frontal sinuses include:

- life-threatening blood loss, and bleeding into the cranial cavity,
- CSF leak with infection of the meninges and brain,
- dysosmia, leading to subjective changes in or loss of the sense of taste,
- defects of vision including blindness,
- infection of the skull base,
- pain and neuralgia in the face and head.

Secondly, it must be explained that the postoperative healing phase may last a long time. Patients often imagine that the disease will be completely relieved once they recover from the anesthetic because they have no postoperative pain, no suture line, no evidence of blood loss or external splints. It must be explained before the operation that an extensive internal organ was chronically inflamed and requires time, patience and tolerance of pain during the healing phase.

Thirdly, every surgeon must be able to answer questions about the likely outcome of the procedure. The author's results are summarized in Chapter 7.

Basic Principles of Endoscopic Surgery of the Paranasal Sinuses: Advantages, Disadvantages and Outcome

Other specialists, such as urologists, internists, etc., introduce their instruments through the endoscope (transendoscopically). Some nasal surgeons, for example Draf (1978), prefer endoscopic manipulations of this type, but the author's bad experiences with the resulting limitation to the use of very small instruments led him rapidly to decide to use a para-endoscopic technique in which the endoscope is reserved for observation only. This option allows instruments of various curves, shapes and sizes, the laser, the cutting diathermy and other instruments to be used.

The binocular operating microscope has contributed so much to the development of ear, nose and throat surgery but has a very limited place in intranasal surgery because it does not provide angular vision allowing a view through antrostomies and into niches.

At the present time simple, rigid, angled telescopes are used by many intranasal surgeons, but they rapidly become obscured by blood or secretions, and need repeated cleaning. Therefore an endoscope has been developed which keeps the eyepiece free by integrated suction and irrigation, and which also keeps the surgical field clear to some extent. However, further technical improvements are required to achieve even better use of the endoscope and special instruments, in particular better manipulation of the instruments alongside the endoscope. Furthermore, very precise removal of tissue is compromised by damage to neighboring mucosa which is worth preserving: punches and forceps that cut rather than tear, must be developed. The ideal would be an effective cutting diathermy that produced no devitalizing thermal effects on the surrounding tissue.

Even without these desirable technical improvements, endoscopic sinus surgery can now be regarded as the optimal method for restoring paranasal sinuses that are free of scar tissue, have a healthy mucosal lining and normal physiology. With an experienced endoscopic surgeon, it is also safer than radical external surgery. Its *advantages* include:

- preservation of the bony contours,
- preservation of viable mucosal surfaces with precise removal of irreversibly damaged mucosa,
- preservation of neighboring structures by optical control of anatomical details,
- abolition of complicated flap procedures on the frontal and maxillary sinuses,
- lower postoperative morbidity.

It has the following *disadvantages:*

- the view into the nose is restricted, even if the septum is first corrected,

- the extent for manipulations is limited, particularly around a bony lesion whereas external access allows radical excisions to be performed,
- suturing, wiring, the use of screws, implantation or reconstruction of entire walls using allogenic materials or ceramics cannot be achieved by endoscopic methods; external exposure is necessary for such types of reconstruction.

Endoscopic intranasal surgery has a limited place in surgery of trauma or tumors of the paranasal sinuses and anterior skull base. However, there is a place for the combination of both procedures, for example dissection of the sinuses by an external approach with endoscopic monitoring or vice versa, so that the external, destructive access does not need to be so extensive as in the classical procedures. Similarly, in severe frontobasal or middle third facial fractures, the structures are better retained if the fracture repair is performed externally whereas the ostia and the cells are debrided endoscopically.

2. Endoscopic Anatomy of the Paranasal Sinuses

Anatomical textbooks and atlases offer very accurate descriptions of the structure and topography of the nose and the paranasal sinuses, but the details have been worked out from macroscopic sections on cadaver dissections. However, the intranasal surgeon must be able to orientate himself looking through straight or angled endoscopes. He must develop a three-dimensional mental image allowing him to know exactly where he is, where the ducts and the danger points lie, and what structures are closely related. Endoscopic topographical anatomy is presented by a discussion of the important regions of the nasal cavity. Three-dimensional anatomy is presented by tomograms and an illustrated dissection of the paranasal sinuses based on photographs and line diagrams.

The Nasal Cavity and its Endoscopic Landmarks

The medial nasal wall, the nasal septum, is simple and smooth, unlike the highly complex lateral nasal wall, the area of interest for the endoscopic surgeon (Figure 2.**1**). The ducts and ostia, covered by the nasal turbinates, form the entrances to the paranasal sinuses. The size and position of the lateral nasal wall vary widely, dictated by the paranasal sinuses. The following endoscopic views should be mentally projected onto the complex of the lateral nasal wall. When the endoscope, usually the 25° telescope, is introduced into the nostril, it impinges immediately on the vibrissae of the nasal vestibule obstructing the view of the nasal valve; therefore these hairs should be trimmed before an endoscopic procedure (Figure 2.**2**). *The nasal valve* is formed by the floor of the nose, the septum and the lower edge of the upper lateral cartilage tilted inwards. Anteriorly the septum and the floor of the nose usually has ridges on both sides arising from the pre-maxilla. The slit-like opening could hinder a view during intranasal surgery, so that preliminary septal correction can be useful; the necessary access may also be widened by a nasal speculum.

Immediately behind the nasal valve lies the second narrow point: the anterior end of the *inferior turbinate* takes up two-third of the field of vision, and divides the inspiratory airstream into an upper and a lower pathway (Figure 2.**3**).

The field of vision can be improved by vigorous decongestion of the musoca by pledgets soaked in 1/1000 adrenalin solution. However, the bone of the anterior end of the turbinate may be large and obstruct the view, requiring limited resection. The body of the turbinate consists of the rigid turbinate bone and erectile tissue (Figure 2.**4**) covering its medial surface. The lateral wall of the turbinate is shaped like a gutter, so that the border between the mucosal surfaces is tilted externally. The inferior meatus lies lateral to the inferior turbinate: its lateral wall is the lowest part of the lateral nasal wall. The line of insertion of the turbinate bone is concave downwards (Figure 2.**5**), and lacks any particular landmarks. Its bony wall is thinnest at the center, just below the

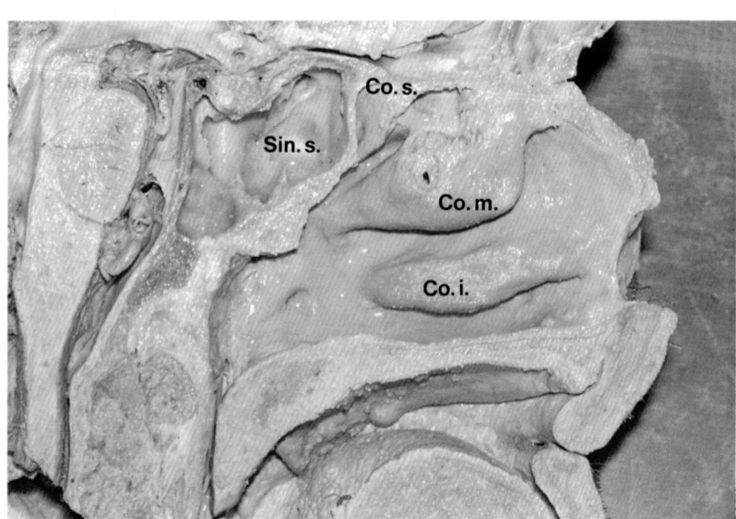

Figure 2.**1** The lateral nasal wall, showing the middle and inferior turbinates and the rudiment of a superior turbinate. The sagittal section through the skull shows the topographical relationships with the anterior skull base, the sphenoid sinus and the nasopharynx. Behind the latter lie the brain stem and the cervical spine.

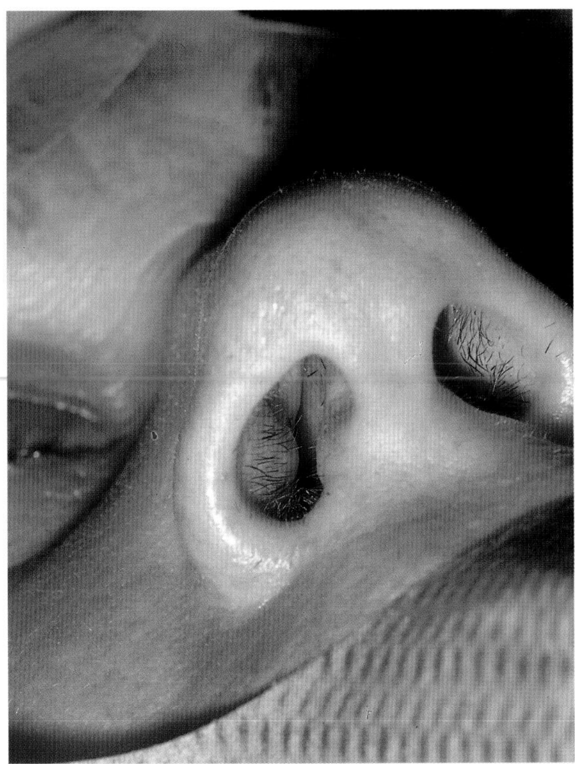

Figure 2.2 The nostrils with narrowing of the nasal vestibule by the process of the ala cartilage (medially) and by the projection of the superior edge of the ala cartilage and the lower edge of the triangular cartilage lying laterally.

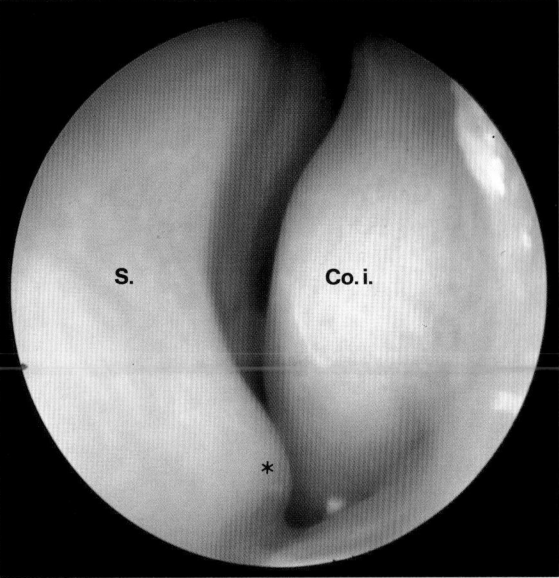

Figure 2.3 The beginning of the common nasal meatus lying behind the nasal valve is narrowed by a septal ridge (*) representing the upper edge of the premaxilla, and by the anterior end of the inferior turbinate.

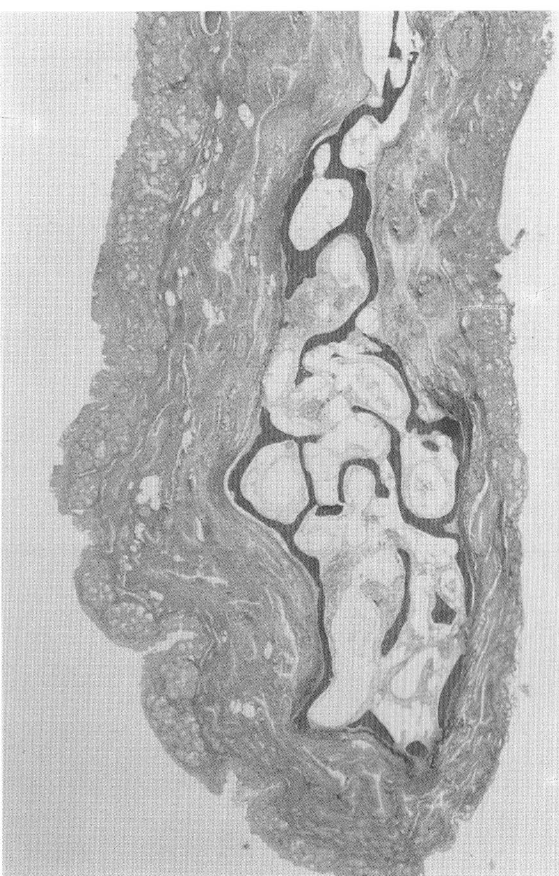

Figure 2.4 Histological appearance of a transverse section through the inferior turbinate. The spongiform erectile tissue is rich in vessels and is covered by rich veins, particularly medially. Numerous mucosal glands lie in the respiratory epithelium (elastic-van Gieson 7×).

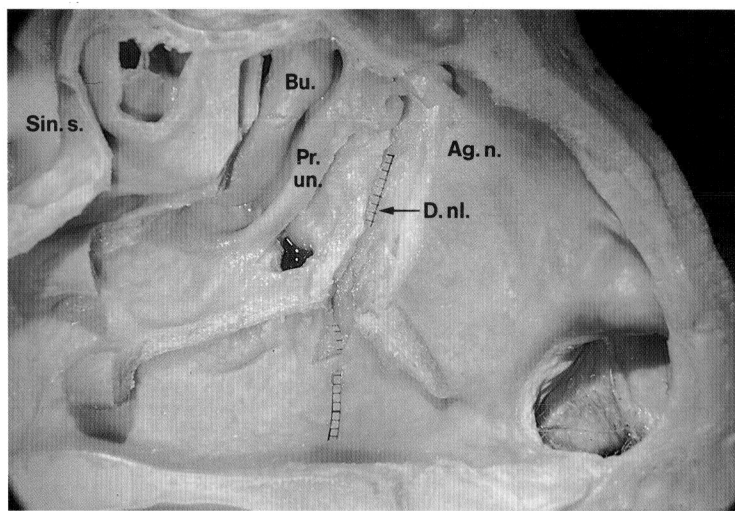

Figure 2.5 The left lateral nasal wall (dissection by Prof. Dr. J. Lang of Wuerzburg). The inferior and middle turbinates have been removed, and the superior turbinate has been fenestrated. The complex consisting of the middle turbinate with the uncinate process, the semilunar hiatus, the bulla and a superior nasal meatus can be recognized. The lacrimal duct has been exposed as far as its opening into the inferior meatus (mm paper). The anterior fontanelle marks a secondary ostium of the antral cavity.

apex of the curve, and antral puncture is most easily carried out at this point. The anterior insertion of the inferior turbinate may lie only 2–3 mm above the floor of the nose, so that an endoscope may only be introduced with difficulty beneath the inferior meatus, leaving little space for an accompanying instrument (Figure 2.**6**). A vertical incision through the mucosa and bone may then be needed at this point to allow the turbinate to be displaced medially and upwards.

The *lacrimal canal* opens immediately behind and about 2 mm below the insertion of the turbinate. Its slit-like opening into the anterosuperior part of the inferior meatus (Figure 2.**7**) must be strictly avoided when creating an inferior meatal antrostomy using the punch. Endoscopic exposure of the lacrimal sac and canal is considerably helped by identification of its nasal ostium. Figure 2.**5** shows the course of the lacrimal canal in the lateral nasal wall of a cadaver (see also Figure 2.**27 f.**)

Extending superiorly from the nasal vestibule, the next structure to come into view is the *agger nasi*, a smooth bony swelling lying in front of the anterior insertion of the middle turbinate (Figure 2.**8**). It may

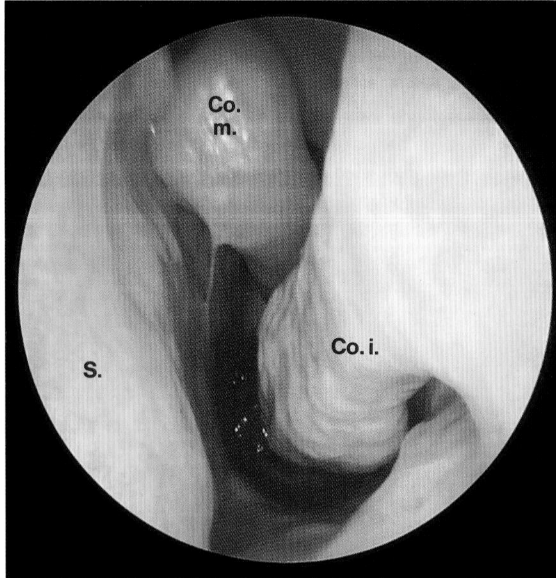

Figure 2.**6** A deep attachment of the inferior turbinate impedes the introduction of the endoscope into the left inferior meatus.

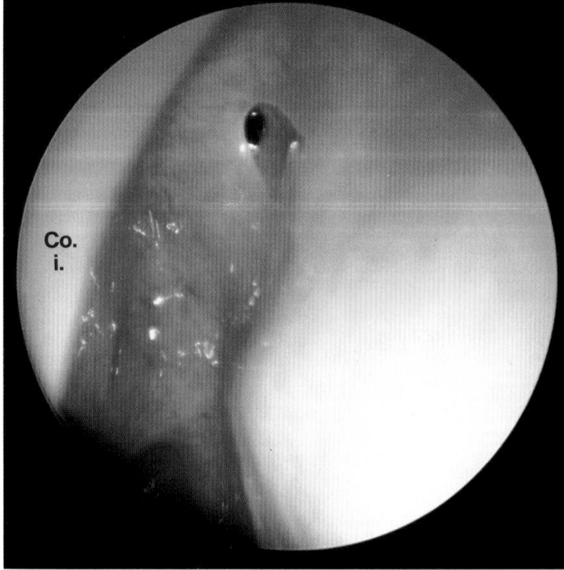

Figure 2.**7** Left inferior meatus with the ostium and the lacrimal duct (70° telescope with a view superiorly).

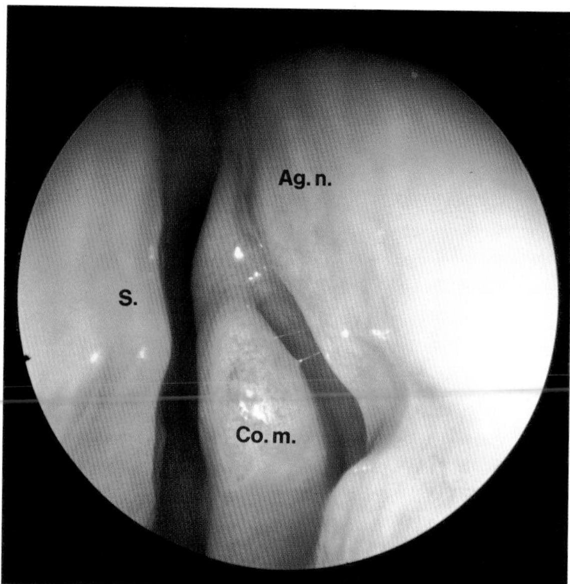

Figure 2.**8** Left nasal cavity with the anterior insertion of the middle turbinate close behind the agger nasi (70° telescope with a view in a superior direction).

be pneumatized and thin walled, and contain the agger nasi cells; more often it has a thick bony wall. Lateral to the agger nasi lies the outflow tract of the frontal sinus, the frontonasal duct. This is normally approached from the semilunar hiatus via the ethmoidal infundibulum, but after ethmoidectomy and clearance of the infundibulum it is entered directly from the nasal cavity. Identification of the agger nasi from the nasal introitus is therefore important. The agger nasi is also an important landmark for endoscopic exposure of the nasolacrimal canal: the canal lies lateral to the lateral nasal wall at the same level as the agger nasi or 1–2 mm in front of it. It runs parallel to the agger, after running medially under some ethmoidal cells. This proximity explains why the lacrimal canal is in danger in the region around the ethmoid cells in massive polyposis with bony erosion. The frontal sinus, the nasolacrimal duct and the agger nasi lie in roughly the same frontal plane.

Passage of the endoscope into the common nasal meatus beyond the narrow area at the anterior end of the inferior turbinate is often hindered further by a *ridge* on the lower edge of the nasal septum. This is formed by the premaxilla and the palatal ridge of the maxilla onto which impinges the lower edge of the septal cartilage. An accessory (Huschke's) cartilage also lies at this point (Zuckerkandl). More superiorly the septum again restricts vision of the nasal roof: an apparent upper septal deviation is actually a widening of the septum (Figure 2.**9a, b**), the turberculum septi (Zuckerkandl). It is present on both sides and

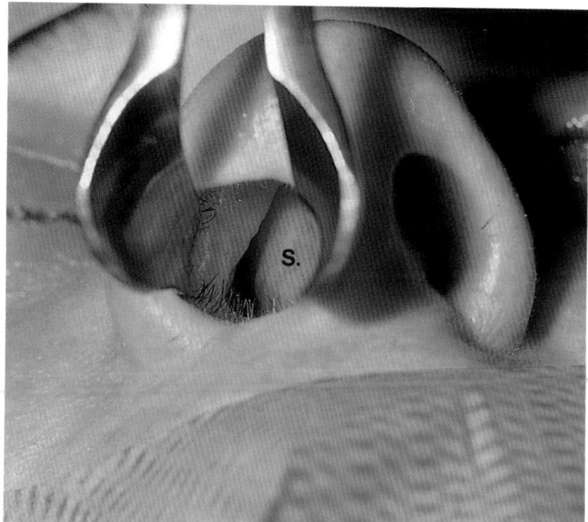

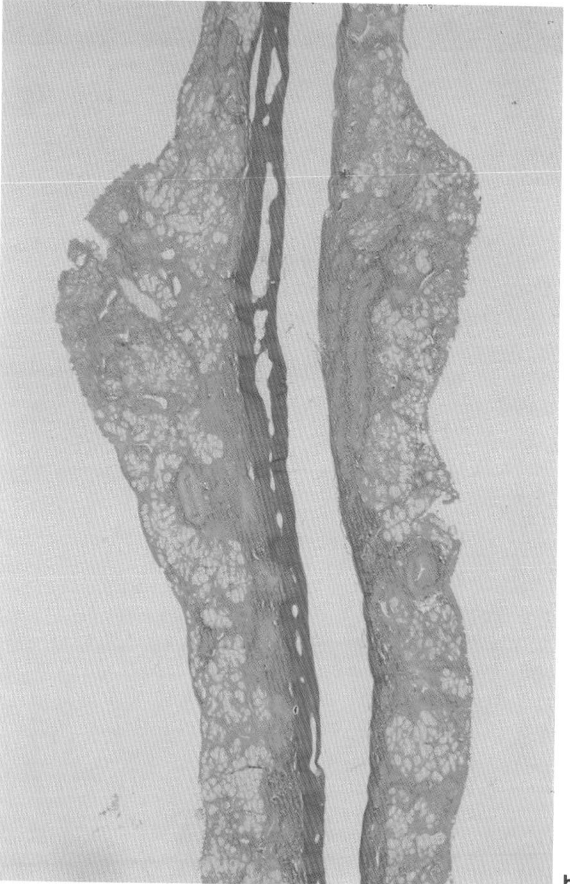

Figure 2.**9** Superior narrowing of the common nasal meatus by the piriform aperture (laterally) and thickening of the septum (medially). **a** Clinical photograph. **b** The histological appearances show that the "pseudodeviation" of the nasal septum is rudimentary erectile tissue body rich in glands and vessels (elastic van-Gieson, 4×).

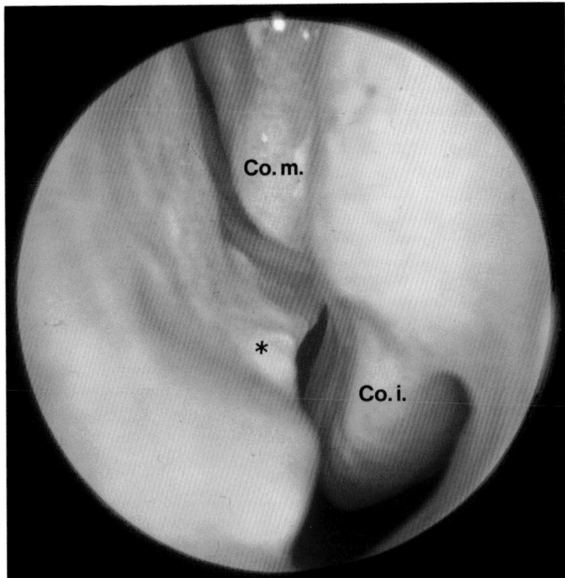

Figure 2.**10** Marked narrowing of the left common nasal meatus by a vomerine ridge running posteriorly and upwards, and impinging upon the atrophic inferior turbinate. The body of the middle turbinate lies on the ridge (75° telescope).

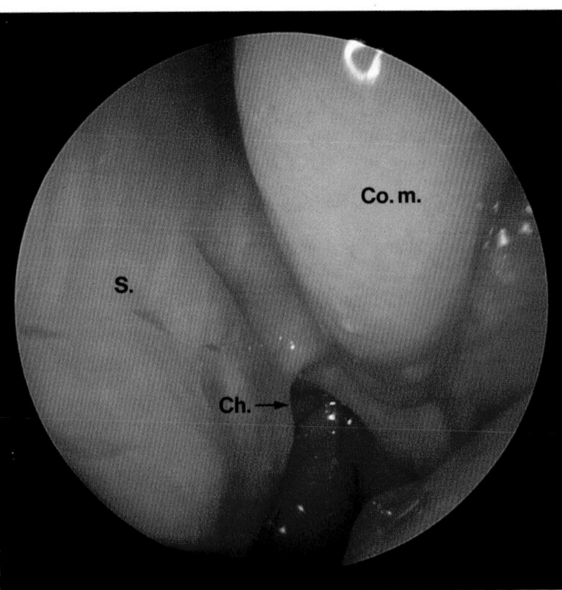

Figure 2.**11** Posterior part of the left nasal cavity. The straight telescope lies between the inferior turbinate and the free edge of the middle turbinate, and the upper edge of the choana can be seen in the center of the field of vision.

histologically it is formed by rudimentary erectile tissue. In addition, a widening of the bony septum may be hidden beneath it. The CT scan in Figure 2.**22**b shows its relation to the base of the skull. It is almost impossible to remove without damaging the mucosa; if it is well developed and is obstructing drainage it may have a very unfavorable influence on the healing of the ethmoid gutter after ethmoidectomy. Synechiae often form in this area where the septum is wide after rough extraction of nasal polyps.

Further back, the endoscope impinges on another obstruction, the oblique *ascending septal ridge* formed by the edge of the vomer and the end of the quadrilateral cartilage extending backwards (Figure 2.**10**). It may even impinge upon the middle turbinate and protrude into the middle meatus affecting the airstream. To bring the nasal choana into view the endoscope must be passed beneath the ascending septal ridge rather than over it. The mucosa along the ridge is usually atrophic and vulnerable to the passage of the endoscope.

The lower *posterior nasal region* and the choanae (Figure 2.**11**) can almost always be inspected with a 0° or 25° rigid or flexible telescope passed along the floor of the nose. In adults the choanae are 1.5 to 2.0 cm high, and form an important landmark (Figure 2.**12**).

The posterior end of the inferior turbinate projects into the lower part of the posterior nasal choana from the lateral side, occupying up to half its height. It is often hypertrophic, resembling a mulberry, and then can considerably narrow the choana. The posterior insertion of the middle turbinate lies in the upper third of the choana, just in front of its anterior edge (Figure 2.**13**). This point of attachment forms a landmark for the front wall of the sphenoid sinus: a thin point in the bony wall of the anterior sphenoidal sinus can be found and perforated lying a little more than 1 cm above and 0.5 cm medially. This point can also be palpated 1 cm above the dome of the choana paramedially. The sphenoidal ostium lies higher and somewhat more medial. It is seldom suitable for access to the sphenoidal sinus. The posterior third of the middle turbinate lies in the same sagittal plane as the lateral wall of the sphenoid sinus. The posterior end of the inferior turbinate and the ostium of the Eustachian tube lie at the same level, and in the same sagittal plane, but separated by the choana (Figure 2.**13**).

The *middle meatus* is the most important region for endoscopic nasal examination: it is the normal entrance to the ethmoid, frontal and maxillary sinuses, and also provides a portal for their surgical exposure. It can only be seen properly after displacing the middle turbinate medially. Figure 2.**14** shows a cadaver dissection after removal of the middle turbinate. The middle meatus extends over two-thirds of the length of the lateral nasal wall between the cut edge of the middle turbinate and the upper edge of the inferior turbinate. After removal of the soft tissues, the bony specimen (Figure 2.**15**) shows the

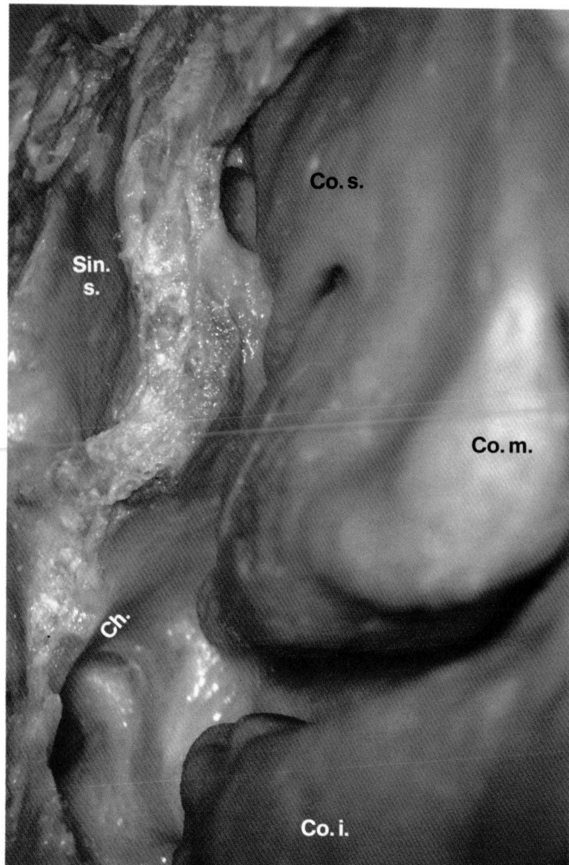

Figure 2.**12** Topography of the posterior part of the left nasal cavity in an anatomical dissection, showing an endoscopic view from in front of the heads of the inferior and middle turbinate. Above this lies a slit-like superior nasal meatus. Medially, next to the rudiment of the superior turbinate, lies the ostium of the sphenoid sinus whose anterior wall has been fenestrated. The posterior end of the middle turbinate, the roof of the choana, the posterior end of the inferior turbinate and the ostium of the Eustachian tube all lie at the same level.

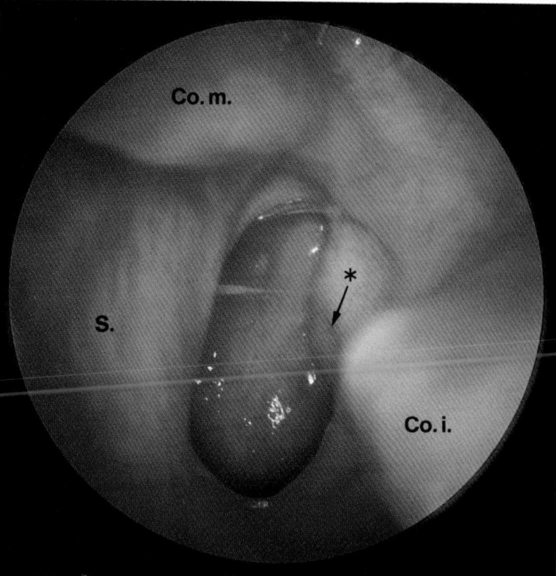

Figure 2.**13** The choana in endoscopic view from in front with a straight telescope on the floor of the nose. The posterior end of the inferior turbinate and the ostium of the Eustachian tube (*) lie at the same level, and require care during posterior turbinectomy. In this case the posterior attachment of the middle turbinate crosses the roof of the choana.

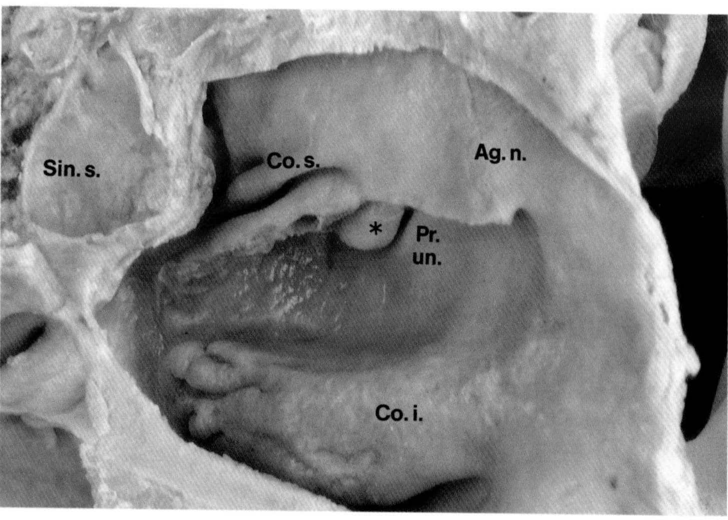

Figure 2.**14** The lateral nasal wall with the sphenoid sinus in an anatomical dissection after removal of the body of the middle turbinate. Between the upper edge of the inferior turbinate and the lower edge of the uncinate process this membranous part of the lateral nasal wall has a height of 1 cm. The ethmoidal bulla (*) hangs into the middle meatus and partially covers the semilunar hiatus. The continuation of the middle turbinate running obliquely upwards and suspended laterally from the lateral nasal wall can be seen. Above it lies a superior turbinate and the rudiment of a supreme turbinate. The ostium of the sphenoidal cavity is visible as a shadow.

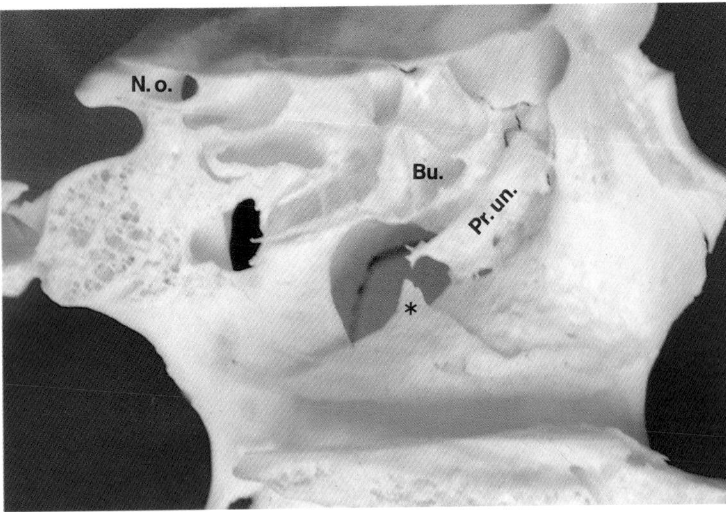

Figure 2.**15** The left lateral wall in a macerated bone. The ethmoid process of the turbinate bone (*) directed superiorly in this case divides the bone-free wall of the antral cavity into a small anterior and a large posterior fontanelle. The uncinate process bounds the semilunar hiatus and the ethmoid infundibulum which is separated from it from below and medial. The ethmoid bulla projecting above the hiatus is opened, demonstrating cells of the anterior and middle ethmoids. Above the basal lamella of the middle turbinate lie the posterior ethmoid cells. The most posterosuperior cells cover the canal for the optic nerve.

relationships in the middle meatus: the ethmoid process ascending from the turbinate bone divides the membranous part of the lateral nasal wall into an anterior and a posterior fontanelle. Usually a small spicule of bone runs toward it from the uncinate process. The endoscopic view (Figure 2.**16**) in the cadaver shows the ethmoid bulla, forming the lower limit of the ethmoid cell system, and the lateral boundary of the middle turbinate. The bulla also forms the upper edge of the semilunar hiatus. The most anterior ethmoid cells, the maxillary sinus and the frontal sinus drain into the hiatus; the frontal sinus opens into the ethmoid infundibulum, the most anterior, upward-pointing and deeply etched prolongation of the hiatus. The hiatus and the infundibulum are usually not visible with the endoscope, so that the primary maxillary ostium cannot be inspected.

Between the curved, anteriorly projecting, uncinate process and the insertion of the inferior turbinate lies a smooth strip of the lateral wall of the middle nasal meatus, 2–4 mm high. This area is part bony and part membranous, the latter being formed by the fontanelles, and it often contains an opening

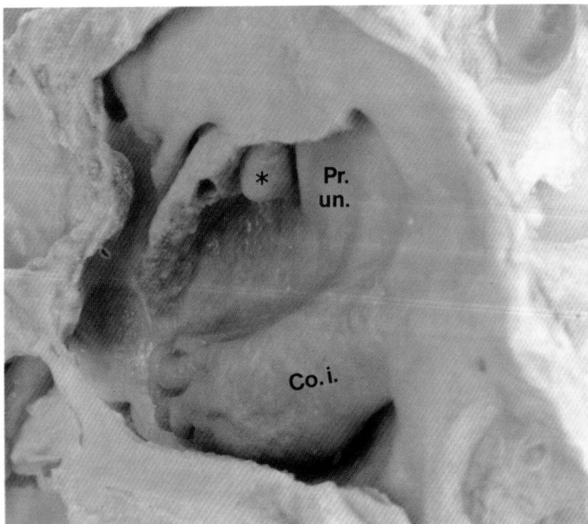

Figure 2.**16** The lateral wall in an anatomical dissection similar to that of Figure 2.**14** viewed from in front.

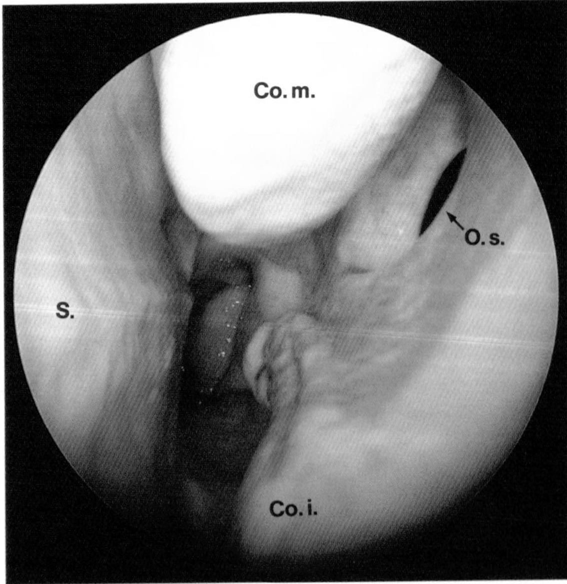

Figure 2.**17** Endoscopic view through a straight telescope of the middle meatus with a secondary ostium in the posterior fontanelle of an anatomical dissection. The middle turbinate conceals the semilunar hiatus.

into the maxillary sinus, the secondary ostium (Figure 2.**17**). The relationships of the middle meatus to the ethmoid sinuses, the maxillary and frontal sinuses, and particularly to the orbit must be studied with great care before beginning intranasal surgery. These are particularly well shown by a series of frontal CT scans (Figure 2.**19** ff.).

The *middle turbinate* is of central importance in endoscopic surgery: its body is integrated into the ethmoid cell system (Figure 2.**18**) so that ethmoid disease extends into the middle turbinate, but not into the inferior turbinate. The medial lamella of the middle turbinate is inserted anteriorly into the skull base: it conducts fibers from the olfactory nerve, is covered with olfactory mucosa, and thus forms part of the olfactory region. In contrast the posterior part of the turbinate is anchored relatively loosely to the ethmoid bone (Figure 2.**19 a, b**), and only its posterior edge is attached to the lateral nasal wall (Figure 2.**13**). As a result good exposure of the pos-

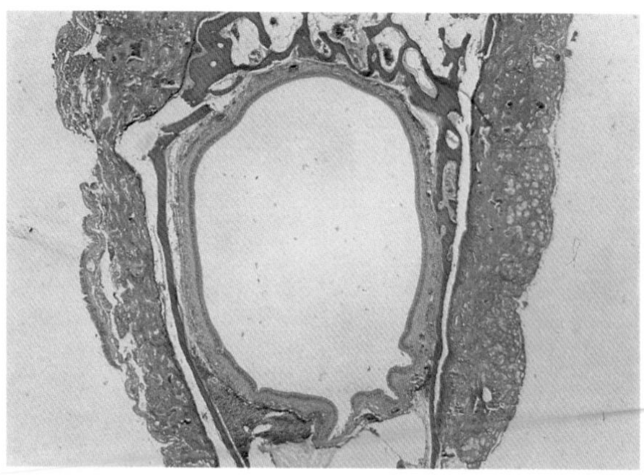

Figure 2.**18** Pneumatized middle turbinate (concha bullosa). The hollow space in the free body of the middle concha is lined by respiratory mucosa (elastic-van Gieson).

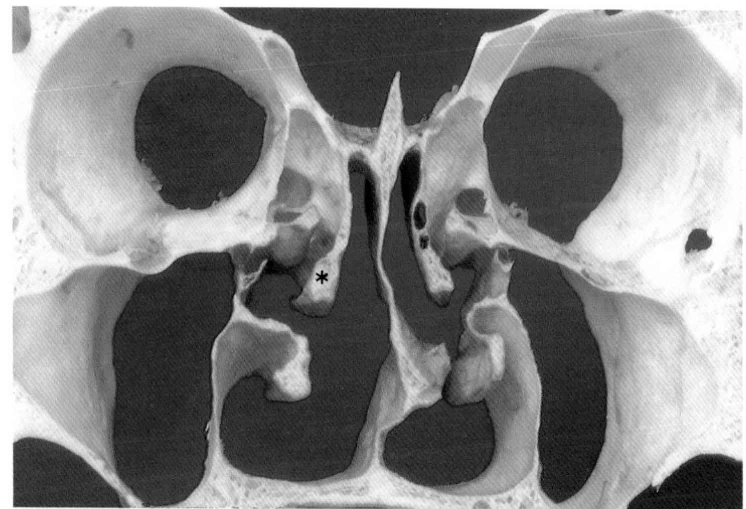

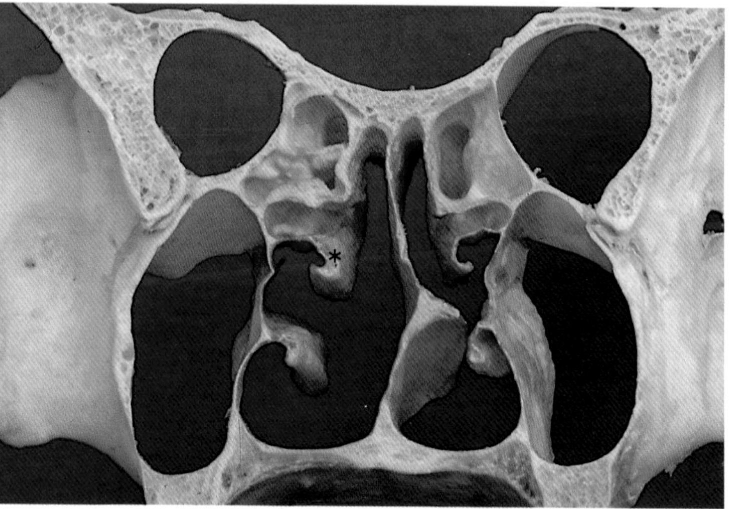

Figure 2.**19** Coronal section through a dissected skull showing the view from in front. **a** The medial lamella of the middle turbinate (*) inserting into the skull base at the level of the crista galli, immediately lateral to the edge of the cribriform plate. **b** The ethmoid roof is thickly ossified at the level of the sphenoid plane, and the medial lamella of the middle turbinate now inserts into the ethmoid or into the lateral nasal wall. Above it, the latter is identical with the orbital wall.

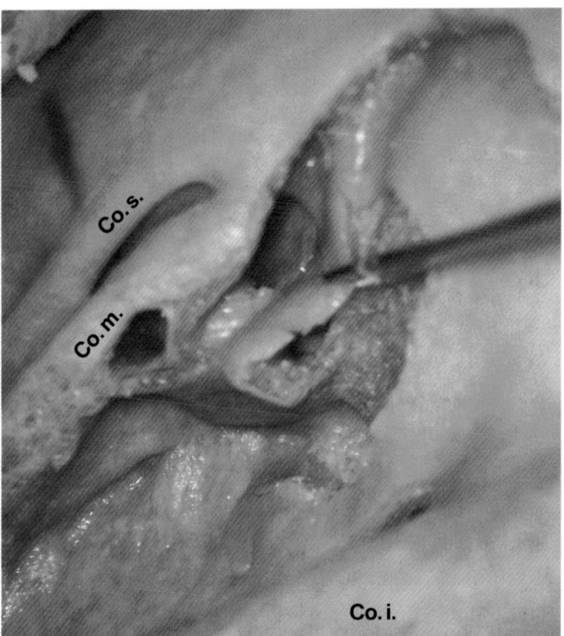

Figure 2.**20** Posterior ethmoid cells in an anatomical dissection. These cells lie behind and above the divided middle turbinate. A needle is pressing the opened bulla downwards. The picture explains why the middle turbinate often floats freely and tears off if it is not removed during an extensive posterior ethmoidectomy.

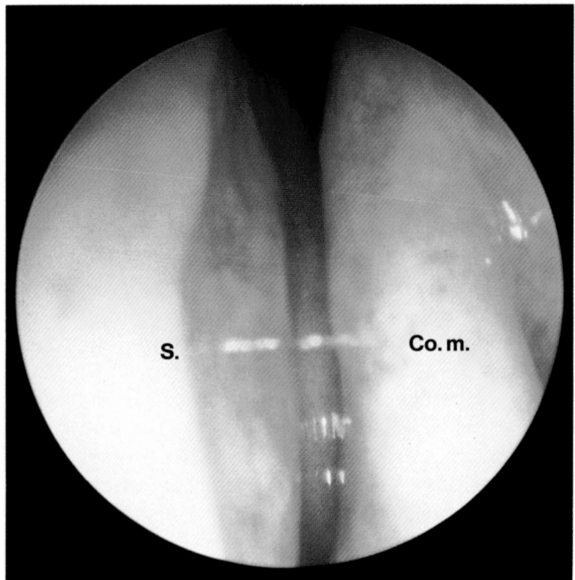

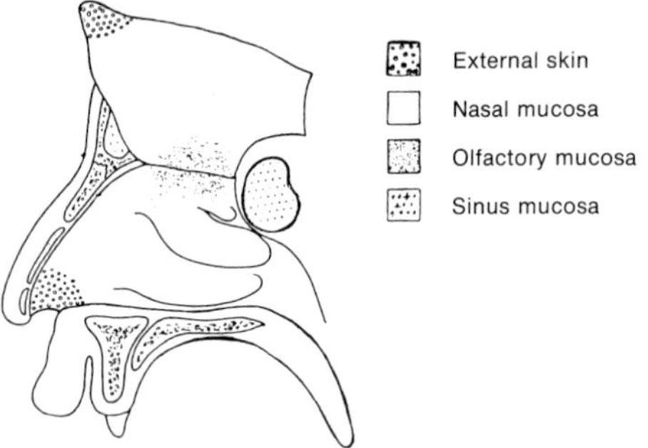

Figure 2.**21** The olfactory cleft. **a** View upwards into the nasal cavity with a 70° telescope. The common nasal meatus narrows medial to the middle turbinate to form the olfactory cleft. **b** Diagram of the olfactory area. The septum has been turned upwards (from Bucher, O.: Cytologie, Histologie und Mikroskopische Anatomie des Menschen, 8th edition, Huber, Bern 1973).

terosuperior ethmoid cells can only be achieved by partial resection of the middle turbinate (Figure 2.**20**). The junction of the part attached to the skull base and the dependent ethmoid bone lies at the posterior edge of the cribriform plate. It can be easily recognized during intranasal endoscopy, and is thus an important landmark.

In front of this junction the middle turbinate carries olfactory fibers, so that destruction of the bony base of the turbinate carries the danger of tearing these fibers leading to a CSF fistula. Behind this junction, on the other hand, the ethmoid roof may be exposed as far as the septum without the danger of a CSF fistula.

The *superior nasal meatus* is difficult to inspect, particularly if the septum is widened or deviated. In front, it contains the *olfactory cleft,* a narrow slit extending superiorly between the middle turbinate and the nasal septum to the roof of the nose (Figure 2.**21 a, b**), and covered on both sides by olfactory mucosa. Posteriorly, the superior nasal meatus is narrowed by the downward-sloping anterior wall of the sphenoid sinus. The superior meatus is similarly narrowed if a supreme nasal turbinate is present, although the latter is usually recognizable only as a smooth swelling (Figure 2.**5**). The natural sphenoid ostium often cannot be recognized at endoscopy, but can occasionally be seen after displacing the middle turbinate laterally, although this may be difficult if the bone is hard (Figure 2.**12**).

A CT Scan Study of the Spatial Arrangement of the Paranasal Sinuses

An important prerequisite for safe endoscopic surgery within the paranasal sinuses is a clear three-dimensional mental picture of their spatial relationships to each other and to the neighboring maxilla, orbit, sphenoid sinus and anterior cranial fossa. This knowledge allows the surgeon to avoid the danger areas while taking full advantage of the endoscopic technique, and gives him the confidence to continue the procedure rather than abandoning it prematurely because of groundless anxieties. The layout of the cell system can best be learnt step-by-step from a series of high resolution CT scans. However, even the most recent three-dimensional reconstructions of CT scan sections do not substitute for a stratigraphic comparison of CT scans and anatomical sections of the skull base as an optimal basis for exploration of these intercommunicating hollow spaces within the anterior skull base.

Vertical Coronal Sections

Examination of coronal CT scans begins anteriorly at the root of the nose. The plane is tilted 10–20° backwards from above downwards, depending on the type of the apparatus and on the patient's ability to extend the head while lying prone. The *frontal sinus* comes into view first (Figure 2.**22 a–c**). Its extension superiorly and laterally varies between subjects, and the sinus is seldom symmetrical on the two sides. Extensive supraorbital niches indicate that an intranasal procedure will not reach the periphery of the sinus without an additional external approach.

The interfrontal septum is seldom in the midline and usually lies lateral to the nasal septum, an important fact in transnasal frontal sinusotomy. The outflow tract of the frontal sinus (the *frontal infundibulum*) tapers inferiorly. It is often directed slightly posteriorly, and runs under the forward convexity of the posterior wall of the frontal sinus. The transition to a true duct or opening into an anterior ethmoid cell may lie very deeply. Superomedial to this point, the nasal roof is formed by the anterior edge of the olfactory cleft, and the crista galli is at its greatest extent at this point. Often the frontonasal duct impinges tightly on the orbital wall, whereas medial to it lie even smaller cell tracts which cannot be inspected.

The *anterior ethmoid cells* are very variable in shape. Sometimes they project into the frontal sinus; rarely supraorbital ethmoidal cells may also run laterally and above the frontal sinus so that the orbit has a doubly pneumatized upper layer. The prebullar

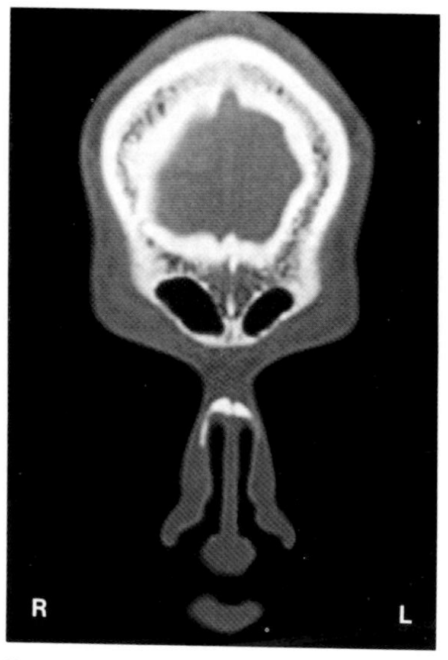

a

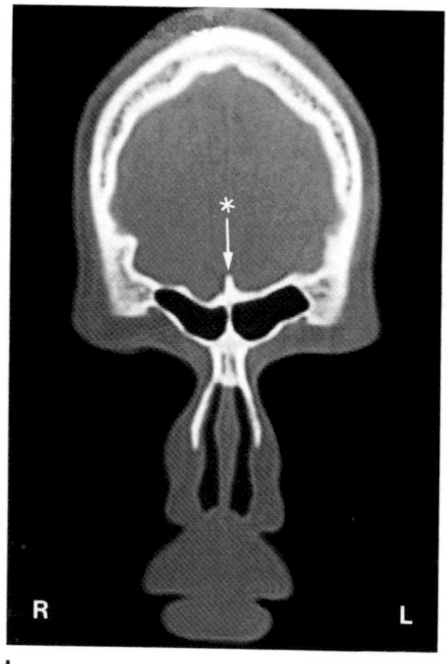

b

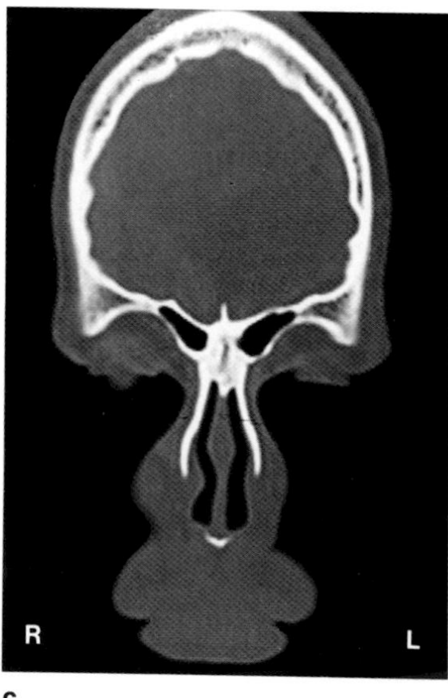

c

Figure 2.**22** The spatial arrangement of the nasal sinuses in a series of quasicoronal high-resolution CT sections. **a** Section through both sinuses just in front of the root of the nose. **b** The interfrontal septum and anterior edge of the crista galli (*) in the midline. Root of the nose. **c** The infundibulum of the frontal sinus.

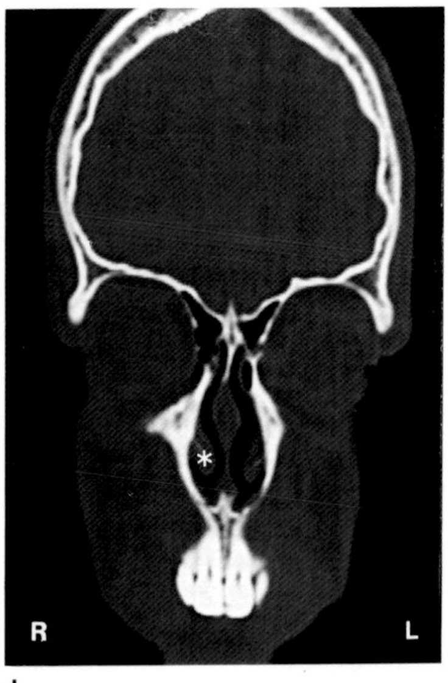

d

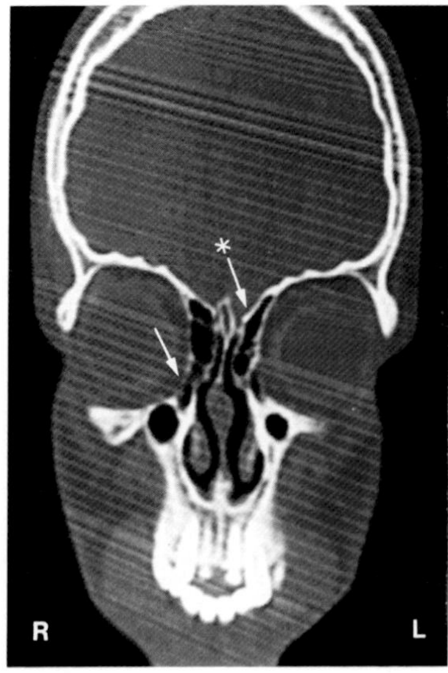

e

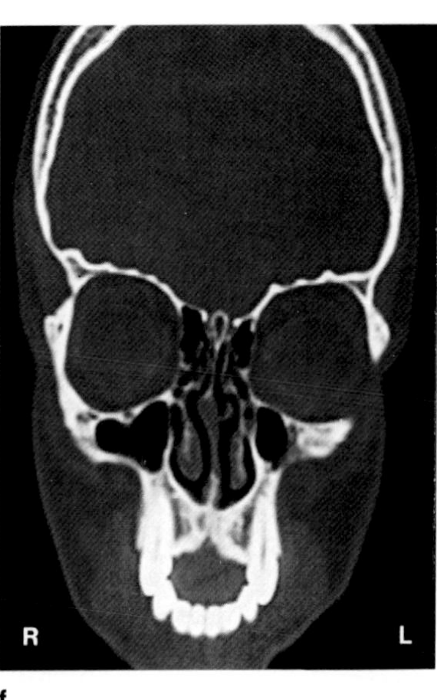

f

d The crista galli, the infundibulum of the frontal sinus and the anterior ethmoid cells are again shown. The end of the inferior turbinate lies in the piriform aperture (*). The upper incisor teeth are shown, and the section cuts across the lacrimal canal. **e** Paramedian oblique section (*) of the anterior skull base (olfactory fossa). Immediately lateral to the agger nasi lies the divided lacrimal canal marked with an arrow. Inferolateral to this lies the prelacrimal recess of the antral cavity. The crista galli is shown as a prolongation above the septum. **f** Pneumatized crista galli, depression due to the cribriform plate, the middle ethmoids, the middle turbinate beginning on the left, and a concave nasal floor.

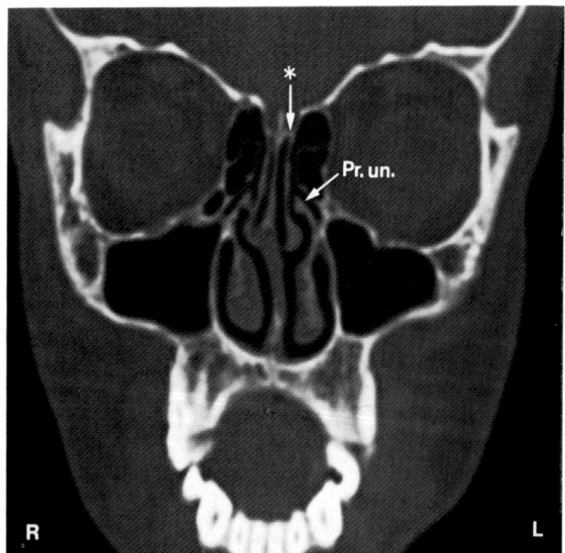

g Coronal plane behind the lacrimal duct. The olfactory region with a steeply hollowed-out olfactory fossa can be seen. The medial lamella of the middle turbinate inserts into the base of the skull (*) and marks the outer edge of the narrow cribriform plate. The uncinate process and a bullar cell are visible on both sides. The lateral ethmoid wall is roughly the same height as the medial wall of the antrum.

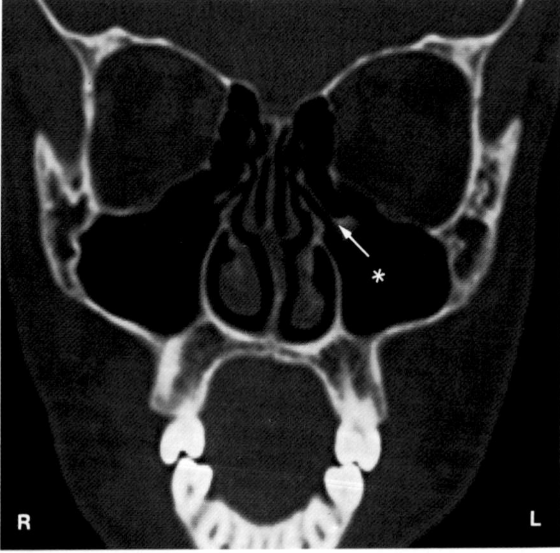

h End of the cribriform plate, with the middle turbinate still extending to the base of the skull. The middle ethmoid cells are shown at the level of the ethmoid bulla. A deep canal from the semilunar hiatus to the maxillary ostium is shown (*) over a high uncinate process. The antral cavities extending laterally now support the orbit completely.

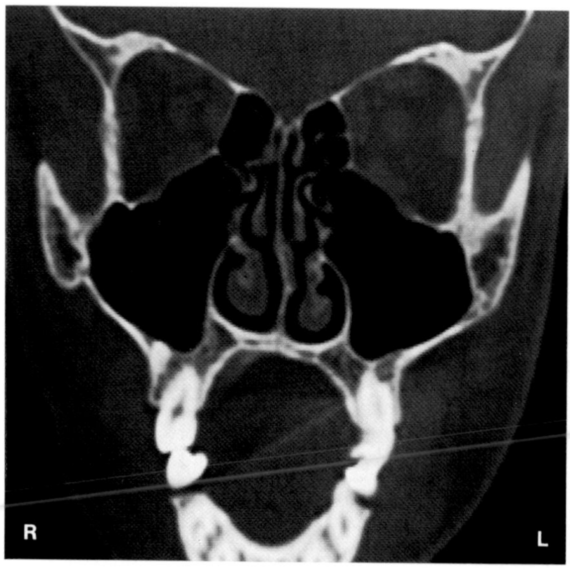

i The middle turbinates now insert into the ethmoids. The end of the ethmoid infundibulum on the left is well visible. The medial wall of the antrum has gained in height at the cost of the lateral ethmoid wall.

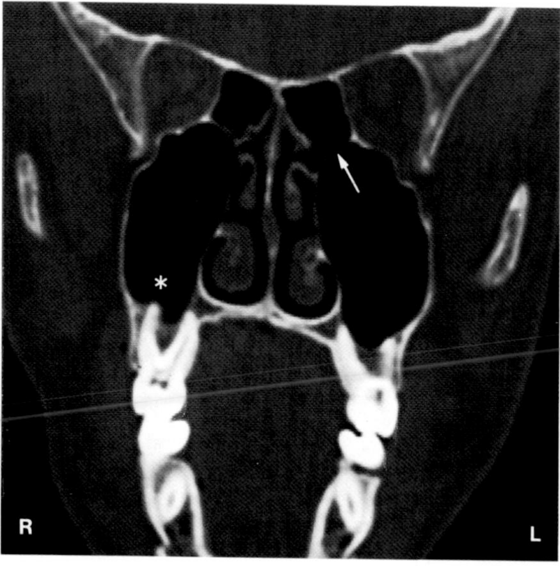

j The posterior end of the ethmoid is considerably wider than the anterior, and its roof is flat and rigid. The root of a molar tooth (*) on the right side projects into the alveolar recess of the now high antral cavity. The party wall between the medial third of the antral roof and the ethmoid compartment is very thin, and is marked by an arrow.

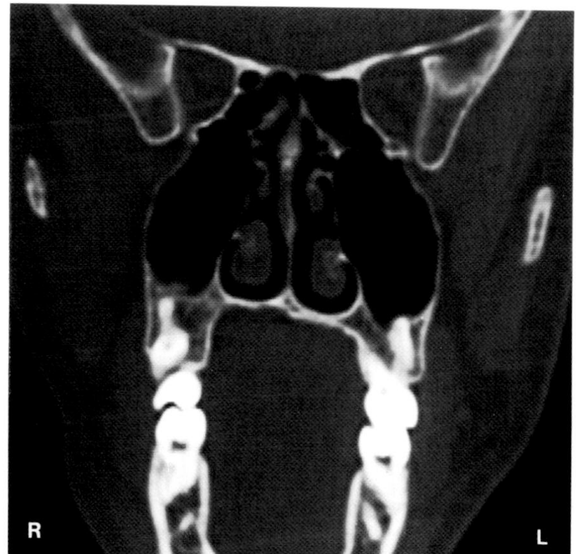

k Posterior ethmoid immediately in front of the sphenoid cavity. The middle turbinate is now slender and shows a thin area of insertion into the lateral nasal wall (i.e. the medial antral wall). The ethmoid in this section is twice as wide as in front.

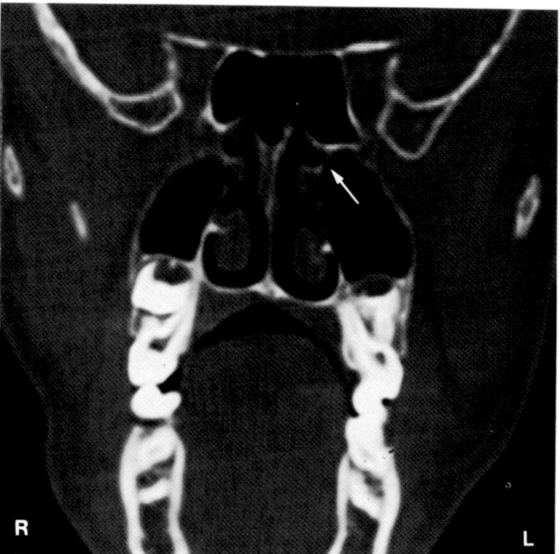

l An asymmetrical sphenoid sinus immediately behind its anterior wall. The intersphenoid septum lies obliquely, above the nasal septum. The end of the antral cavity lies in front of the pterygoid process. The medial wall of the antrum is marked with an arrow.

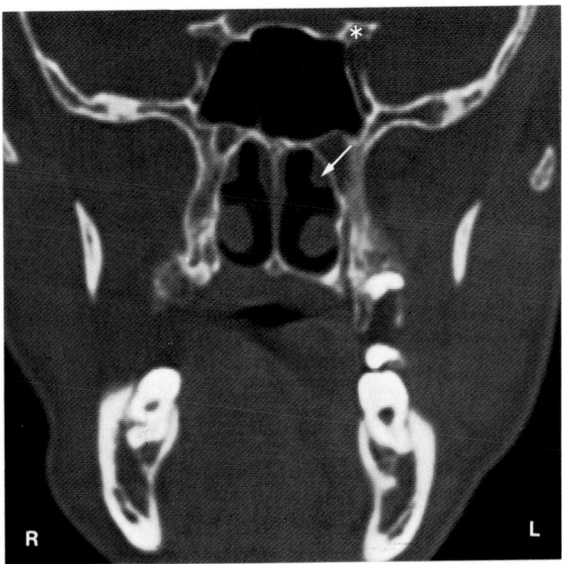

m A small right and a large left sphenoid sinus, and the clinoid process (*). The externally directed insertion of the middle turbinate lies on each side on the pterygoid process, marked with an arrow.

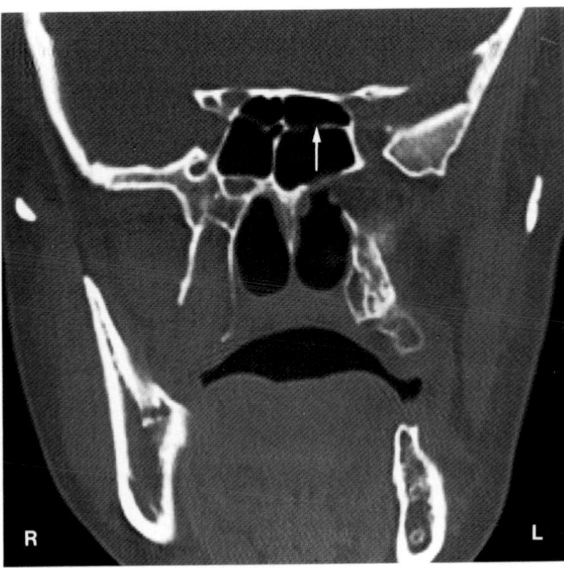

n Sphenoid sinus lying over the posterior end of the nose and the posterior edge of the vomer. Its height is about the same as that of the choana. Ridges present in the posterior wall marked with an arrow (different patient to that shown in Figures 2.**22 a–n**).

cell system is divided up even more precisely (Terrier 1987) as follows:

- uncinate cells with upper, anterior (agger) and posterior cells,
- anterior and posterior meatal cells.

Classically the upper uncinate cell opens into the frontal sinus, but the frontal sinus may also drain via the meatal cell. Bagatella and Guirado (1983) name these cell groups as follows:

- pre-infundibular cells (0–1 cell) with the agger nasi cell,
- lateral infundibular cells (0–2 cells),
- post-infundibular cells (0–2 cells).

The varying development of these cells is the cause of the differences in the outflow tract of the frontal sinus.

The *nasal septum* can always be recognized easily on CT scans. Its height increases from anteriorly to the middle, reaches its maximum beneath the crista galli where it contacts the base of the skull in the midline and then decreases towards the choana, to not quite half of its original size. The anterior soft tissue widening of the septum lying close to the anterior end of the inferior turbinate can always be recognized, and its varying cartilaginous and bony construction can be recognized over its entire length as far as the vomer.

The interfrontal septum in front and the intersphenoidal septum behind do not always lie in the same plane as the nasal septum. This is important information in transeptal sphenoidotomy. The asymmetrical insertion of the septum into the palate, and the varying level of the floor of the nose can also be seen easily on CT scans.

The *lateral nasal wall* must be examined systematically. Below it is typically convex, corresponding to the concavity of the medial antral wall, and above concave corresponding with the lateral ethmoid wall. The edge is convex into the nose and concave into the orbit (Figure 2.**22 f**). This relationship is usually constant between sides and between subjects, giving the surgeon confidence during sphenoidal-ethmoidal operations. Whereas the lateral wall of the ethmoid and nasal cavity thus forms a lazy S in frontal section, the continuation of the lateral ethmoid wall into the roof of the maxillary cavity forms a continuous curve without a step, an important point during intranasal maxillary operations and middle meatal antrostomy.

The point of intersection of the lateral nasal contour with the orbitomaxillary arch is an important landmark: 1 to 3 mm beneath it lies the primary maxillary ostium. This outflow tract often runs very close to the orbit, almost exactly in the same frontal plane in which the medial lamella of the middle turbinate swings away from the base of the skull to insert into the ethmoid (Figure 2.**22 h** and **i**). This point represents the posterior end of the olfactory cleft.

Whereas the point of intersection of the roof of the maxilla with the lateral wall of the nose or of the ethmoids lies about halfway up the nose at the center it inclines upwards due to the tapering of the orbit, until it breaks up in the root of the pterygoid process. Further posteriorly the lateral wall of the ethmoid is continuous with the lateral wall of the sphenoid cavity without a step. This slightly bulging but smooth transition between the lateral sphenoid and ethmoid wall can be easily recognized on axial CT scans. This detailed knowledge of anatomy facilitates complete removal of cells during intranasal ethmoidosphenoid operations.

The shape of the *maxillary cavity* changes from anterior to posterior. In front it is triangular, in the middle kidney-shaped, and posteriorly it resembles a large almond with rounded contours. Familiarity with its upper (ethmoid) and lower (alveolar and palatine) recesses (Figure 2.**23**) is important since they must be reached by instruments introduced through an inferior or middle meatal antrostomy.

Before intranasal procedures, particularly revision surgery, it is worthwhile estimating the relationship of the *inferior turbinate* to the nasal and maxillary cavities on serial three-dimensional sections. The extent of the obstruction of the common and inferior meatus by the turbinate bone is clear, although its absolute size varies with the nasal cycle. The turbinate extends along the entire length of the lateral nasal wall as far as the posterior choana, two-thirds of which can be obstructed by the thick posterior end of the turbinate.

The varying height of the inferior meatus and of the groove that it forms in the turbinate are particularly marked in frontal sections. Usually the free edge of the turbinate is tilted externally. The turbinate bone may also be curved externally but sometimes it forms only a narrow ridge in the center of the turbinate. A limited turbinectomy may be needed in some cases.

The *middle turbinate* is a key structure in intranasal surgery. Beneath and immediately lateral to it in the middle meatus lie the most important outflow tract of the paranasal sinuses, the ostia and the ducts for the frontal, maxillary and anterior ethmoid sinuses. Its shape is very variable: sometimes it is high and narrow with few or no cells, on other occasions it is plump and permeated by many cells which are difficult to assign either to the turbinate or the ethmoid, as the two merge with each other. Anteriorly, the medial lamella of the middle turbinate always extends to the dome of the nose, thus forming the lateral wall of the olfactory cleft (Figure 2.**8**), but posteriorly it deviates from the roof of the nose, curves more deeply and inserts into the ethmoid (Figure 2.**19 b**). Above it the superior turbinate lies in the posterior half of the nose; alternatively the ethmoid cells reach this point. The point at which the middle turbinate deviates from the anterior skull base is thus an important landmark which must be identified during ethmoidectomy, otherwise the medial surface of the turbinate can be torn off by a rough technique, damaging the olfactory fibers and producing a CSF fistula.

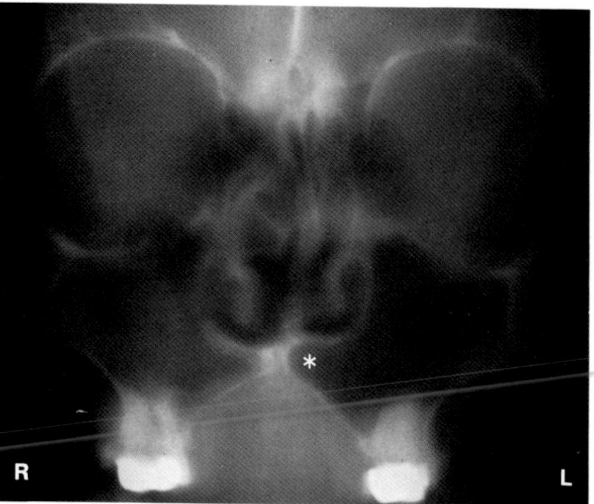

Figure 2.**23** Pronounced palatine recess (*) of both antra running under the floor of the nose. Coronal cut through the sinuses (polycyclic tomography).

The posterior attachment of the middle turbinate can be readily identified on a CT scan, lying on the lateral nasal wall just in front of the floor of the sphenoid sinus, at the point where the wall becomes thicker due to the base of the pterygoid process.

The *superior turbinate* is often overlooked by the surgeon, and it may be represented only by a slight swelling, in which case the superior meatus is difficult to define. However, the superior turbinate is often well developed and can be confused with the medial turbinate on rapid examination. The CT scan illustrates its slender structure and its suspension from the dome of the nose at the point where the medial turbinate is running more deeply to insert into the ethmoid, at the level of the posterior edge of the crista galli. Occasionally a supreme turbinate is also present.

Understanding of the three-dimensional structure of the *ethmoid* is mandatory for the intranasal surgeon. The main features are constant, but the individual shape of the ethmoid varies so much that it is scarcely worthwhile identifying or naming individual cells. The most important landmarks are the following:

- the semilunar hiatus and its rostral prolongation, the ethmoid infundibulum,
- the uncinate process,
- the ethmoid bulla forming the foundation wall of the anterior ethmoid cells,
- the posterior wall of the bulla forming the anterior boundary (basal lamella) of the posterior ethmoid cells,
- the middle turbinate,
- the olfactory region, particularly its anterior and posterior limits,
- the agger nasi,
- the frontonasal duct or its equivalent in the form of ethmoid duct cells,
- the primary maxillary ostium.

The endoscopic image of the *semilunar hiatus* has already been described above. Its gutter is moon shaped, curving forwards and upwards, and is usually only visible on a CT scan if 2 mm slices at 2 mm intervals are used. Posteriorly it is 1–2 mm high, but anterosuperiorly it often forms a 3 mm deep ethmoid infundibulum (Figure 2.**24**). Posteriorly it extends a good 3 mm in a trough shape. The canal between the infundibulum and the antral cavity is shown in the sections in Figure 2.**22i** (right) and Figure 2.**22h** (left): it is not a true ostium but rather a tunnel several millimeters long.

The inferior wall of the hiatus is formed by the *uncinate process* whose thickness and height vary (Figure 2.**22g–i,** right, and in Figure 2.**22h–i,** left). During middle meatal antrostomy it forms a barrier, at least in the posterior half of the middle meatus, and must often be removed to allow an antrostomy to be created large enough to permit manipulations within the antral cavity.

The *ethmoid bulla* projects in an inferomedial direction over the semilunar hiatus (Figure 2.**22g** right, Figure 2.**22h** left). Several ethmoidal cells of varying size lie above the hiatus and drain into it, and are thus classified as anterior ethmoid cells. However, they do not form the lateral boundary because ethmoid cells are present lateral to the bullar cells and lateral to the semilunar hiatus (Figure 2.**22h** left). This fact is easily overlooked during overtimorous removal of the bulla anteriorly, so that complete ethmoidectomy is better achieved by concentrating on the lateral nasal wall as a landmark. The length of the bulla varies between 4 and 8 mm. At its posterior edge there is said to be a bony wall running obliquely in an anterosuperior direction, the basal lamella of the middle turbinate, or the floor of the posterior ethmoid cells. However, in practice this party wall is often not found, so that the posterior ethmoid cells are also opened during anterior ethmoidectomy.

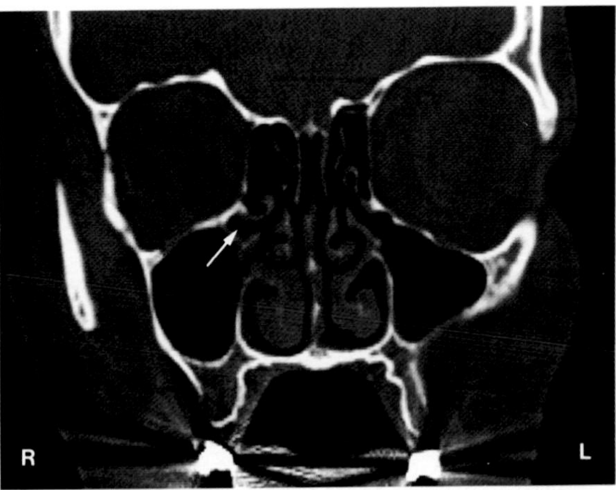

Figure 2.**24** Depression of the semilunar hiatus forming the ethmoid infundibulum (marked with an arrow) in a coronal cut on the right side. The uncinate process projects beyond the gutter by 2 mm.

Defining a boundary between the intraconchal cells of the middle turbinate, the bulla cells and the posterior ethmoid cells is of theoretical rather than practical importance. Complete removal of this boundary zone can easily damage the medial lamella of the middle turbinate resulting in damage to the olfactory region. The turbinate cells (most anterior medial ethmoidal cells) can be easily seen lying under the lateral olfactory region in the sections in Figure 2.**22f** and **g.** Their removal must therefore greatly weaken the anterior suspension of the middle turbinate.

Endoscopic identification of the relation of the *anterior ethmoid cells* to the frontal sinus is vital. This boundary zone often varies between the two sides, and particularly between different subjects (Figure 2.**22d**); ethmoid cells sometimes penetrate far laterally. It is impossible to expose this area without resecting the agger nasi. Anteriorly at this point can be seen the medial boundary of the ethmoids formed by the lamella inserting into the skull base (Figure 2.**22g**). The frontonasal duct can occasionally be recognized on sagittal sections, but not in frontal projections. Figures 2.**22d** and **e** illustrate the distance from the semilunar hiatus of small ethmoid cells surrounding the duct. It is easier to distinguish the *posterior ethmoid* cells from the sphenoid sinus. It is usually possible to recognize the party wall easily on a CT scan by following the lateral ethmoid and nasal wall, and taking the end of the middle turbinate as a landmark. This point will not be mistaken either by endoscopy or under the microscope if the surgeon sticks to the posterior end of the middle turbinate as a landmark. Occasionally an Onodi cell extending laterally under the optic nerve may render orientation difficult, and careless radical removal with the sharp punch may endanger the optic nerve.

A CT scan of the *sphenoid sinus* may demonstrate the wide variation of size between the two sides and individual recesses extending deeply into the pterygoid process (Figure 2.**25**). A pronounced inferolateral recess can be found in about one-third of all subjects, lying immediately adjacent to the bone over the nerve of the pterygoid canal and the maxillary nerve. The floor of the sphenoidal sinus has no significant structures except bone, and the only complication of excessive resection is bleeding from branches of the sphenopalatine artery: in contrast, the lateral wall of the sinus carries the optic nerve, the internal carotid artery and the cavernous sinus. Its position relative to the sinus cavity can be readily seen on CT scan. A well developed superolateral recess between the optic nerve and the internal carotid artery is found in about 20% of sphenoid sinuses.

Before undertaking his first endoscopic ethmoid operation on patients, the surgeon must be intimately aware of the shape of the *anterior base of the skull,* as it appears on intranasal exposure. The CT scan is helpful, because it shows clearly the danger zones during intranasal manipulations. Anteriorly the dome of the nose projects towards the nasal bone, but the septum does not yet meet the skull base (Figure 2.**22 a–c**). Even the plane in which the anterior end of the middle turbinate arises from the agger nasi is not free from danger because the frontal sinus lies above the septum (the frontal section in Figure 2.**22 d** is not absolutely perpendicular). There is no dura lying anterior to the frontonasal duct, so that the bone in front of the duct can be resected.

However, the base of the skull reaches its deepest point behind the frontonasal duct: at this point begins the olfactory fossa. This boundary is marked by the anterior edge of the crista galli lying immediately upon the septum (see Figure 2.**22 e**). The depth of the olfactory groove varies widely between different subjects, and between the two sides in the same subject. Furthermore, its width increases as it extends posteriorly. The cribriform plate is perforated by olfactory fibers, and it usually lies obliquely rather than horizontally, so that the skull base and its overlying dura can lie medial to the upper ethmoid cells (Figure 2.**22 e**). The roof of the ethmoids may sometimes present a dangerous construction; the olfactory region is always dangerous! Behind it the slope flattens out and the sphenoid plane projects over the posterior ethmoid cells as a thick horizontal plate (Figure 2.**22 k**).

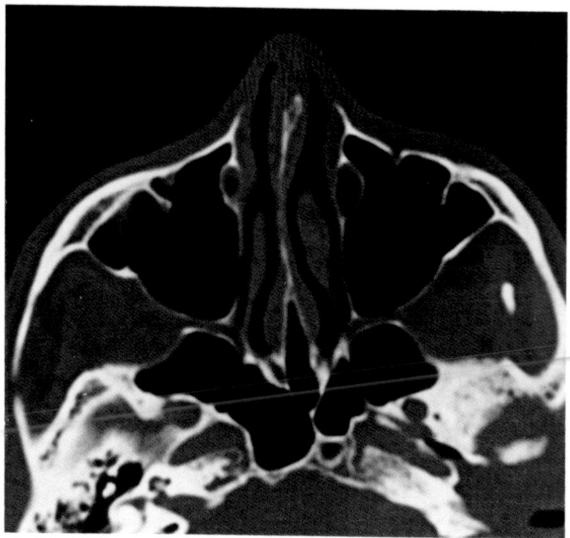

Figure 2.**25** Extensive lateral recess of the sphenoid sinus reaching into the pterygoid process in an axial CT scan.

Horizontal Axial Sections

Axial slices (Figure 2.**26 a–i**) are less informative than coronal, because they do not always clearly demonstrate the relative positions to the endoscopist as he enters the nose from the nostril. The endoscopist orientates himself to vertical landmarks, and the horizontal sections are less helpful. Also the skull base may be confused with opaque cells (Figure 2.**26 d**). Furthermore, asymmetry of the sections produces a greater effect on axial than on coronal tomograms. The value of axial tomograms is that they outline continuous contours such as the lateral nasal wall or the lateral wall of the sphenoid sinus. They may be very useful in the identification of recesses or of pathological expansion by mucoceles or tumors. As an example, Figure 6.**51** highlights the optic canal projecting from the lateral wall of the sphenoid sinus: removal of bone with the punch to expose the lateral recess would have devastating results.

The examination begins above and continues downwards. The upper part of the frontal recess and the cavity of the frontal sinus are clearly seen in the first sections. As the infundibulum of the frontal sinus is usually not demonstrated, the anterior ethmoid cells are reached quite abruptly (Figure 2.**26 c**), although it is usually not clear whether the air spaces extending laterally are small supraorbital ethmoid cells or whether they belong to the frontal sinus. The uniformity of the ethmoid compartment can be easily seen in the center of the ethmoid (Figure 2.**26 e–f**). All ethmoid sections and the shape and properties of the sphenoid sinus are best assessed in this position.

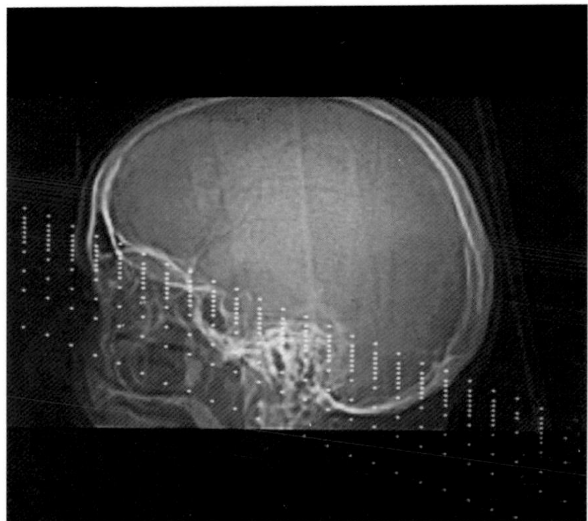

Figure 2.**26** The spatial arrangement of the nasal sinuses in a series of axial cuts on high resolution CT scan.
a Position of the cuts in relation to the skull base.

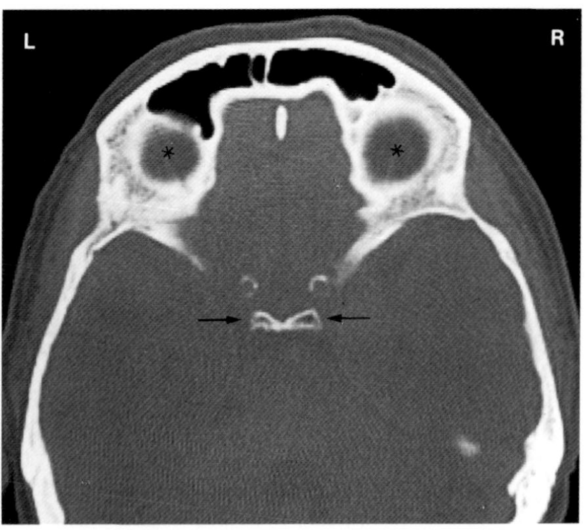

b The uppermost cut shows the upper recess of the frontal sinus above, behind it the orbital roofs (*) and the clinoid process marked with an arrow. The ethmoid roof is not yet visible. The interfrontal septum appears to be hollow because of a paramedian ridge of bone.

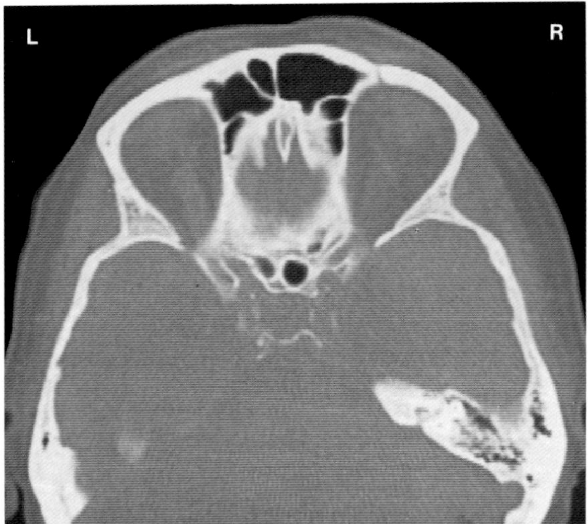

c The frontal infundibulum on the right side, the anterior ethmoid cells and the superior sphenoid recesses are now visible posteriorly. Centrally lies a horizontal section through the ethmoid roof.

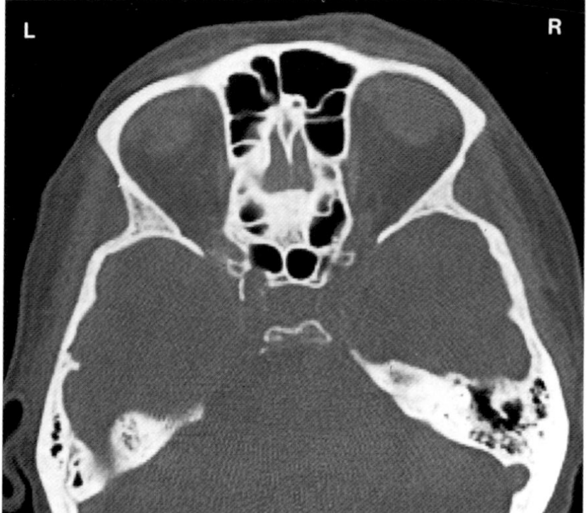

d Whereas the anterior and posterior ethmoid cells are now visible the central part is still formed by the bone of the anterior skull base. The orbital walls are well defined.

Cells extending laterally are only seen in sections below the level of the floor of the orbit (Figure 2.**26 h**): At this point the lumen of the antral cavity on a horizontal CT scan shows a typical rhomboid outline (Figure 2.**26 g–h**). The nasolacrimal duct is usually well seen in the neighboring cuts. These sections are also suitable for demonstrating circumscribed changes of the middle nasal meatus.

The deepest sections show clearly the relation of the walls of the antral cavity to the facial soft tissues, to the retromaxillary space (Figure 2.**26 i**) and to the alveolar process of the upper jaw.

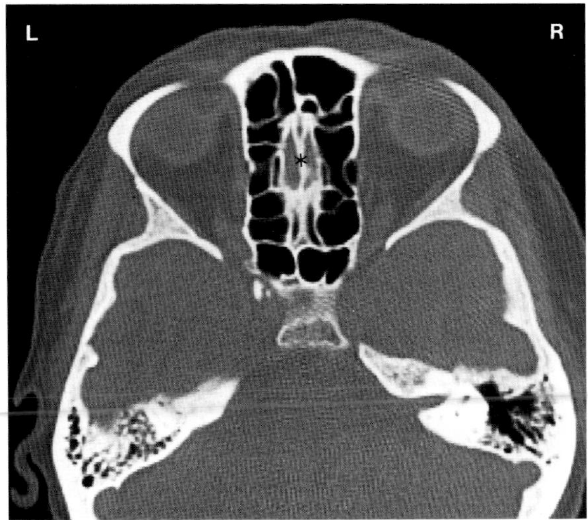

e The entire ethmoid cells and the sphenoid sinuses can now be seen. Fine cell septa are also well defined. The bone of the low-lying olfactory fossa (*) can still be seen in this section.

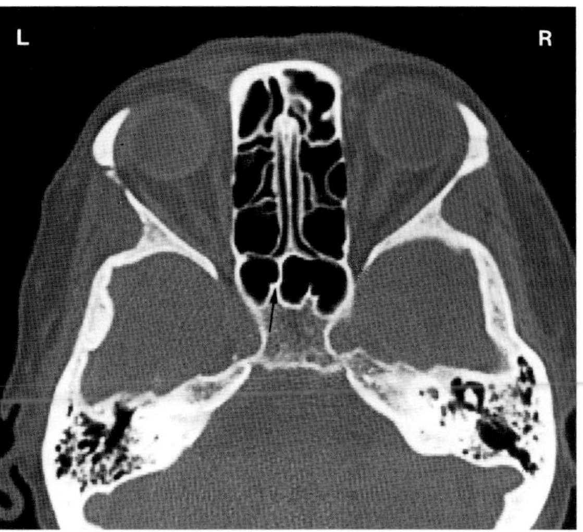

f The upper edge of the septum has now come into view. Close by it lies the medial lamella of the middle turbinate. The asymmetrical sphenoid sinus is divided by an intersphenoid septum marked with an arrow lying to the left, and not in the plane of prolongation of the vomer.

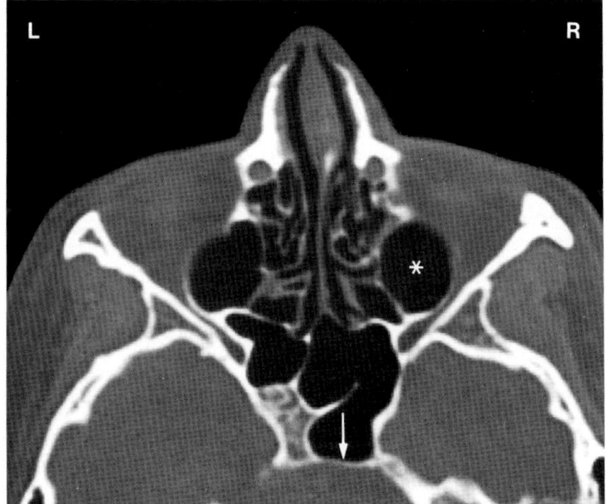

g Cut through the upper part of the antra (*). The rhomboid figure of the anterior cells of the base of the skull project downwards from this plane. Thin posterior wall of the clivus (marked with an arrow) and right sphenoid cavity extending far posteriorly to the left across the midline.

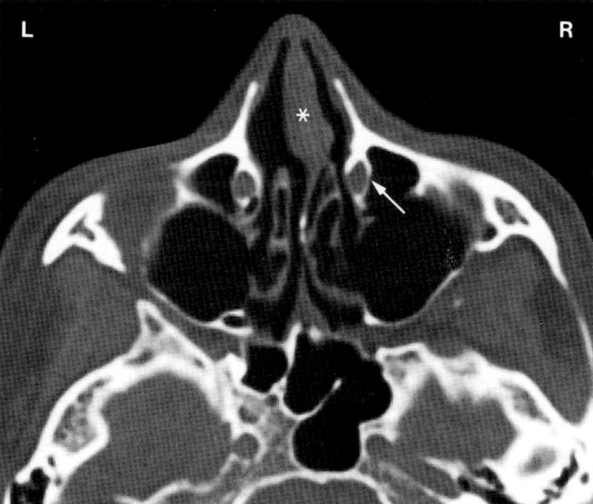

h The antral cavity is now visible lying beneath the floor of the orbit. The lacrimal ducts (marked with an arrow) can be recognized easily lying between the anterior recess of the antrum and the nasal cavity. There is a marked widening of the septum causing a pseudodeviation (*).

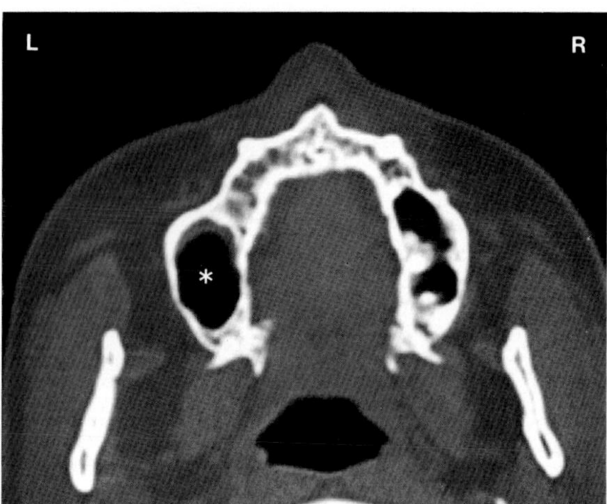

Figure 2.26 i The lowest cut shows the expansion of the alveolar ridge by the alveolar antral recess (*).

Typical Operative Steps on a Cadaver

We have now completed the endoscopic view of the nasal cavity supplemented by CT scans allowing the surgeon to build up a three-dimensional image of the paranasal sinuses. An illustration of several typical operative steps on an anatomical dissection now follows. The steps should be studied before being performed on patients, and if possible should be practiced on a skull. A safe topographic perspective and a feeling for bimanual endoscopic dissection in the confined spaces closely related to the orbital cavity and the anterior cranial fossa should be developed.

We begin with various dissections of the lateral nasal wall, and practice inspection with the microscope and angled telescopes.

Dissection of the Lateral Nasal Wall in Eight Steps

W. Hosemann

First Step

The nasal septum has been completely resected. In the center of the exposed lateral nasal wall (Figure 2.**27 a**) lies the medial surface of one ethmoid bounded by a middle and a superior nasal turbinate. Below lies the independent inferior turbinate. In the midline, the saw cut passes through the opposite sphenoid cavity, providing a view of the intersphenoid septum.

In just under two-thirds of cases a supreme nasal meatus is present. The ethmoid is 4–5 cm long, 2.5–3.0 cm high, 1.5 cm wide posteriorly and 0.8 cm wide anteriorly. Its volume of 8–10 cm^3 is occupied by as many as fifteen ethmoid cells. On the lateronasal wall in the fetus lie up to six isolated swellings (main turbinates) lying behind each other as an uncinate mass resembling the free edge of the later middle turbinate. Posteriorly these fetal main turbinates merge completely, whereas anteriorly the medial ethmoid wall of the adult arises from the dome of the swelling. However, from four to five remnants of the main and accessory fetal turbinates can be recognized in the ethmoid labyrinth. These are the basal lamellae:

- basal lamella 1: uncinate process (remnant of a nasal turbinate),
- basal lamella 2: lamella of the ethmoid bulla (remnant of a nasal turbinate),
- *basal lamella 3: basal lamella of the middle nasal turbinate,*
- basal lamella 4: basal lamella of the superior turbinate,
- basal lamella 5: basal lamella of the supreme turbinate.

The third lamella, the basal lamella of the middle turbinate, is the best developed and the most important. In a lateral view of the dissection it lies obliquely (Figure 2.**27 f**), behind the ethmoid bulla, uniting the medial part of the middle turbinate to the lamina papyracea and the roof of the ethmoid. It often appears very marked on axial CT scans: it can be found on CT scans at the anterior point of contact of the maxillary sinus and the ethmoids from which it deviates at a right angle. This basal lamella divides the ethmoid anatomically into an anterior and a posterior part. The cells of the posterior ethmoid are large but few in number: the anterior cells are smaller but more numerous. However, there is no constant relationship of the size of the anterior to the posterior ethmoid. The compartments between the basal lamellae show an individual variation of invasion and expansion of the ethmoid cells, so that the lamellae may be displaced or deformed. For example, the posterior ethmoid may be narrowed by a pushed-back basal lamella due to an enlarged an-

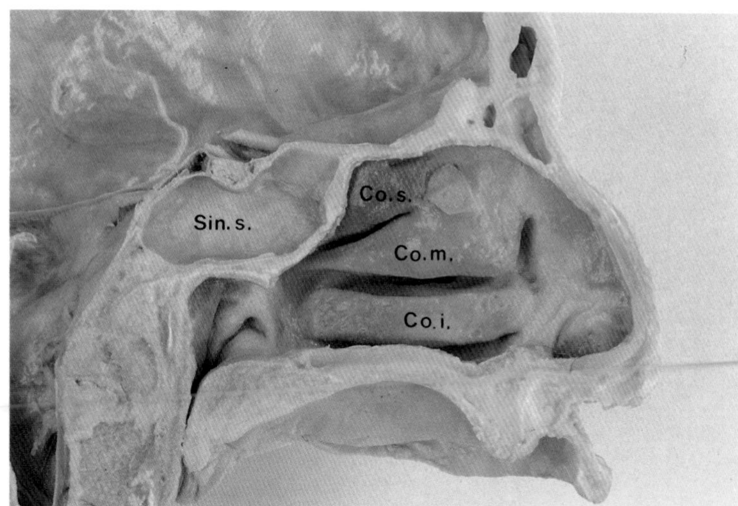

Figure 2.**27** Dissection of the lateral nasal wall. The details are given in the text.

a Dissection of the skull on the left side after the first cut of the dissection.

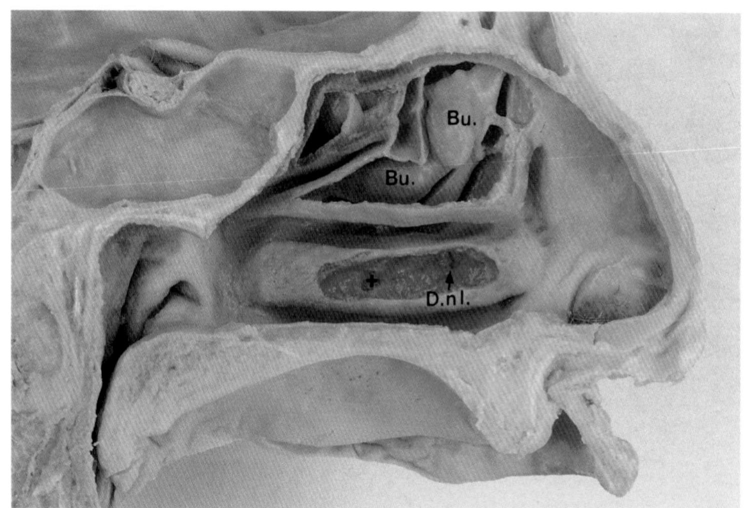

b Second cut of the dissection of the nasal sinuses.

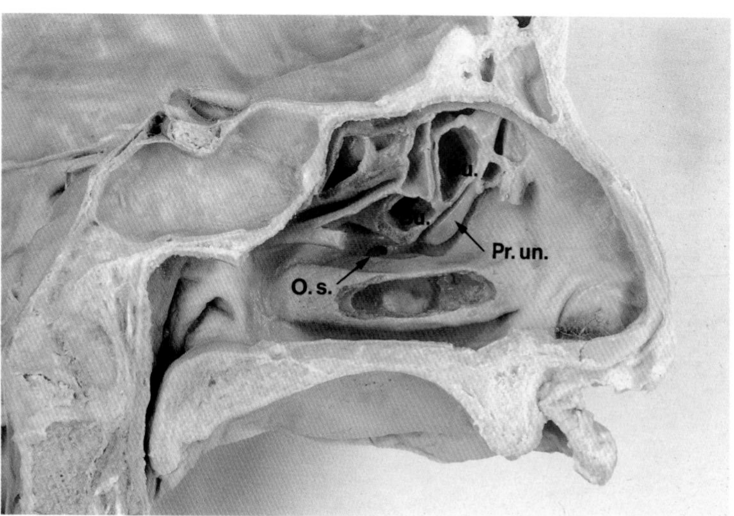

c Third cut of the dissection of the nasal sinuses.

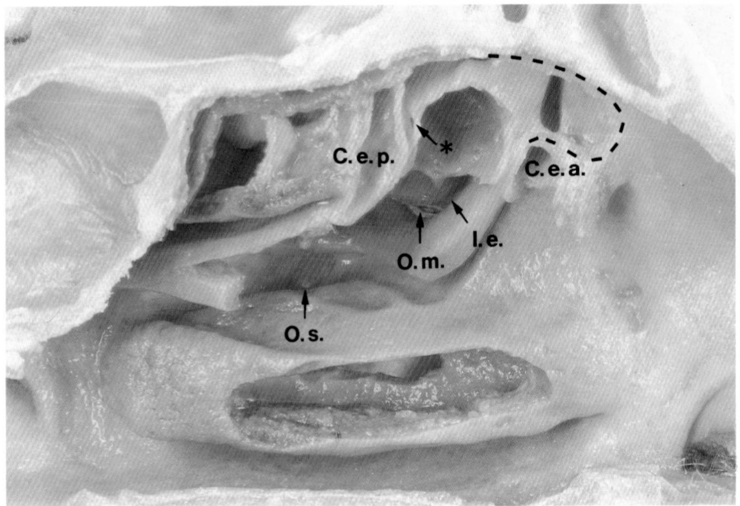

d Fourth cut of the dissection of the nasal sinuses.

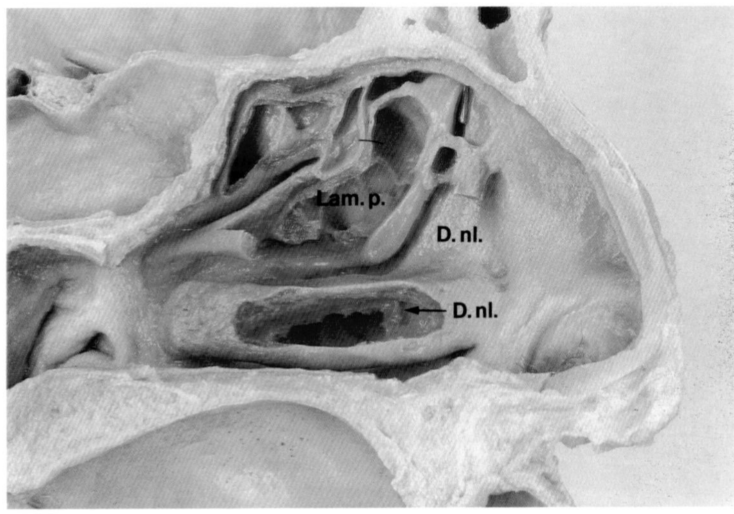

e Fifth cut of the dissection of the nasal sinuses.

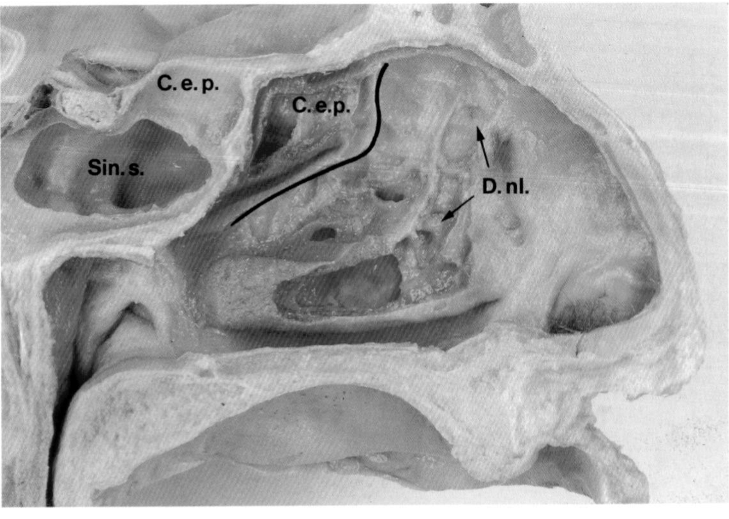

f Sixth cut of the dissection of the nasal sinuses.

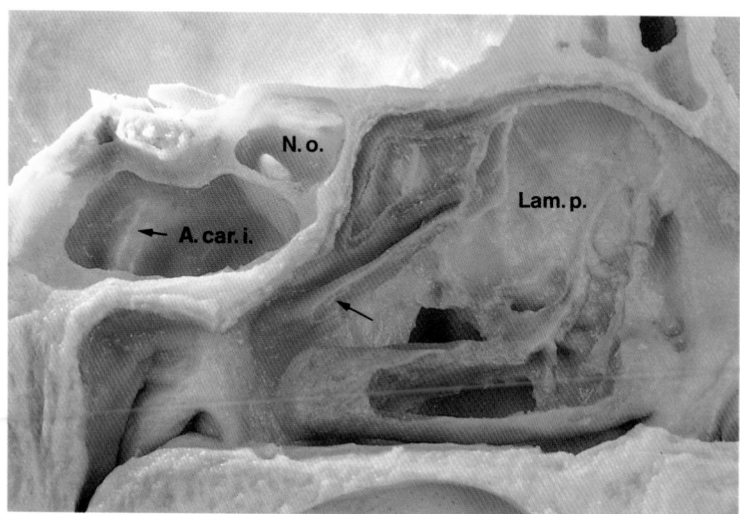

g Seventh cut of the dissection of the nasal sinuses.

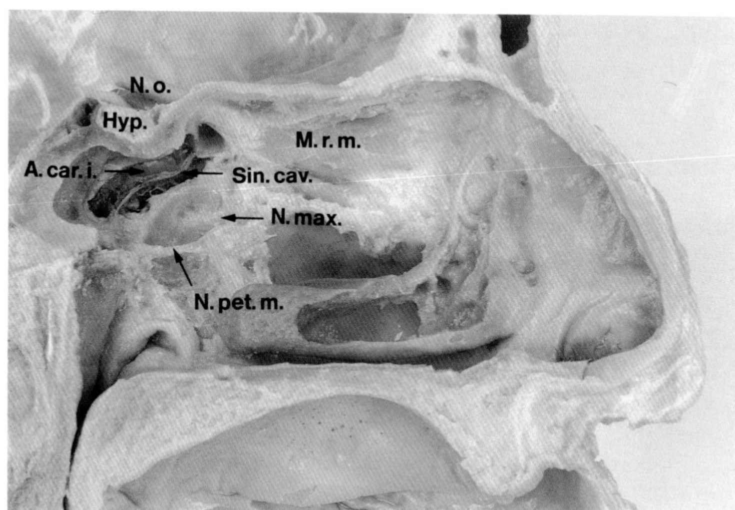

h Eighth cut of the dissection of the nasal sinuses.

terior cell compartment. Posterior ethmoid cells may in this case encroach upon the anterosuperior sphenoid cavity (Figure 2.**27 g**): The reverse relationship is also possible. The basal lamella of the middle turbinate forms a functional landmark: the mucociliary apparatus of the anterior ethmoids discharges its secretion into the middle meatus, whereas the posterior ethmoids and the sphenoid cavity drain via the superior or supreme nasal meatus.

Second Step

The anterior and posterior ethmoid cells come into view after uncovering the medial ethmoid wall (Figure 2.**27 b**). Palpation with a fine probe provides additional information about the position of the ostium of the cells (determining their developmental origin) and the sinus.

In this dissection the cell complex of the ethmoid bulla is voluminous, consisting of two cells with a wide connection. The ostium of the bulla cells usually lies posteriorly (star with arrow in Figure 2.**27 d**). The inferior turbinate has been fenestrated so that the ostium of the nasolacrimal duct can be seen. A star marks the site of puncture of the antral cavity for endoscopy of the antral cavity, using a flexible or rigid telescope.

A detailed classification of the cells into subgroups within the compartments determined by the basal lamellae is not always possible because of the marked variation of the ethmoid cells. Furthermore, there is variation in the literature about the classification and the anatomical nomenclature.

The following terms may be defined:

The **semilunar hiatus** is a gap in the shape of a half moon up to 3 mm wide, between the ethmoid bulla and the upper free edge of the uncinate process. The hiatus is thus a cleft which opens into the ethmoid infundibulum.

The *ethmoid infundibulum* is the gutter lying between the ethmoid bulla and the uncinate process.

The *frontal infundibulum* is the upper end of the frontal outflow tract (the frontonasal duct or the ostium) lying within the frontal sinus.

The *frontal recess* is a space within the anterior ethmoids. It lies in a plane which is an anterosuperior continuation of the direction of the semilunar hiatus. It can reach the base of the skull between the lateral nasal wall and the middle turbinate (Figure 2.**27 d** outlined in black). It is bounded in front by the agger nasi, and behind by bony swellings in the region of the ethmoid bulla, for example.

The *maxillary ostium* is more a tunnel than a simple opening; it may be straight or curved and lies between the ethmoid bulla, the uncinate process and the orbital plates of the maxillary and the ethmoid bones. It unites the antral cavity with the ethmoid infundibulum.

If the *frontonasal duct* forms a true duct, the term *frontal ostium* indicates both the opening into the lumen of the frontal sinus and that into the nasal cavity or the ethmoid.

Third Step

Removal of the edge of the middle turbinate provides a free view of the secondary ostium of the antral cavity in the region of the posterior fontanelle, (Figure 2.**27 c**), but the uncinate process and the projecting bulla cells still obstruct the view of the maxillary ostium.

The term *fontanelles* indicates those parts of the medial wall of the antral cavity in the middle meatus consisting of membrane only with no bony support. The anterior fontanelle lies beneath the uncinate process and in front of the ethmoid process of the inferior turbinate; the posterior fontanelle extends between the uncinate process and the palatal bone. About one-quarter of specimens demonstrate secondary accessory ostia of the antral cavity through these membranes, especially posteriorly.

Fourth Step

Removal of the walls of the bulla renders the maxillary ostium visible (Figure 2.**27 d**). The ethmoid infundibulum continues anterosuperiorly giving off ethmoid cells in the direction of the agger nasi. The anterosuperior part of the frontal recess is marked by a broken line. The most anterior of the posterior ethmoid cells extends anteriorly into the resected body of the middle turbinate. A star with an arrow marks the ostium of the upper bulla cell.

In about three-quarters of cases the maxillary ostium opens into the posterior third of the ethmoid infundibulum. However, due to the varying width of the uncinate process the maxillary ostium can be assessed without endoscopy in less than 10% of cases.

The anterior ethmoid cells, delineated as infundibular cells, arise from the ethmoid infundibulum. In particular, a cell extending towards the agger nasi is found in 80% of cases. The ethmoid infundibulum itself often ends blindly above as the terminal recess, or in a further infundibular cell, the terminal cell.

The frontal recess demonstrates characteristic frontal accessory turbinates on its lateral wall during the course of its development. Local cells of the frontal recess develop in about 50% of cases from the intervening frontal grooves which may be up to four in number; furthermore, the frontal sinus is pneumatized from this point in up to 60% of cases. The frontal sinus arises by direct extension of the ethmoidal infundibulum in only 5% of cases, and it is much more often pneumatized via the intermediate stage of infundibular cells.

The free part of the middle turbinate can conceal an air-filled hollow space due to a pronounced inrolling of its free edge laterally and superiorly. This hollow turbinate sinus drains into the middle meatus. On the other hand posterior ethmoid cells lying behind the basal lamella or anterior ethmoid cells arising from the frontal recess can pneumatize the body of the turbinate to form a bullous turbinate ("concha bullosa"). Either cavity (a bullous conchal sinus or a concha bullosa) may become diseased separately, but in both cases the principle of surgical treatment is resection of the lateral part of the wall of the cavity (turbinate).

Fifth Step

The outflow tract of the frontal sinus is demonstrated by pushing a probe from within the sinus inferiorly (Figure 2.**27 e**). The duct opens into the frontal recess independently of the ethmoid infundibulum. The bulla cells have been partially removed, and part of the lamina papyracea is shown. The inferior meatal antrostomy has been suitably extended for an adequate distance from the ostium of the nasolacrimal duct. The lacrimal duct can be seen in the anterolateral nasal wall extending in an anterosuperior direction from the ostium. The duct of the frontal sinus and any supraorbital cells can be palpated with a probe.

The ethmoid bulla is the most constant ethmoid cell in shape. It almost always reaches the lateral boundary of the ethmoids, thus filling their entire width. An anterior bulge in the floor of the frontal sinus produced by an anterior ethmoid cell is termed a frontal bulla. It is found in 10% of cases, but is in reality only a particularly well developed cell lying in the floor of the frontal sinus, whereas smaller cells are found here in 50% of specimens. Duplication of the frontal sinus and its duct is found in 8% of cases. The varying anatomy of the floor of the frontal sinus can be assessed during surgery by rigid 70° endoscopes.

One anomaly is a recess of the middle nasal meatus extending into the antral cavity. The lateral nasal wall fuses at this point with the orbital process of the maxillary bone for some distance. In this way a part of the orbit extends into the nasal cavity, demanding care during the creation of a middle meatal antrostomy.

In about 20% of specimens from one to four ethmoid cells extend into the orbital roof.

Sixth Step

The anterior ethmoid cells and the greater part of the uncinate process have been removed (Figure 2.**27 f**). The basal lamella of the middle turbinate (shown by a black line) divides the resected area from the preserved posterior ethmoid. The medial wall of the maxillary antrum is preserved in the region of the middle nasal meatus; it encloses the natural maxillary ostium, the accessory ostium with its membranous fontanelles and bony wall consisting of the uncinate process, and the ethmoid process of the inferior turbinate. The nasolacrimal duct is shown with its medial wall removed. The bulge due to the anterior ethmoid artery lies in the roof of the ethmoids. The intersphenoidal septum has been removed providing a free view into the left sphenoid cavity. A posterior ethmoid cell projects above the sphenoid sinus. A probe is passed into the ostia of the posterior ethmoid cells and the sphenoid sinus.

The volume of one sphenoid sinus varies widely between 0 and 14 cm^3. In 10% of cases the posterior ethmoid cells invade the sphenoid sinus. The sphenoid ostium lies in the upper half of the anterior wall in the sphenoethmoid recess. The ratio of the breadth of the nasal part of the anterior wall of the sphenoid sinus to that of the ethmoid part is 3:5.

The bulge of the anterior ethmoid artery runs close to the line of attachment of the second or third basal lamella along the anterior skull base. Small defects in the bone of the ethmoid roof can be shown in 10% of cases.

The nasolacrimal duct lies in a similar angle to the frontonasal duct (about 110° to the Frankfurt horizontal).

Seventh Step

The ethmoid cell lying over the anterior part of the sphenoid sinus has been uncapped (Figure 2.**27 g**); it encloses the optic nerve and is known as an Onodi cell. The internal carotid artery projects from the lateral wall of the sphenoid sinus. A black arrow marks the sphenopalatine foramen.

The term Onodi cell is used to describe any posterior ethmoid cell related to the optic nerve. The bone surrounding the nerve is usually 0.5 mm thick, but is dehiscent in 4% of cases. Those cells which completely enclose the optic nerve are of particular importance. Onodi cells are found in 10% of cases, but an optic nerve lying freely within such a cell is less common.

Haller's cell is an ethmoid cell which arises by splitting of the medial part of the floor of the orbit, and should thus be classified as an ethmoid cell penetrating the anterior or posterior orbital floor. Haller's cells overlooked during surgery can be a source of persistent mucopurulent secretion, but can be demonstrated easily by endoscopy.

Eighth Step

Wide removal of the posterior ethmoids, the lamina papyracea and the orbital periosteum brings the rectus muscles of the orbit into view. The sphenopalatine foramen has been dissected. The optic nerve can be followed by removing its bony wall; the greater petrosal (Vidian) and maxillary nerves are followed similarly. The lateral wall of the sphenoid sinus is resected, providing a view of the slit internal carotid artery and the cavernous sinus. The pituitary gland has been divided.

The sphenopalatine foramen usually lies just behind the posterior end of the middle turbinate.

The internal carotid artery bulges into the lateral wall of the sphenoid sinus in more than half the specimens. In two-thirds of cases the optic and maxillary nerves are also outlined. The sphenoid sinus may have wide recesses, firstly a superolateral recess between the optic nerve and the internal carotid artery in 25% of cases, secondly an inferolateral recess running towards the pterygoid process or the greater wing of the sphenoid bone in 25% of cases.

Inferior Meatal Antrostomy

The shape of the antral cavity has already been described (Figure 2.**28 a** und **b**). Its height varies with the floor of the orbit: it is higher anteriorly and posteriorly than in the middle, and it is higher medially than laterally where it tapers off to form the zygomatic recess. It has a roof, an anterior, a posterior and a medial wall. The first three are smooth, flat and convex, but the medial wall is complex (Figure 2.**29**). The lacrimal duct produces a vertical bulge in the anterior third. In front of that the prelacrimal recess leads upwards, whereas behind it the maxillary ostium lies above a small horizontal bulge. The maxillary sinus ostium lies very close to the roof of the antral cavity; its antral opening varies widely in shape (Figure 2.**30**).

An inferior meatal antrostomy can be created without an endoscope. The inferior turbinate is displaced by a Killian's speculum, and the lateral nasal wall is perforated by a sharp dissector in the middle third of the exposed inferior nasal meatus. The dissector is angled outwards, and used to lever the piece of bone into the nose, where it is removed with forceps. An endoscope can be introduced to inspect the antral cavity after smoothing the edges of the defect. An opening 3 × 5 mm is enough for transnasal antroscopy. The antrostomy can be enlarged with forward- or backward-cutting punches; a diameter of 6–12 mm usually suffices (Figure 2.**31**). The antrostomy can be extended inferiorly and anteriorly to allow introduction of instruments into the antral cavity.

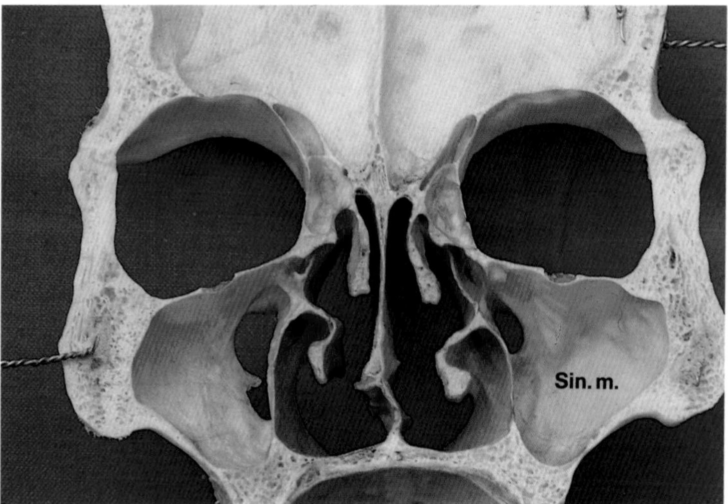

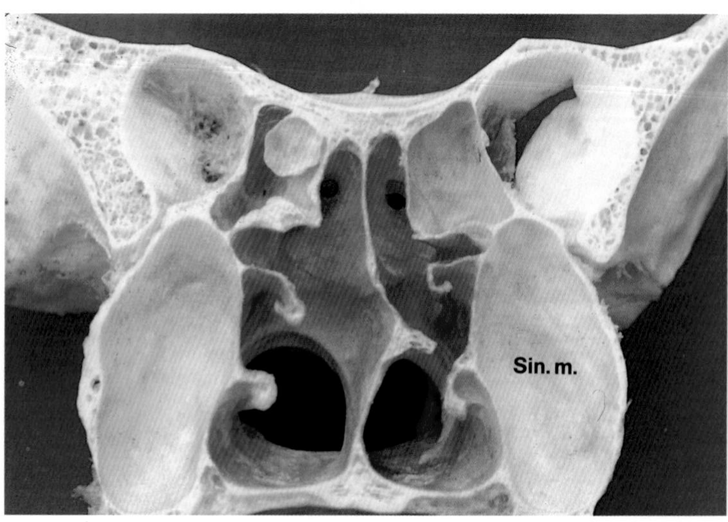

Figure 2.**28** Frontal section through the antral cavity in the plane of its greatest diameter. **a** View of the internal surface of the anterior wall from behind. **b** View in a posterior direction of the posterior wall showing the topographical relationships to the middle turbinate, the ethmoid cells, the orbital cavity and the floor of the nose.

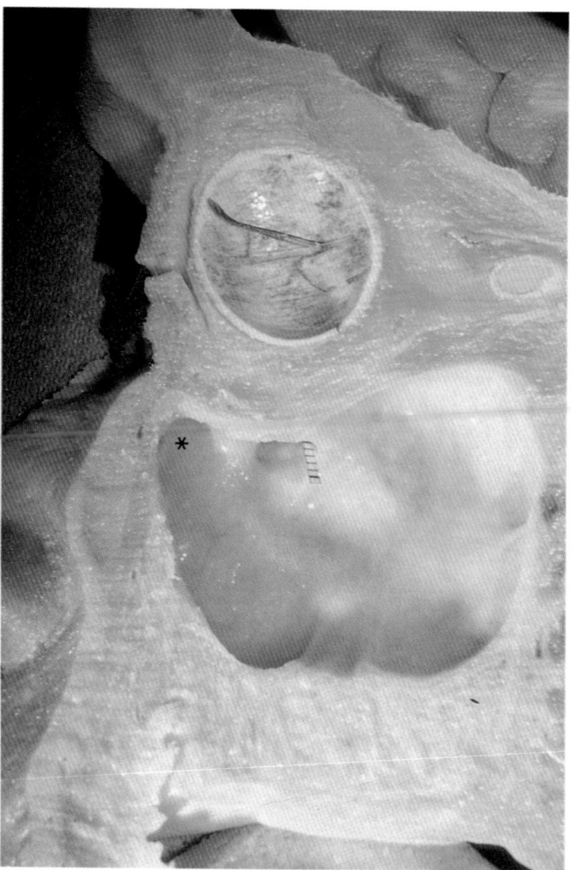

Figure 2.**29** Medial wall of the antrum in an anatomical dissection (Prof. Dr J. Lang, Würzburg). The prelacrimal recess (*) protrudes in an anterosuperior direction, in front of the bulge of the nasolacrimal canal. It is difficult to assess by intranasal endoscopy. A millimeter paper lies in the maxillary ostium, and the internal maxillary artery is marked in red.

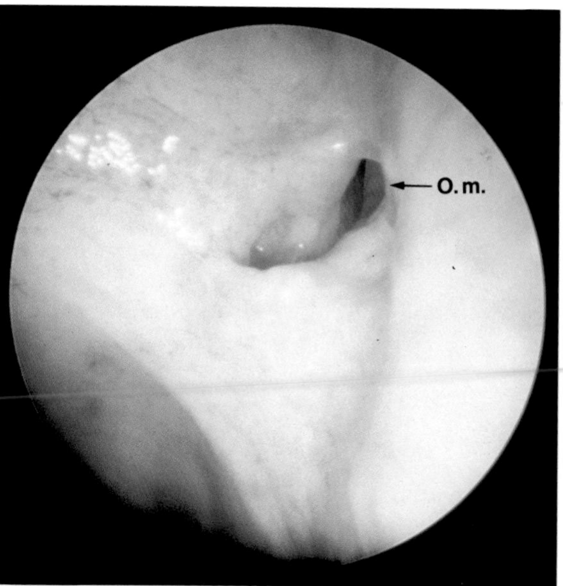

Figure 2.**30** The natural primary antral ostium is usually not round, but split up and very variable in shape (straight telescope with a view through a left-sided anterior antral window).

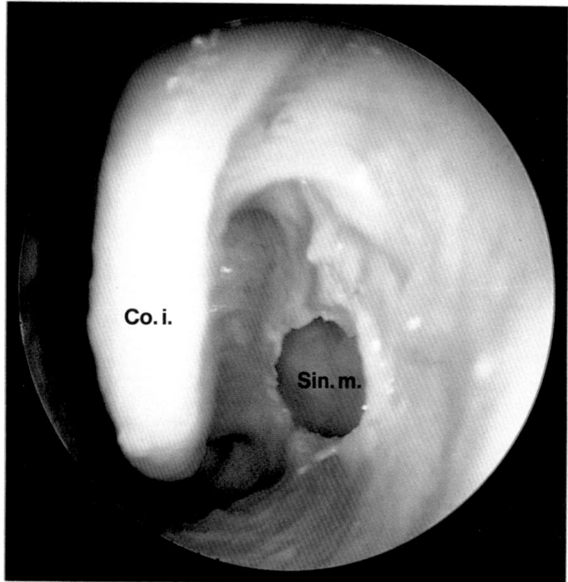

Figure 2.**31** Inferior meatal antrostomy on the left side, showing a small window and the posterior wall of the antrum lying behind it (30° telescope).

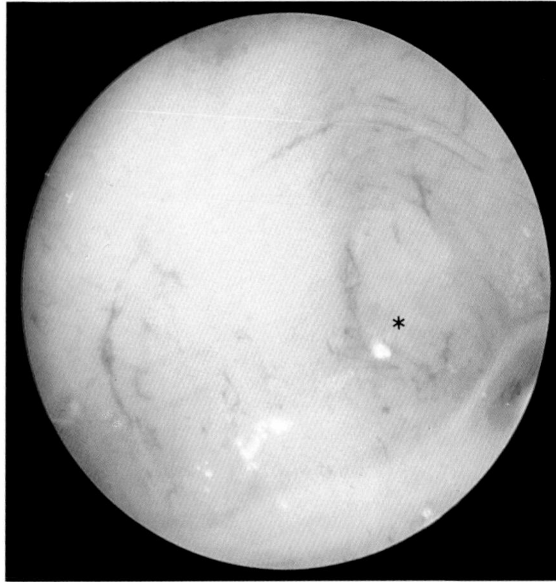

Figure 2.**32** Endoscopic view of the left posterior wall of the antral cavity through an inferior meatal antrostomy. The zygomatic recess lies on the right side (*) (70° telescope).

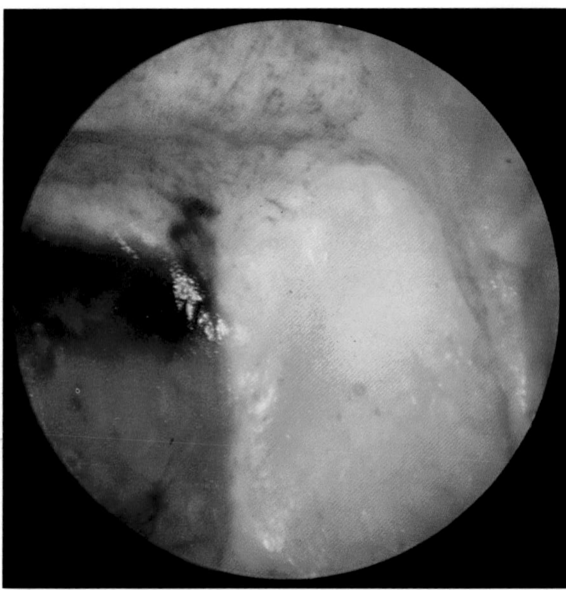

Figure 2.**33** The left anterior antral wall shown in yellow, bordering onto the roof shown in pink, and the posterior wall in blue. The zygomatic recess lies at the point of intersection of the three different colored regions. A 70° telescope introduced through a window in the inferior meatus.

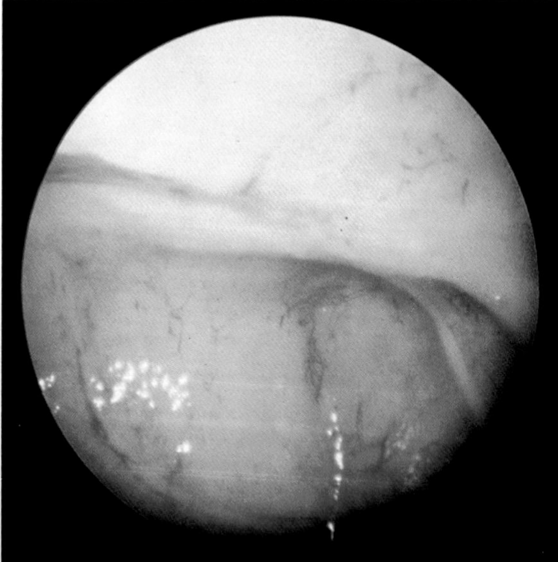

Figure 2.**34** Left antral roof with prominent canal for the infraorbital nerve. View with a 70° telescope through an inferior meatal antrostomy.

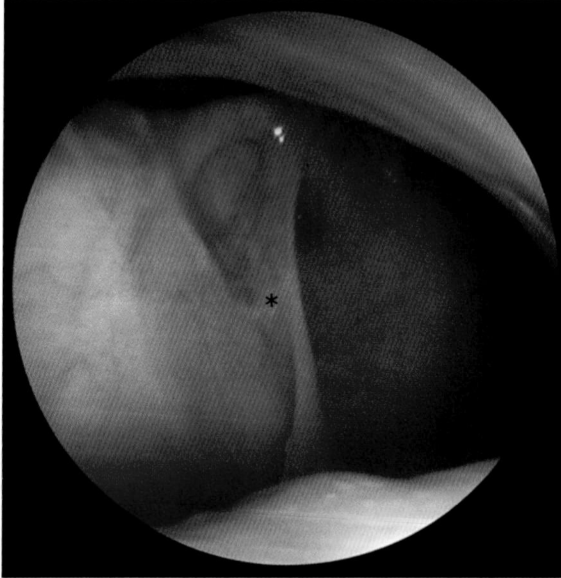

Figure 2.**35** Mucosal fold (*) in a left antral cavity. View with a 70° telescope through an inferior meatal antrostomy.

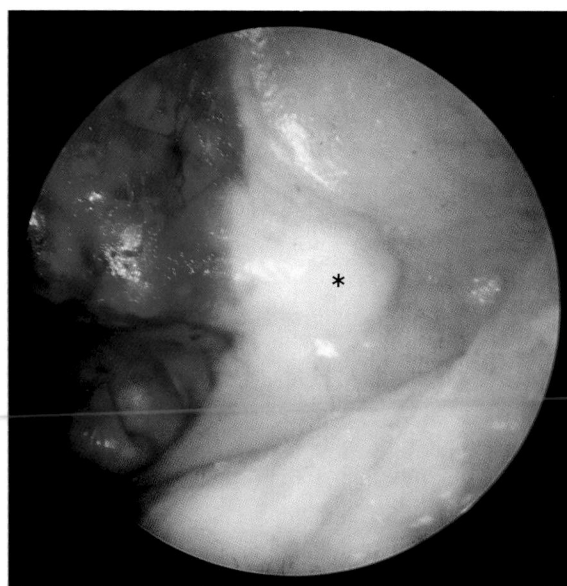

Figure 2.**36** Alveolar recess of a left antral cavity with the root of a molar tooth (*). The posterior wall of the antrum is marked in blue, the anterior wall in yellow. View with a 70° telescope through an inferior meatal antrostomy.

Orientation within the antral cavity is not always simple. The posterior wall is relatively easy to inspect (Figure 2.**32**) using a forward-viewing telescope, but a wide-angled 70° telescope is needed to inspect the anterior wall and the prelacrimal recess lying anterosuperiorly. A prominent landmark is the *zygomatic recess,* the most lateral recess. From this point a flat groove can be followed as it runs upwards and medially to form the boundary between the posterior wall and roof of the antral cavity. The junction between the roof and anterior wall is usually smooth. The surgeon learns to recognize the typical contours usually bilaterally symmetrical in order to preserve the thin wall of the orbit during sharp dissection. The anterior wall of the antral cavity slopes outwards, and tapers inferiorly (Figure 2.**33**).

The bony canal of the infraorbital nerve may form a sagittal bulge running anteriorly in the roof of the antral cavity providing a valuable landmark (Figure 2.**34**). It must not be confused with mucosal bands which often run from the medial to the lateral walls of the antral cavity under its roof (Figure 2.**35**).

The entire *medial wall of the antrum* can only be inspected satisfactorily through an infraturbinate portal using a telescope with an angle of at least 70°. Since disease very often begins medially and at the ostium, it is always necessary to check the medial wall, including the ethmoid recess.

Rotation of the endoscope illuminates the lowest antral recesses, the alveolar recess and a palatine recess if present (Figure 2.**36**). Often these recesses are partially walled off from each other or the main antral cavity by bony septa.

Safe surgery depends on familiarity with the topographical anatomy of the danger areas, and this facility must be developed by practice on the skull. Firstly, the *nasolacrimal canal* is demonstrated by extending the inferior meatal antrostomy anteriorly until the nasolacrimal ostium is exposed. Then the anterior end of the inferior turbinate is removed with a scalpel, demonstrating the position of the ostium relative to the insertion of the inferior turbinate.

The *posterior relations* can be demonstrated by cutting off the inferior turbinate completely from the lateral nasal wall using the large nasal scissors. The posterior edge of the antrostomy is now extended backwards using a punch under endoscopic vision until nothing more remains. The proximity of the sphenoid sinus and the exit of the sphenopalatine artery can now be recognized and impressed on the memory.

Piecemeal resection of the uncinate process and of the lateral ethmoid cells finally demonstrates the construction of this part of the medial wall of the antral cavity. This step leads to practice of middle meatal antrostomy.

If a dissected skull is available it is usuful to punch out the anterior antral wall at the same time, to be able to monitor the endoscopic field of vision through the inferior meatus by the naked eye anteriorly.

Middle Meatal Antrostomy

Once the surgeon is familiar with infraturbinate endoscopy of the antrum, middle meatal antroscopy using a 70° telescope is not difficult.

There are two possible methods of middle meatal antrostomy: firstly exposure via the semilunar hiatus, the ethmoid infundibulum, and the primary maxillary ostium, and secondly through the lateral nasal wall beneath the uncinate process. The following description is concerned solely with the second, more usual, method of access.

Typically the antrostomy is created immediately above the insertion of the inferior turbinate (Figure 2.**37a, b**). A 45° upward-cutting Blakesley punch is used to perforate the wall; it must be introduced horizontally along the upper edge of the turbinate, to the center of its long axis (Figure 2.**38**). This point is also marked by the lower part of the semilunar hiatus which can usually be recognized endoscopically anteriorly as a very well marked channel running anterosuperiorly between the uncinate process and the ethmoid bulla (Figure 2.**39**). Normally a circumscribed antrostomy with a diameter of about 8 mm suf-

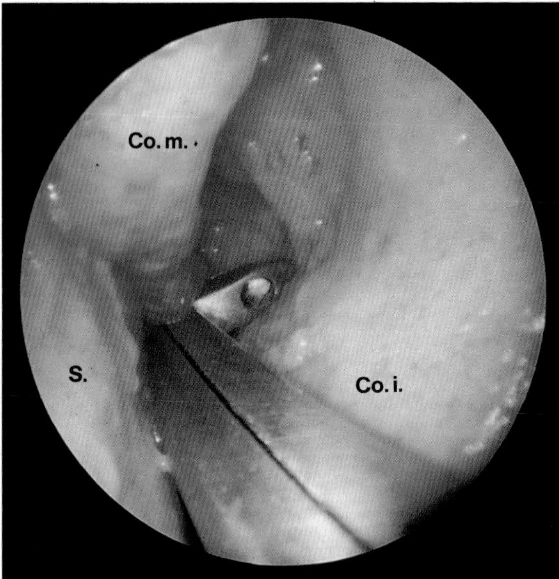

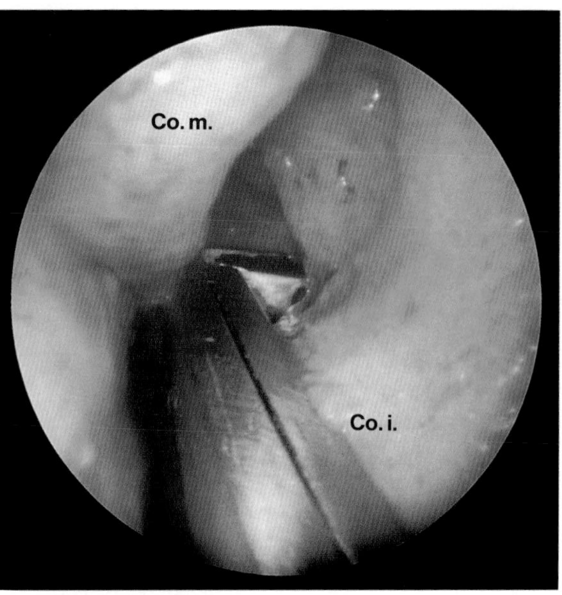

Figure 2.**37** Intranasal middle meatal antrostomy. **a** First step: application of a pointed 45° upward-cutting ethmoid forceps immediately above the center of the inferior turbinate.

b The punch is pushed in a strictly horizontal direction with the jaws slightly open. A small window is created by closing the forceps and removing fragments which are grasped.

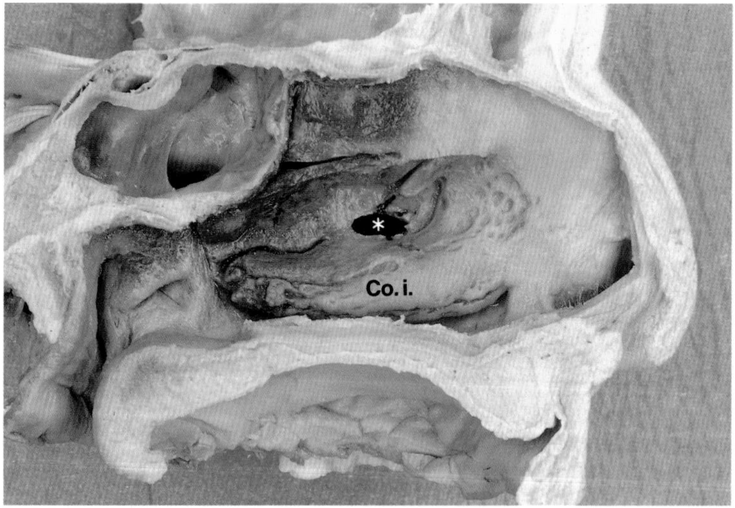

Figure 2.**38** The left lateral nasal wall of an anatomical dissection with a small middle meatal antrostomy (*) at the typical site above the center of the inferior turbinate, immediately above its upper edge, directly under the posterior end of the uncinate process. The window may be considerably widened above, anteriorly, and posteriorly from this point.

fices to drain the antrum (Figure 2.**40**); in this case only the membranous wall (the fontanelle) is resected. A hole as small as 5 × 5 mm may suffice for simple endoscopy, but for more extensive procedures within the antrum the antrostomy must be enlarged by resection of the uncinate process, and be extended to the wall of the orbit above (see Chapter 6). Figure 2.**41** shows, in an anatomical frontal section, the position of the lateral nasal wall which is to be fenestrated relative to the maxillary ostium, the turbinate bone and the orbital wall. It also emphasizes how the endoscopic view using a 70° telescope through the middle meatal antrostomy always falls first on the posterior antral wall. The other antral walls must then be viewed with telescopes of appropriate angles.

Figures 2.**42 a–c** show the position of the middle meatal antrostomy relative to the four main surfaces of the antrum. The alveolar recess is the most difficult area to inspect, since the view from above is often obstructed by a convex projection of the me-

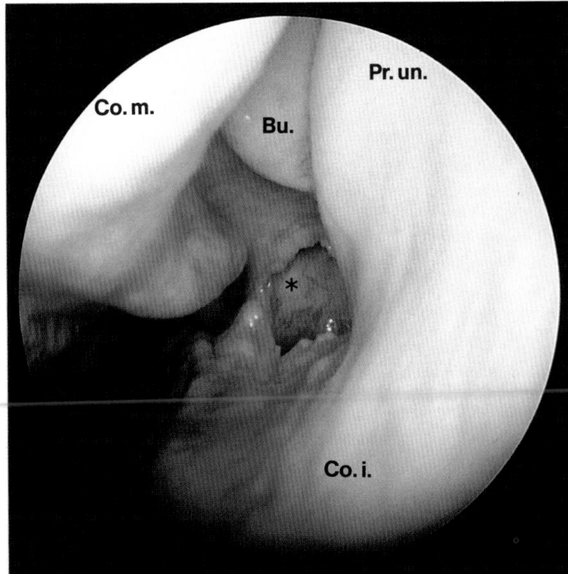

Figure 2.**39** A small middle meatal antrostomy (*) seen through a straight telescope from in front. The middle turbinate has been pushed slightly medially and upwards. The uncinate process and the ethmoid bulla are visible.

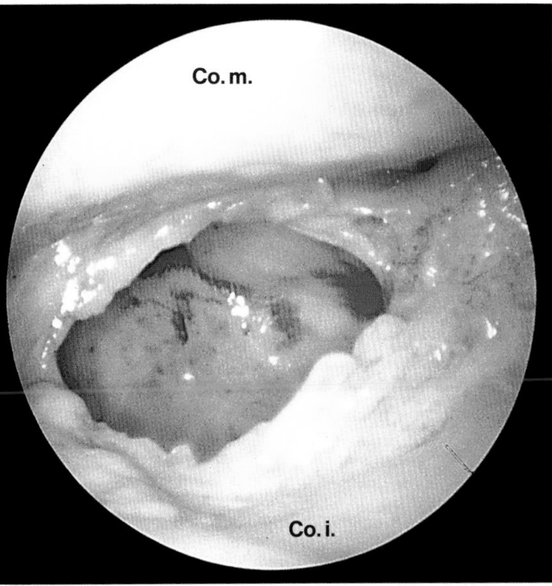

Figure 2.**40** A large middle meatal antrostomy as seen through a 70° telescope, and the posterior wall of the antrum beyond it. The overhanging middle turbinate conceals the uncinate process and the bulla.

Figure 2.**41** Topography of the supraturbinate part of the lateral nasal wall which is to be fenestrated in a frontal section of a dissected specimen. The antral opening of the maxillary ostium lies very close to the floor of the orbit above a fold. If the nasal wall is always perforated in a strictly horizontal direction above the dorsum of the turbinate bone, the orbit is always out of reach of the instrument.

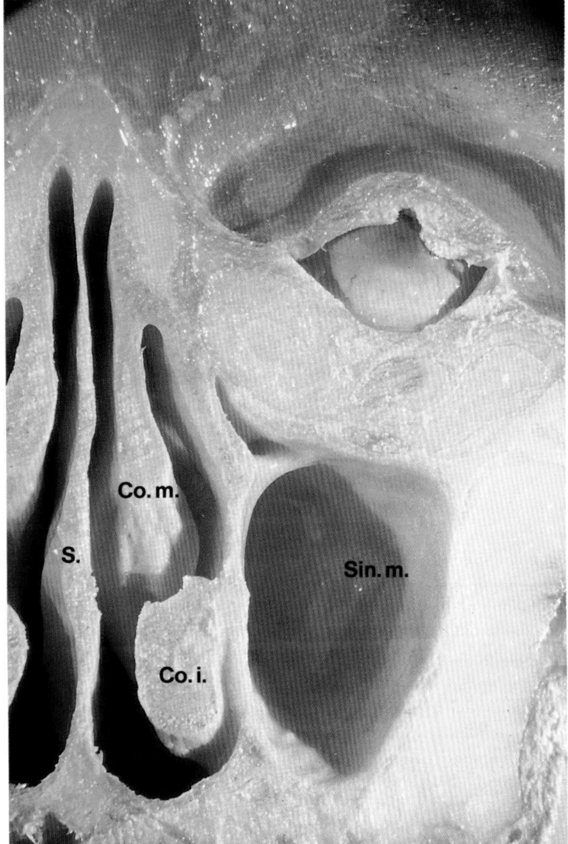

dial antral wall. In contrast, examination of the upper part of the antrum is easy, and the anterior and posterior walls can be seen better than by the infraturbinal access because the view is not obstructed by the inferior turbinate. The surgeon should now practice introducing a curved instrument into all recesses to develop familiarity with orderly inspection of the antral cavity, and purposeful endoscopic manipulations within it. If a dissected skull is available an additional portal through the canine fossa is useful to allow the endoscopic maneuvers to be monitored.

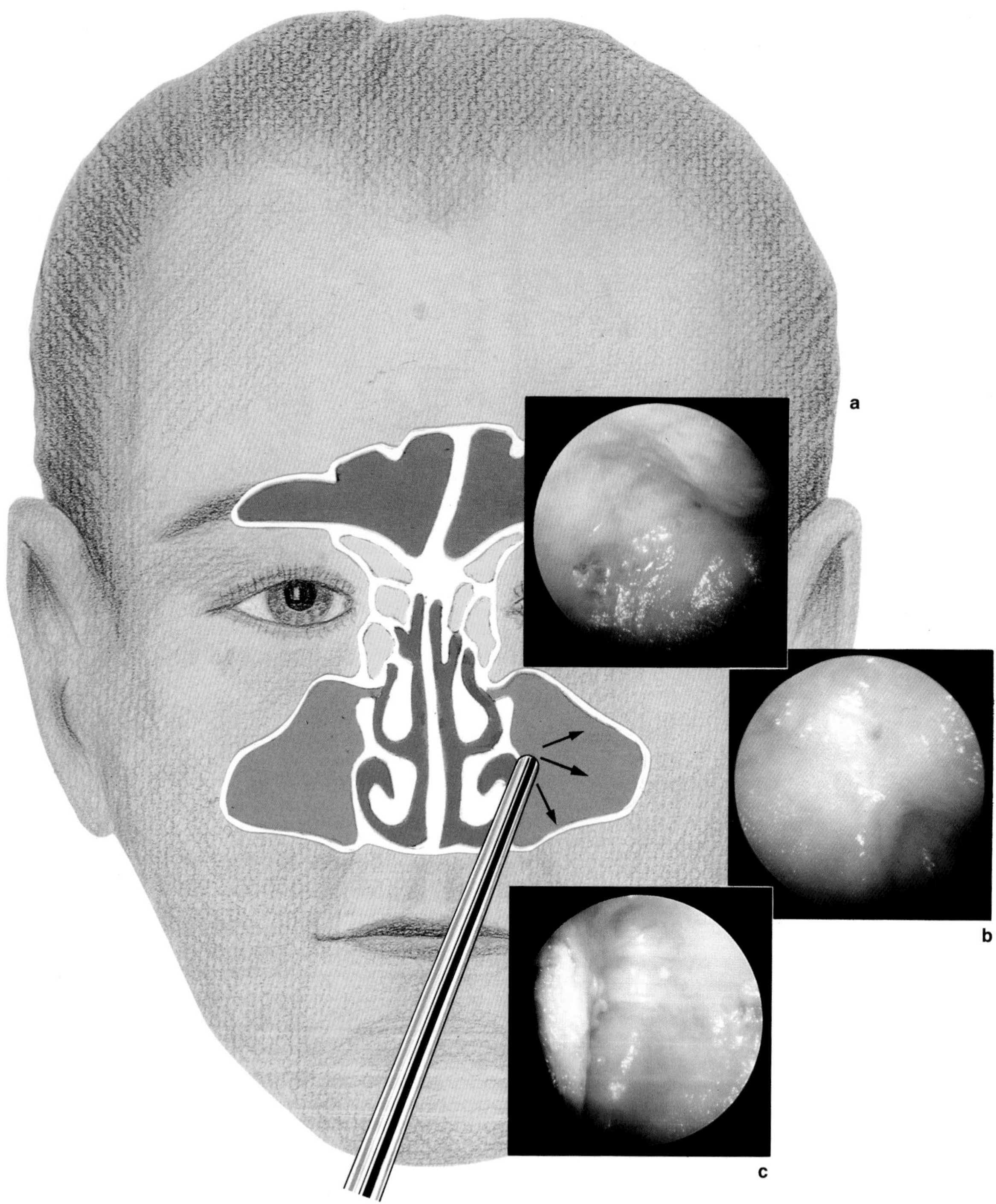

Figure 2.**42** Diagram of antral endoscopy. **a** View of the roof of the left antrum. **b** The anterior wall shown after slight clockwise rotation of the 70° telescope. **c** A view in an inferior direction along the medial wall of the alveolar recess in which several root sockets can be recognized.

Anterior Ethmoidectomy

Familiarity with the topographical anatomy of the ethmoids is essential for understandig the pathogenesis of chronic sinusitis, and for safe surgery in this dangerous area. The steps of a typical operation are now described on a dissected skull. These steps need not be followed slavishly in the order given during an operation; the surgeon should rather be guided by the wide individual variation of the pneumatization of the ethmoids.

Step I: Middle Meatus: Opening of the Semilunar Hiatus

Using a forward-viewing telescope (usually with an angle of vision of 25°) the first structure to come into view is the middle turbinate projecting medially (Figure 2.**43 a**). The sharp edge of the uncinate process curving anteriorly and upwards forms the lower edge of the semilunar hiatus, and the ethmoid bulla its upper edge. The ethmoid cells and the maxillary ostium opening within it cannot be seen initially. However, a secondary antral ostium in the anterior or posterior fontanelle is often visible below the uncinate process (Figure 2.**43 b**). Superiorly a transverse bony bar can be seen closing off the hiatus in front (Figure 2.**43 c**). The cells opening into the hiatus can be demonstrated by removing the lower edge of the hiatus, the upper edge of the uncinate process, using a sharp fissure knife and slender forceps. The ethmoid tunnel running under (occasionally over) the bar of bone described above, and towards the frontal duct now comes into view above and anteriorly (Figure 2.**43 d**). Several ostia do not open into the narrow groove of the hiatus (called the inferior semilunar hiatus by Hajek), but they communicate with the middle nasal meatus via a superior semilunar hiatus. This superior semilunar hiatus (Gruenwald) runs in a curve parallel to the lower semilunar hiatus above the ethmoid bulla. It also opens into the middle meatus, and it drains part of the anterior or middle ethmoid cells, particularly the bulla cells, and may expand superiorly and laterally to form a lateral sinus (Gruenwald).

Because of the wide variation in pneumatization of the ethmoids it is usually futile to define a "typical" arrangement of ethmoid cells: in practice the pathology of the lesion is more important. However, one must always try to remove as many cell walls as necessary from the inferior semilunar hiatus in an anterosuperior direction until the ethmoid infundibulum is reached. This dissection can be termed ethmoid infundibulotomy (Stammberger).

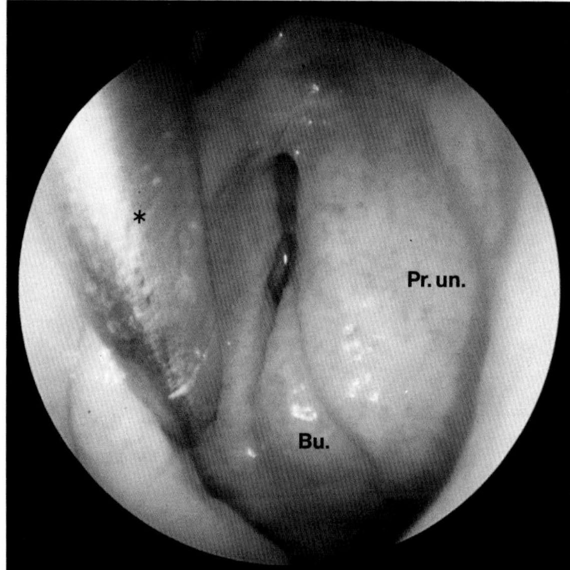

Figure 2.**43** Endoscopic ethmoid dissection on an anatomical specimen.
a Left middle meatus: middle turbinate on the left under the retractor (*), a voluminous uncinate process and the half-concealed bulla (straight telescope).

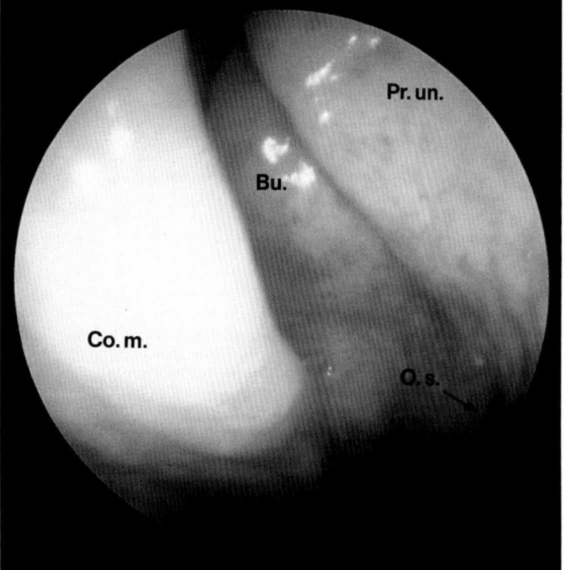

b Secondary ostium in the anterior fontanelle (straight telescope).

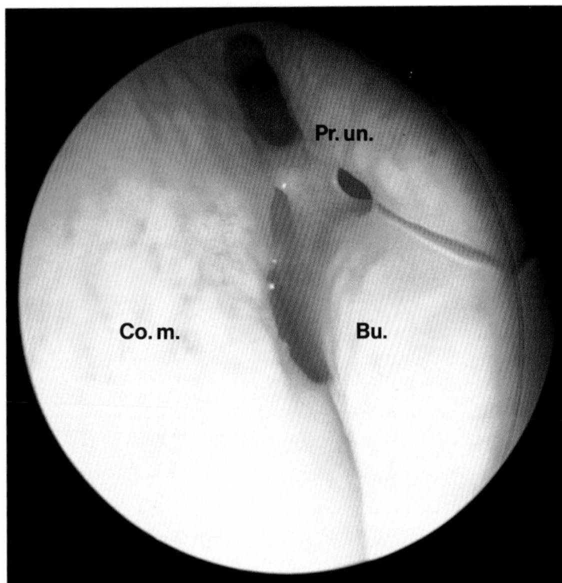

c View of the anterior end of the semilunar hiatus with the 70° telescope. A small bridge joins the middle turbinate, the bulla and the uncinate process to form one complex.

d View after resection of the upper edge of the uncinate process. The bulla is now completely visible, and the nasal opening of the maxillary ostium into the ethmoid infundibulum can be seen (25° telescope).

Step II: Opening of the Ethmoid Bulla

The lower wall of the bulla can now be removed using a sharp elevator and a narrow-pointed ethmoid punch (Figure 2.**43 e**). The anterior and middle ethmoid cells are thus partially opened. It is true that the cell septa are arranged according to a specific plan, but the individual arrangement is so variable that uniform nomenclature is not possible. The cells are serially opened, and the party walls removed precisely until the position of the cell tunnel running to the frontal and antral cavities is visible, and the pathology can be assessed. Figure 2.**43 f** shows the junction of the bulla cells and those of the middle turbinate.

Step III: Clearance of the Anterior Ethmoid

A telescope with an angle of not less than 70° is used for optical control of dissection of the anterior ethmoidal cells. In this phase of dissection on the cadaver it is possible to preserve the middle turbinate completely, but this cannot be achieved in all cases of chronic ethmoid polyposis. The turbinate, or the medial bony ethmoid lamella, bounds the cleared ethmoid compartment medially, and the lamina papyracea separates it from the orbit laterally. Both boundaries are exposed by stepwise semi-sharp resection of the cell septa using the smallest Blakesley punch or double forceps, under endoscopic control. The roof of the ethmoids above is often concealed by an upper layer of shallow ethmoid cells. The canal of the anterior ethmoid artery forming a shallow bulge running across the roof of the ethmoids should be identified carefully.

Step IV: Resection of the Agger Nasi, and Frontal Sinusotomy from below

It is usually not possible to expose the most anterior ethmoid cells and the connecting ducts to the frontal cavity by endoscopy without opening up the nasal cavity in front by removing the overhanging bone of the agger nasi. However, once 3–6 mm of this obstructing bony ridge has been removed with a cutting punch, the entire anterior ethmoid comes into view (Figure 2.**43 g–i**). The superolateral cell recesses can now be inspected, the medial lamella of the middle turbinate up to its union with the base of the skull identified, and the frontonasal duct inspected.

If a frontonasal duct is absent, but the radiographs have shown a frontal cavity to be present, then frontal sinusotomy is carried out with a sharp, curved curette or with a diamond burr from the nasoethmoidal cavity under endoscopic control. In both cases the direction of dissection runs from the skull base anteriorly: initially a dark, transparent, party wall usually lying 3–8 mm in front of the easily recognizable bulge of the anterior ethmoid artery is identified, and perforated carefully. It is occasionally dif-

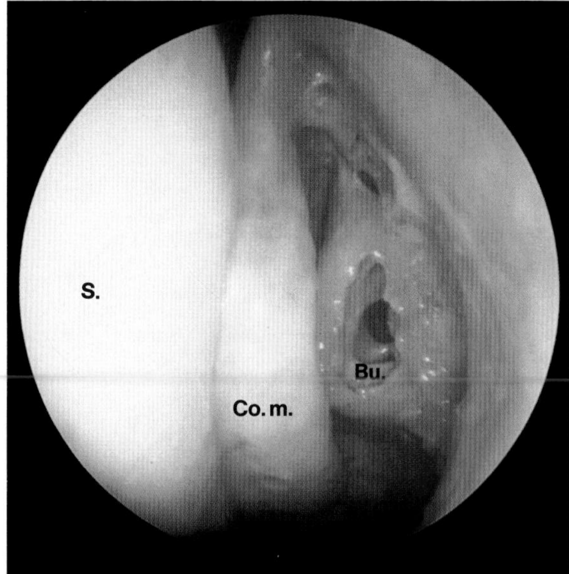

e The bulla opened. The bulla cells lead in an anterosuperior direction into the terminal recess (25° telescope).

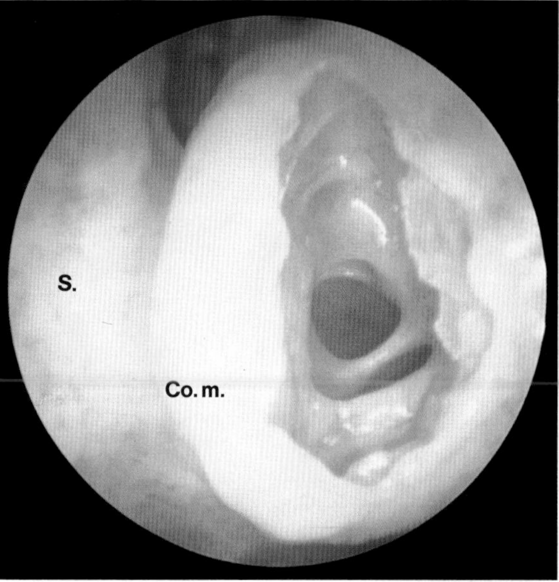

f The bulla exenterated. The basal lamella of the middle turbinate has been perforated (straight telescope).

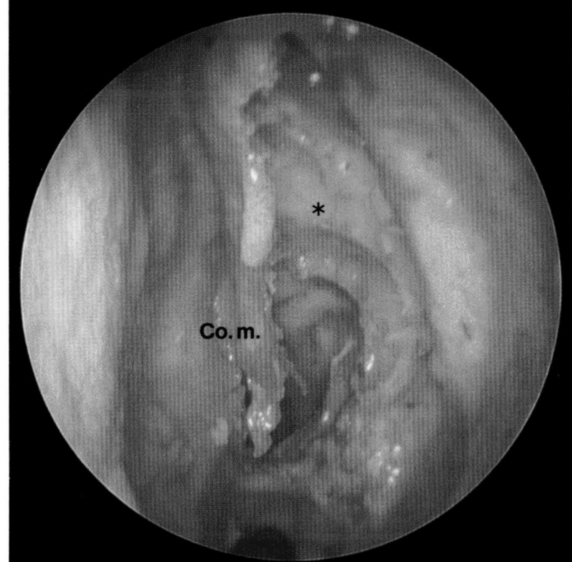

g Anterior and middle ethmoids and the intraconchal cells of the middle turbinate dissected. The base of the skull (*) can be seen (70° telescope) (a different specimen to that shown in Figure 2.**43 a–f**).

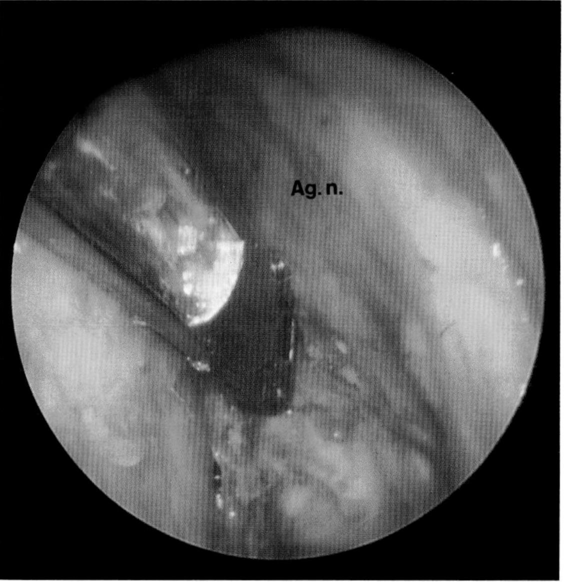

h Resection of the agger nasi with the upward-cutting 90° punch (70° telescope) (same specimen as in Figure 2.**43 g**).

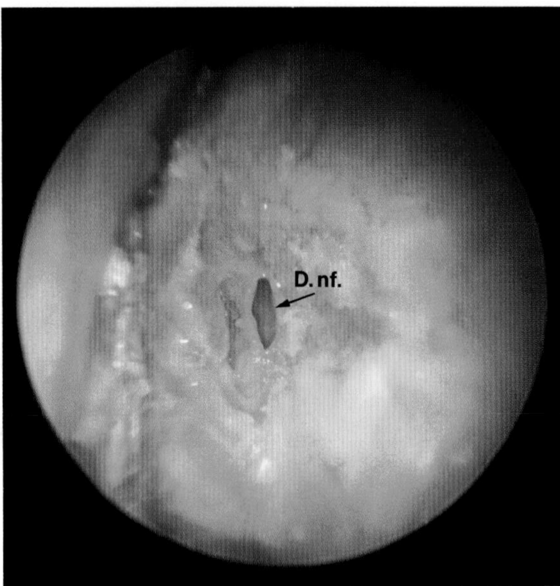

i The slit formed by the nasofrontal duct is now visible after resection of the agger nasi and removal of the anterior ethmoid cells (70° telescope) (same specimen as in Figure 2.**43 g**).

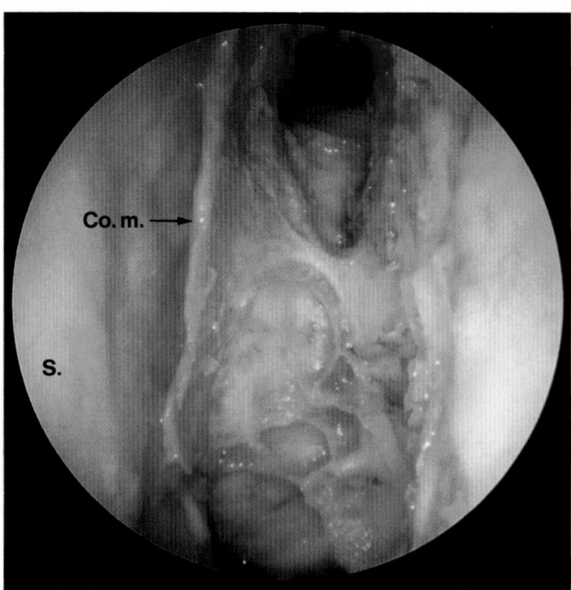

j Showing the view after endoscopic exenteration of the anterior ethmoid cells and widening of the frontal duct. The middle turbinate has been resected including the lower third of its medial lamella. The ethmoid artery can be identified as a clear horizontal bar (70° telescope) (same specimen as in Figure 2.**43 g**).

ficult to be sure whether the delicate membrane lying behind it is dura or mucosa, but the experienced endoscopic eye can usually distinguish the two. Figure 2.**43 k** shows a limited frontal sinusotomy. Continuity of the roof of the ethmoid with the convex curve of the posterior wall of the frontal sinus is a definite landmark for successful exposure of the frontal sinus. For practice, the floor of the frontal sinus can now be removed extensively, removing the anterior circumference of the small sinusotomy using sharp curettes.

Mastery of anterior ethmoidectomy and the creation of a sufficiently wide access to the frontal sinus is of decisive importance in the surgical treatment of severe polypoid pansinusitis. The ethmoid narrows anteriorly, and it is this area which determines healing or recurrence, and where the tendency to formation of scar tissue, and the danger of injury of the olfactory cleft is highest. Practice of correct manipulations under endoscopic control is therefore particularly important for this area of dissection.

The surgeon must assure himself on the dissected skull that all the cells have been removed, by going one step further and dissecting more widely in the surrounding area. The following are recommended:

- removal of the middle turbinate entirely in stages, and study of its attachment to the base of the skull,
- identifying the anterior ethmoid artery and exposing the surrounding dura,
- removal of the lamina papyracea to demonstrate the spatial relationships with the orbit,
- removal of further bone from the agger nasi until the nasolacrimal canal and lacrimal sac are completely exposed,
- opening the floor of the frontal sinus completely from below, and inspecting the posterior wall of the frontal sinus and its recesses.

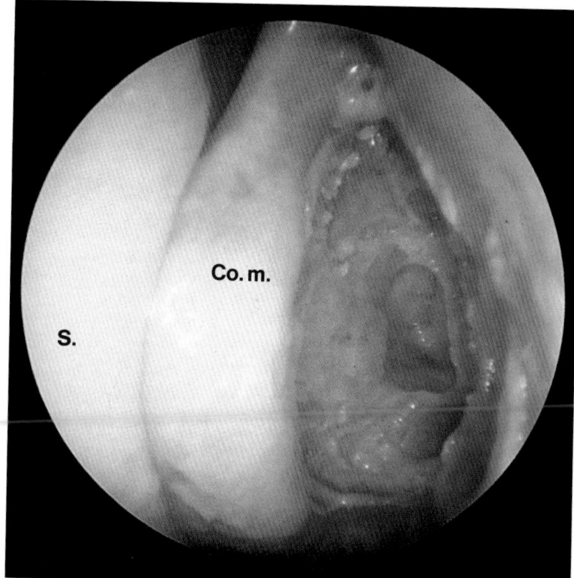

k View after exteneration of the middle ethmoid cells (straight telescope) (same specimen as in Figure 2.**43 a–f**).

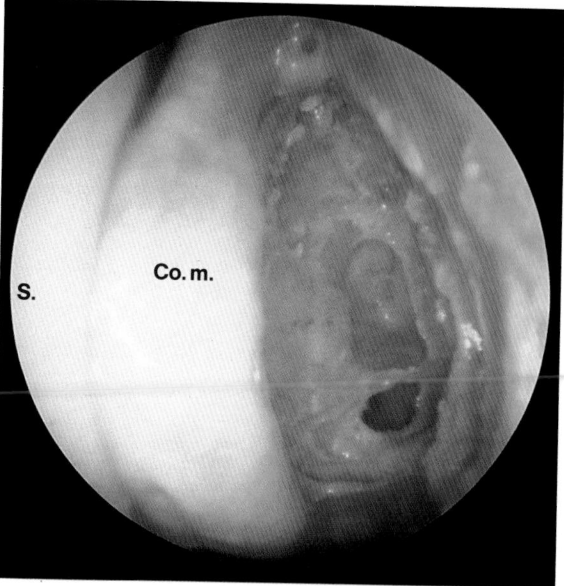

l Posterior ethmoid cells partially cleared (straight telescope) (same specimen as in Figure 2.**43 a–f**).

Posterior Ethmoidectomy

A bony party wall between the anterior and posterior ethmoid cells formed by a continuous basal lamella cannot always be recognized as is indicated in anatomical texts. Therefore the surgeon cannot always build up a mental image through the endoscope of separate anterior ethmoid cells draining into the middle meatus and posterior cells opening into the superior meatus (Figure 2.**43 l**). Dissection backwards from the bulla, preferably using a narrow ethmoid punch after removing the anterior ethmoid cells, brings the picture about to be described into view after resection of the posterior ethmoid cells. Examination can be carried out with the naked eye, but more effectively with the straight telescope or the operating microscope (Figure 2.**43 m**).

Laterally the ethmoid compartment has now reached its greatest extent, because its external wall, that is the medial wall of the orbit, runs laterally to form the orbital apex. Room can also be gained medially by dividing the middle turbinate from the skull base. Its upper insertion lies further laterally at the center of the ethmoids (that is the posterior end of the cribriform plate) and runs deeply to insert into the ethmoid and reach the lateral nasal wall more posteriorly, where its posterior point of attachment lies at the level of the floor of the sphenoid sinus (see Figure 2.**13**).

If the ethmoid is well pneumatized, tracks of cells may run laterally alongside the inferior turbinate (paraturbinal cells), either posteroinferiorly into the pterygoid process, or in a posterolateral and superior direction as Onodi cells beneath or lateral to the canal for the optic nerve. They are all of great importance in complete ethmoidectomy.

Exposure of the Sphenoid Sinus

Smooth and safe surgery on the ethmoidosphenoidal complex depends on thorough understanding of the topography of the sphenoid sinus and its relations. During total ethmoidectomy, a partial resection of the posterior ethmoid is carried out first, with subsequent broad fenestration of the sphenoid sinus. After this maneuver, a complete posteroanterior exenteration of the ethmoid follows. Exposure of a sphenoid sinus following complete ethmoidectomy on a cadaver is described here. Figure 2.**43 n** shows an endoscopic view through the nose after complete ethmoidectomy, with the anterior wall of the sphenoid still intact and with its natural ostium lying

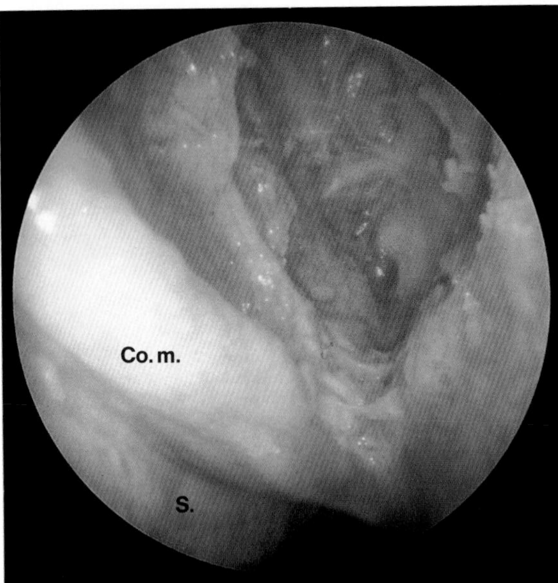

m Posterior ethmoid cells removed completely; the anterior wall of the sphenoid sinus is now visible (straight telescope) (same specimen as in Figure 2.**43 a–f**).

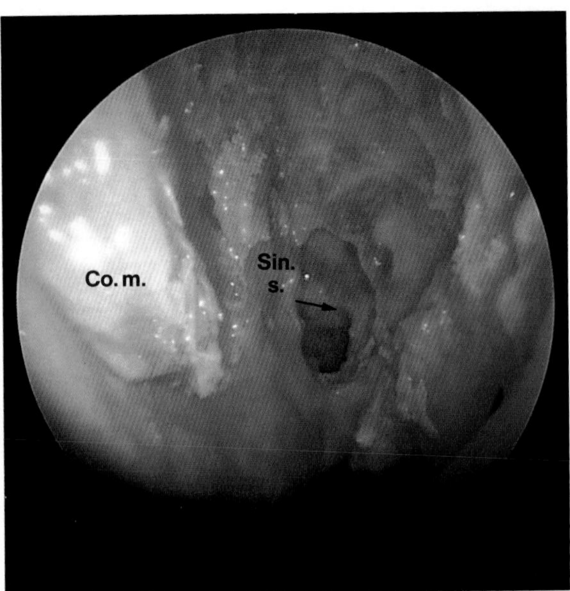

n Anterior wall of the sphenoid sinus removed. The posterior insertion of the middle turbinate lying at the level of the lower edge of this new opening has been partly removed (straight telescope) (same specimen as in Figure 2.**43 a–f**).

superiorly. The mental picture of topographical relationships gained from CT scans should be projected onto this situation, and the distance from the orbital wall, the optic nerve, the anterior cranial fossa and the carotid canal, should be remembered. It is also worthwhile considering the expected position of the sphenopalatine fissure and both the canalis rotundus and the canalis pterygoideus.

The anterior wall of the sphenoid sinus is fenestrated and removed completely with a punch. All walls of the sphenoid sinus are illuminated using a forward-viewing or a 30° telescope, and the preoperative concept of the topography of the structures named above is compared with the endoscopic view which ist now available (Figure 2.**43 o**). The distortion of the image due to the wideangled telescope should be remembered: close objects are magnified whereas distant objects appear too small.

If the sphenoid ostium cannot be found, and the view of the posterior ethmoid is narrow and obstructed by the middle turbinate, the posterior third of the middle turbinate should be resected with scissors (see Figure 6.**48**). The most posterior ethmoid cells can be removed easily and the transparent sphenoid wall can be seen (Figure 2.**43 p**) and perforated with a probe or with a fine closed ethmoid punch. In the author's experience, the cavity will always be found if the site of perforation lies about 1 cm above the roof of the posterior nasal choana (Figure 2.**43 q**). The entire anterior wall of the sinus is now removed with a 90° punch, allowing the sphenoid cavity to be examined with the straight telescope or with an operating microscope (Figure 2.**43 r**).

The roof of the sphenoid cavity sloping obliquely downwards and backwards is marked by the bulging wall over the pituitary. The sphenoid septum seldom lies in the midline, and often is not strictly sagittal. The lateral wall may be largely formed by the projections produced by the canals of the optic nerve and the carotid artery. Sphenoid recesses extending laterally and inferiorly can be of great importance in complete clearance of the sphenoid sinus (see Figure 2. **26 h**). The floor of the sphenoid sinus also varies. Usually the bone is too hard to allow removal with the punch. Arterial bleeding from the bony branches of the sphenopalatine artery indicates the level of the floor of the sphenoid sinus.

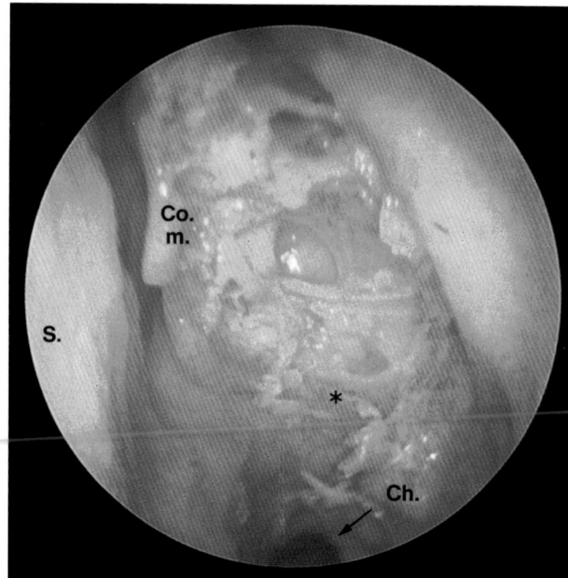

o Posterior ethmoid exenterated. The anterior wall of the sphenoid sinus (*) is transparent. The middle turbinate including the lower third of its medial lamella has been resected. Its posterior insertion has also been removed. The upper edge of the choana is visible (70° telescope) (same specimen as in Figure 2.**43 g**).

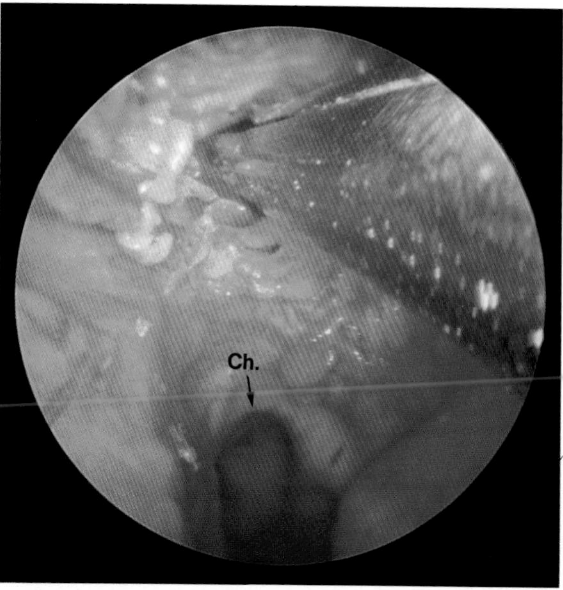

p Perforation of the anterior wall of the sphenoid sinus with the suction tube about 1 cm above the upper edge of the posterior nasal choana, paramedially immediately above the point of attachment of the resected middle turbinate (70° telescope) (same specimen as in Figure 2.**43 g**).

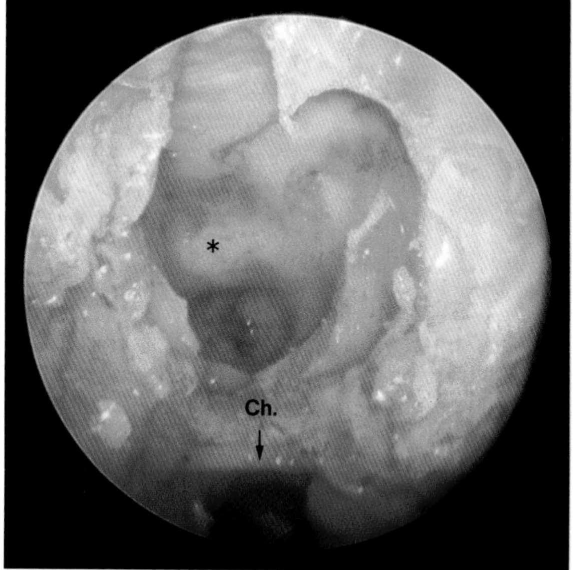

q The sphenoid sinus widely opened. The asterisk shows the sella turcica after subtotal resection of its anterior wall downwards almost 3 mm towards the roof of the choana (marked with an arrow) (straight telescope) (same specimen as in Figure 2.**43 g**).

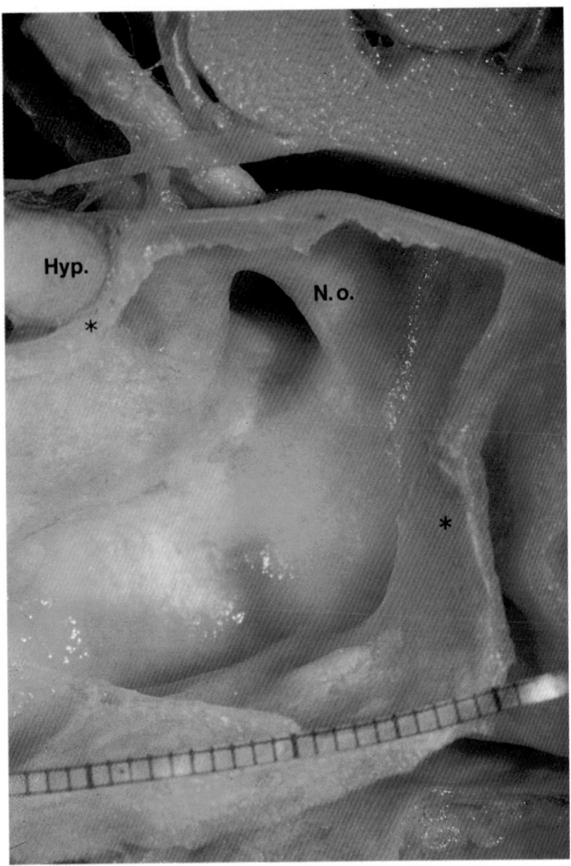

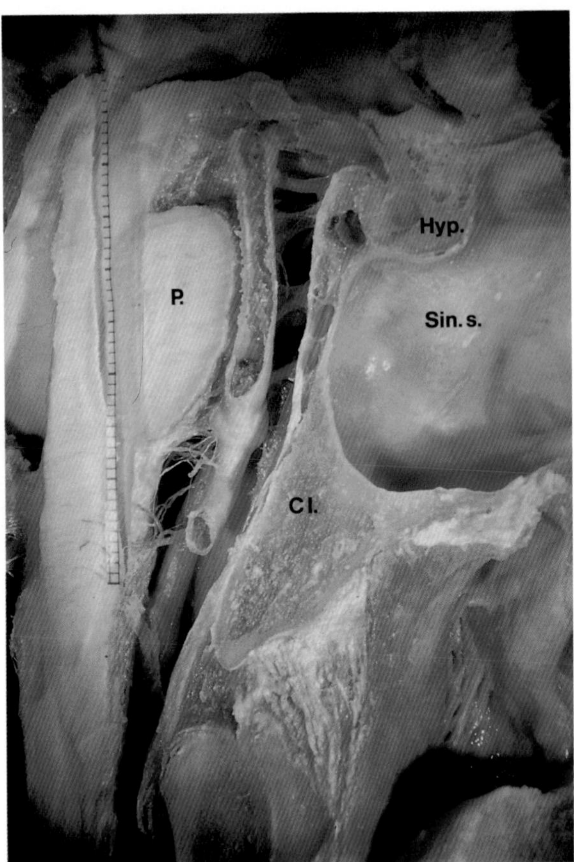

Figure 2.**44** Left sphenoid sinus in an anatomical preparation (Prof. Dr J. Lang, Würzburg). **a** The anterior half, showing the anterior wall, the bulge formed by the canal for the optic nerve, and the sella turcica (*).

b The posterior half with the pituitary gland, and the thin posterior wall behind which lie the basilar artery and the pons.

During endoscopic procedures within the sphenoid cavity, for example for treatment of a CSF fistula or for removal of papillomas, the bone of the lateral wall, roof or posterior wall must on occasion be thinned, using endoscopically monitored diamond burrs. Knowledge of the topographical relationship of the structures in the wall to the anterior and middle skull base, and the contents of the neighboring cranial fossa is very important (Figure 2.**44.a** and **b**). The distance between the anterior wall of the sphenoid sinus and the optic canal, the carotid canal and the pituitary gland, demand particular care but attention should also be drawn to the relative fragility of the posterior wall of the sphenoid sinus and the proximity of large basal blood vessels.

3. Preoperative Diagnosis

Endoscopic surgery of the paranasal sinuses is indicated for the treatment of tumors or trauma, the removal of foreign bodies, but mainly for chronic sinusitis and recurrent acute infection of the sinuses and its complications. A diagnosis of chronic hyperplastic sinusitis is not always an automatic indication for surgery, since not all these lesions need surgical treatment. Only a small proportion of patients with inflammatory mucosal lesions present to the otorhinolaryngologist. If a symptom-free sinusitis is discovered coincidently, careful assessment is required to determine whether surgery is advisable, because it carries risks and complications which may make the patient worse. On the other hand, symptom-free chronic sinusitis contributes more often than is commonly thought to the genesis of a wide range of serious diseases including lesions of the orbit and the optic nerve, otitis, laryngotracheobronchitis, and inflammation of the heart, the joints, the urinary tract and the skin.

Table 3.1 Main symptoms in chronic sinusitis. Data from 234 patients before operation.

Symptom	%
Nasal obstruction	64%
Facial pain, pressure or headache	51%
Troublesome nasal discharge	44%
Discomfort in the throat and hawking	9%
Bronchitis and cough	9%
Globus	9%
Disorders of smell	7%
Eustachian tube dysfunction	7%
Hay fever	5%
Bronchial asthma	5%

History Taking

The typical symptoms of sinusitis (Table 3.**1**) include anterior nasal discharge, postnasal drip, catarrh and nasal obstruction. The cause and effect often overlap: septal deviation may cause nasal obstruction, which is made worse by the resulting hypertrophy of the turbinates and thickening of the mucosa due to sinusitis. Pain, a feeling of pressure and loss of the sense of smell, are not universal symptoms, and are more common in acute than in chronic sinusitis. Questioning should be systematic and encompass the most important symptoms, and should also cover the symptoms of ear disease (such as variable hearing loss, crackling and itching in the ears, feeling of pressure, etc.) pulmonary symptoms (cough, spit, wheeze, etc.) diseases of the teeth and jaws, allergic symptoms, inflammatory disease of the joints, the urogenital system, the orbital apparatus, the skin and autonomic disorders, dizziness and fatigue. Chronic throat symptoms such as pain and dryness in the throat, hawking, globus and hoarseness are often due to discharge from a chronic sinusitis flowing down the pharynx. Thus the ear, nose and throat area should always be examined carefully.

Rhinoscopy and Nasal Endoscopy

Inspection of the nose by anterior and posterior rhinoscopy, preferably with a 30° angled telescope, may show a stream of pus running from the semilunar hiatus over the inferior turbinate (Figure 3.**1**), tenacious plugs of mucus lying in the ostium of the antrum, or polyps. These cases are almost always associated with a polypoid ethmoiditis if small granulations or large polyps are found protruding from under the middle turbinate or lying in the superior meatus in the region of the posterior ethmoids (Figure 3.**2**). Isolated nasal polyposis without sinusitis is exceptional, although edematous swellings of the end of the turbinate can occur. The pedicle of a choanal polyp often arises in the antral cavity, but can originate from the posterior ethmoid. Nasal mucosa that appears normal does not exclude chronic sinusitis: conversely it is not possible to deduce anything about the sinus mucosa from the swelling or color of the nasal mucosa. Nevertheless, reddening, lichenification or eczyma of the nasal vestibule and the external skin at the nasal introitus strengthen suspicions arising from the history.

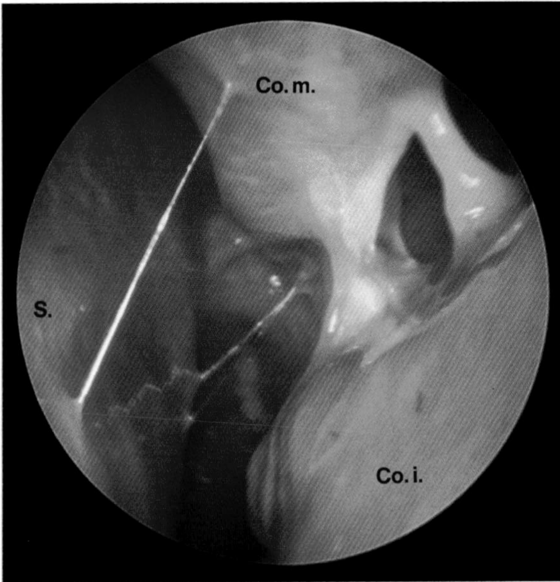

Figure 3.**1** Pus in the left middle meatus between the inferior and middle turbinate (30° telescope).

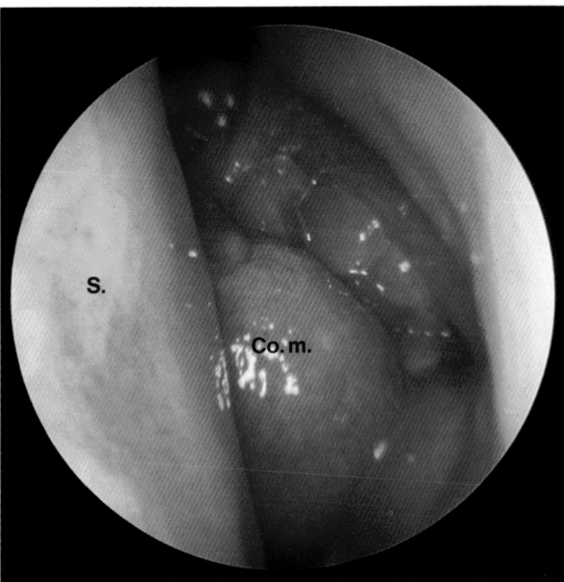

Figure 3.**2** Polyp in the left middle meatus. Only the head of the middle turbinate can be seen (straight telescope).

Ultrasound Scan

Although ultrasound using A scan can prove useful in identifying an empyema or an isolated antral cyst and in follow-up, it has proved unreliable for the assessment of maxillo-ethmoidal polyposis. Furthermore a B scan has not proved useful for precise localization of a circumscribed or diffuse mucosa hyperplasia nor for demonstrating the recesses of the frontal and antral cavities. However, ultrasound is indicated for follow-up after conservative treatment of sinusitis, particularly of patients who should not be subjected to irradiation, such as pregnant women and children.

Radiography and Computer Tomography (CT)

Precise information about the type and extent of chronic sinusitis is usually obtained from radiography. The *occipitomental view* is very suitable for demonstrating mucosal swellings or round shadows (Figure 3.**3a, b**) of the antral and frontal sinuses. Imaging of the sphenoid cavity is unsatisfactory and of the ethmoid is unreliable. For this purpose, plain films in other planes can be used, for example posteroanterior sagittal views with highlighting of the ethmoid, Rhese's projection, and the tilted axial views described by Hirtz and Welin. Lateral views of the frontal sinus are seldom useful. A concave or straight edge shadow indicates fluid, whereas round or half round convex shadows indicate mucosal hyperplasia, cysts or polyps. These findings should be taken into consideration when deciding whether a puncture alone, a sinusotomy for drainage or ventilation, or removal of a pedicled mass is indicated. Diffuse, complete opacity of one frontal or antral cavity may indicate a collection of fluid, hyperplasia or both. In

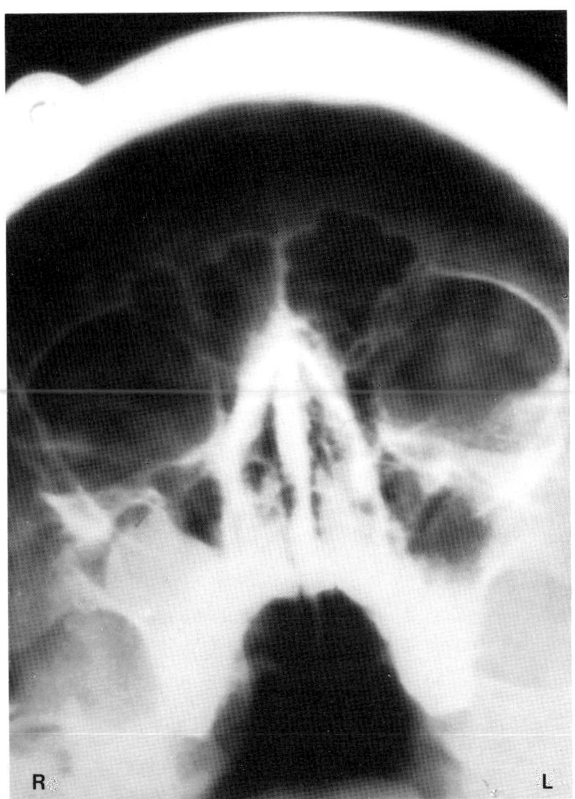

Figure 3.3 Opacity in the antral cavity in the occipitomental view. **a** Round shadow in the right antrum.

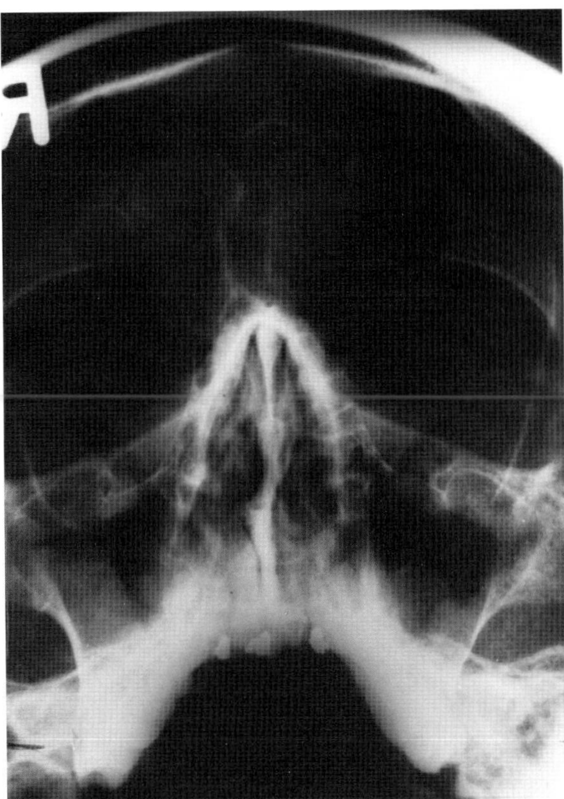

b Faint peripheral shadow in the right antral cavity.

this case puncture or endoscopy can help to establish the cause. In the author's experience isolated disease of the antral or frontal cavity is unusual, and imaging of the superimposed ethmoid is always necessary.

Imaging of the cells by plain films in various projections is of limited value because of the unavoidable overlap of the shadow of the turbinate on the ethmoids. Tomography provides more information per unit of radiation dosage.

Precision polycyclical tomography is very useful. For many years the author has depended on polycyclical tomography using four 1.5 cm sections from the root of the nose to the sphenoid sinus. This technique provides excellent images of all three dimensions and is very reliable for the assessment of disease of the sphenoid and ethmoids. It is also the most suitable for assessment of fractures and tumors of the facial skeleton and the anterior base of the skull; it can be refined by intermediate cuts. This view has taught us that an apparently normal plain film does not exclude massive polyposis of the antral cavity and ethmoids (Figure 3.**4a, b**).

Computer tomography provides incomparably clearer information with relatively low radiation exposure, particularly using coronal sections, which allow excellent comparison between the sides. Axial sections with suitable aperture settings provide an almost perfect imaging of the bony party walls and of the thickness of the mucosa. The rhinologist must therefore familiarize himself with the basics of computer tomography, the settings and avoidance of artifacts. For example he must know the slice thickness and intervals most suitable for special conditions and that a soft tissue setting rather than bone settings must be used to demonstrate subtle mucosal lesions.

Figure 3.**5a–d** serve as an example of the ability of computer tomograms to demonstrate discrete lesions. The patient had undergone several radiographic investigations over a long period for post-traumatic anosmia, but the results were always negative. A *coronal CT scan* clearly showed bilateral circumscribed ethmoiditis and opacity of one frontal sinus, requiring ethmoidectomy and exposure of the frontal duct. Coronal sections also provide important

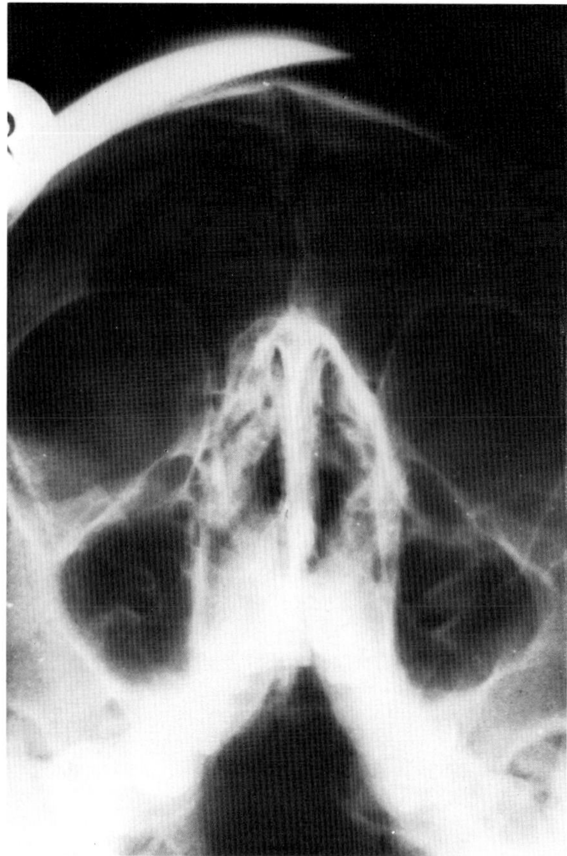

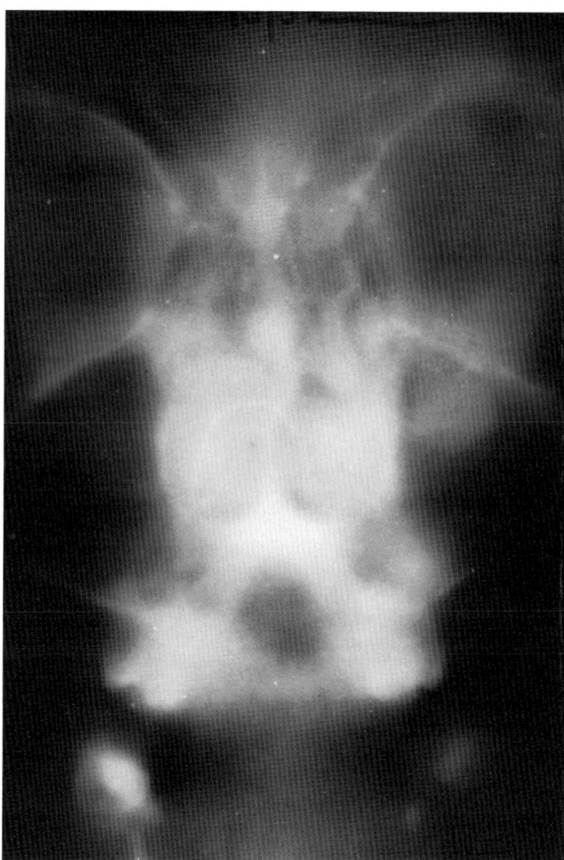

Figure 3.4 Occult ethmoiditis demonstrated by radiology. **a** Apparently normal occipitomental view. **b** Massive opacity of the ethmoid and ethmoid recess of the antrum shown by polytomography.

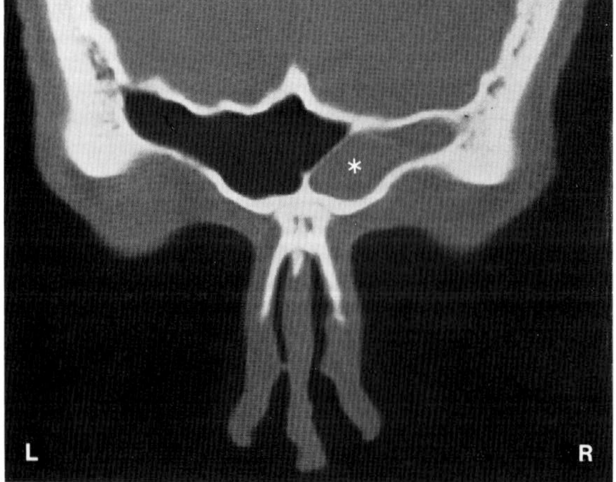

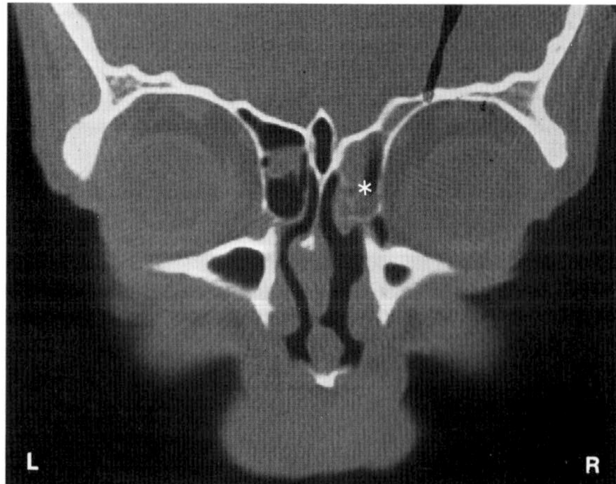

Figure 3.5 Circumscribed ethmoiditis in coronal CT scan.
a Opacity of the right frontal sinus due to a mucoempyema (*).
b Circumscribed opacity of the left anterior ethmoid and a diffuse opacity on the right (*).

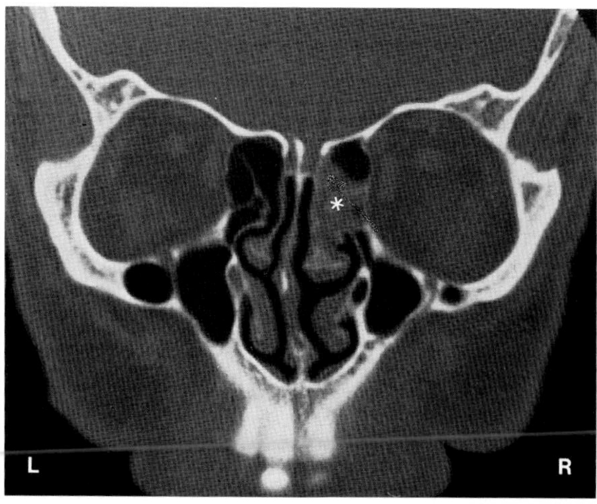

c Circumscribed opacity of the right middle ethmoid (*) whereas the left side is clear in this section.

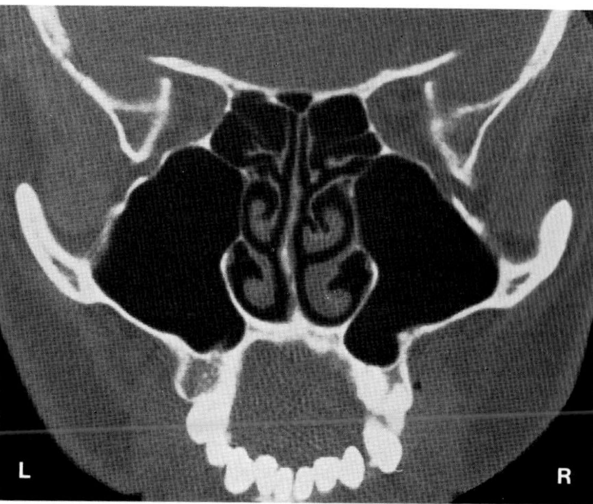

d Both ethmoids are healthy posteriorly.

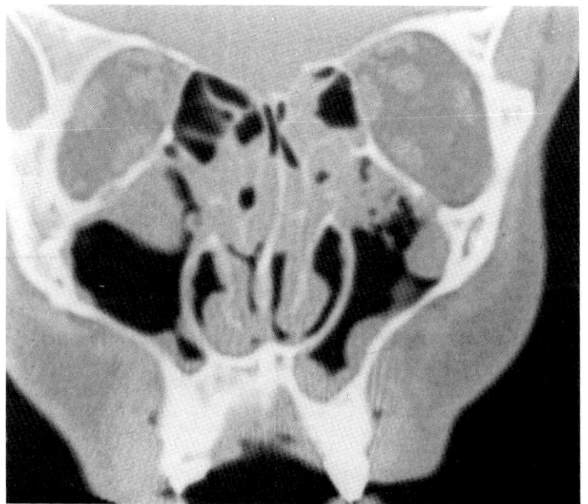

Figure 3.**6** Polypoid pansinusitis in coronal CT scan. Dependent round shadows in the antral cavity can be clearly seen. Only a few posterior ethmoid cells are still aerated.

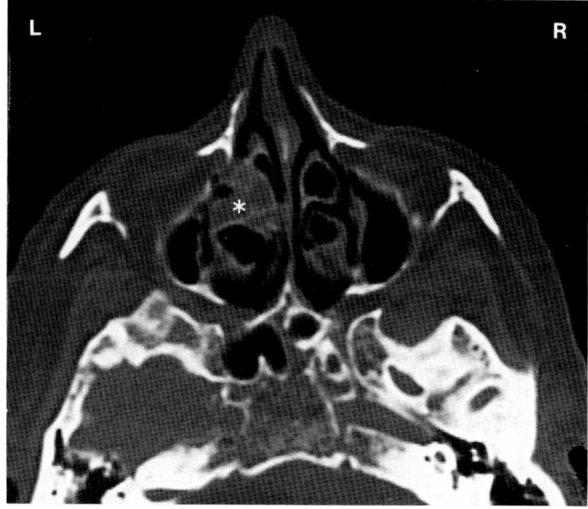

Figure 3.**7** Disseminated ethmoiditis in axial CT scan. On the left side there is a dense opacity of the middle ethmoid cells (*). The main symptom was boring left-sided facial pain.

information about the variable involvement of the nasal cavities in diffuse polypoid pansinusitis (Figure 3.**6**).

The *axial CT projection* is also suitable for demonstrating localized ethmoid disease (Figure 3.**7**). However, since the skull base which forms the roof of the ethmoids is flat it can be confused with opaque cells. Coronal sections are therefore indispensible for assessment of the anterior skull base. Also the ostia and the maxillo-ethmoidal outflow tract into the ethmoid infundibulum are less well shown in axial than in coronal cuts. The latter demonstrate the lateral extent of pneumatization and anomalies of the floor of the nose clearly (Figure 3.**8**). However, both projections are equally useful in the demonstration of diffuse pansinusitis.

The rhinologist must master this relatively new imaging technique, so that he can make precise requests to the radiological department and provide information about the questions to be answered and the choice of settings (Table 3.**2**). Otherwise a general radiology department will deliver overexposed bone images which do not show the mucosa, and provide many useless views of the calvaria, the skull

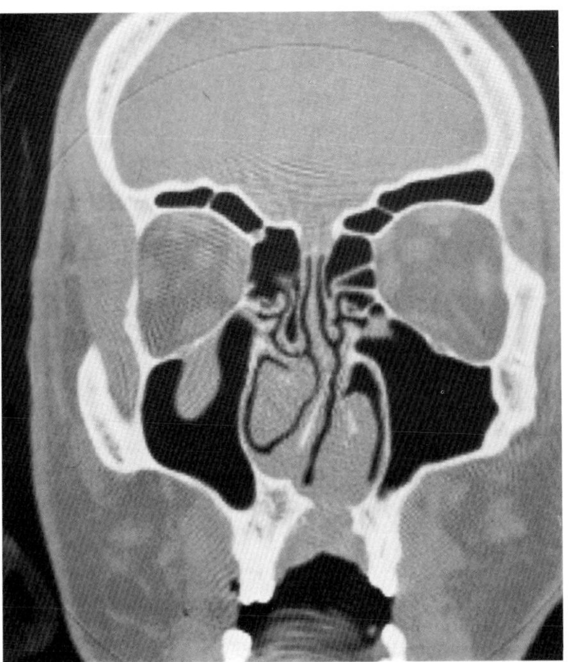

Figure 3.**8** Isolated antral polyp, and surgically corrected cleft palate in coronal CT scan. The ethmoid cells are aerated.

Table 3.**2** Settings for coronal CT scans to show the mucosa and bony walls of the nasal sinuses.

Coronal section, quasi-frontal	
Bony window	
High resolution	
Slice thickness	2 mm
Slice interval	5 mm

base and the brain, and too few of the nasal sinuses. The glut of unsuitable exposures in conventional radiography could be reduced by more expertly chosen CT scans, to the great benefit of our patients and the economy.

The value of tomography in the recognition of disease of the paranasal sinuses cannot be overestimated. It uncovers many cases of occult sinusitis, and places the treatment of disease due to focal infection on a sound basis. In view of the often long-standing unsuccessful treatment of mucosal disease of the upper and lower airway including chronic bronchitis and asthma, the additional costs of more frequent CT imaging of the paranasal sinuses is fully justified.

Magnetic Resonance Imaging (MRI)

This technique is still in its developmental phase, and personal experience of a limited number of cases does not allow any conclusions to be drawn. However, the poor bone signal is a grave disadvantage in the diagnosis of inflammatory lesions of the paranasal sinuses, although MRI appears to be useful in the assessment of tumors.

Functional Tests

Nasal respiration and the paranasal aeration are not always correlated. Improvement of the nasal air passage, however, will basically contribute to the recovery of the sinuses from sinusitis. Besides that, a correction of the septum or a conchotomy must often be combined with endoscopic sinus surgery in order to widen the surgical field for necessary manipulations. Functional measurements of nasal viability are, therefore, welcome for the planning of therapy.

Active anterior *rhinomanometry* is a valuable accessory method for assessing the patency of each side of the nose at a given instant. The curve is very dependent on difference of pressure between the nasal introitus and the choana, but it does not give any detailed information about the ventilation of indivudal parts of the nasal cavity and the paranasal sinuses. Ostial manometry demands a puncture of the sinuses, and is little used clinically.

Often the symptoms of nasal obstruction conflict with the findings of endoscopy or radiology. If a CT scan demonstrates narrowing of the nasal passages (Figure 3.**9**) with deformity of the middle turbinate, and the patient has symptoms such as headache, recurrent acute sinusitis, chronic ethmoiditis, etc., a septal correction should be considered.

Pre- and postoperative olfactometry is very valuable for assessing disorders of function of the olfactory mucosa and the results of ethmoid operations in

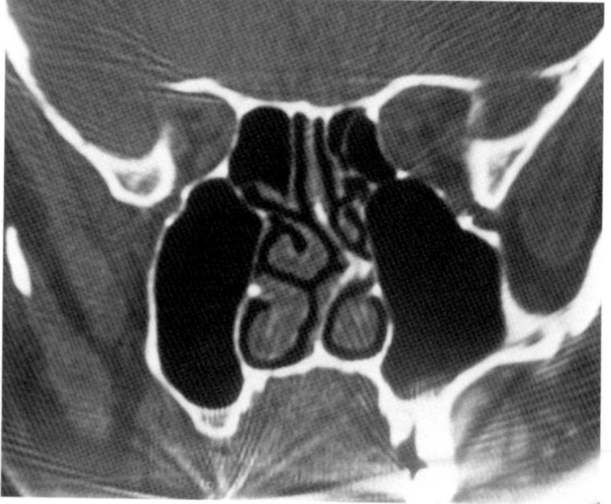

Figure 3.**9** Very marked septal spur in coronal CT scan. Marked narrowing of the middle meatus with atrophy of the middle turbinate. The patient had recurrent maxillary sinusitis.

diffuse polyposis. Dysosmia is often caused by inflammation, and improves after opening up or reconstruction of the olfactory cleft. Recurrent dysosmia is the first, and very sensitive, indication of recurrent swelling or adhesion of the mucosa or of recurrent polyps demanding endoscopic management or revision surgery.

Semiquantitative olfactory testing by Elsberg's method using increasing concentrations of the olfactory substance has been valuable. The results are displayed in an olfactogram (Figure 3.**10a**), showing the disorder of olfaction and its extent (Figure 3.**10b**). After ethmoidectomy, olfactometry can be very useful in assessing the loss of olfactory mucosa, aeration of the olfactory cleft, the value of conservative treatment, and in detecting recurrence.

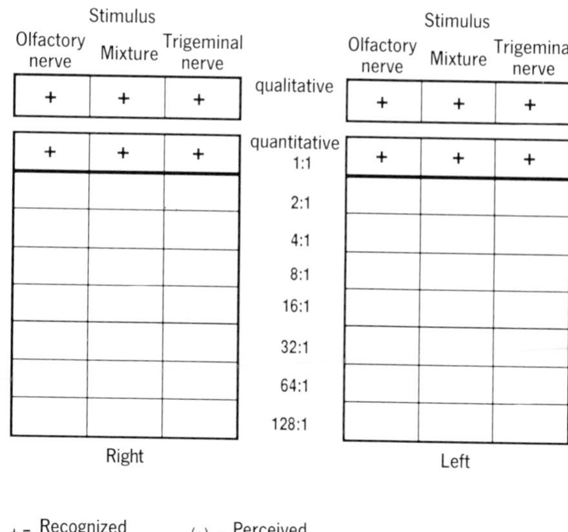

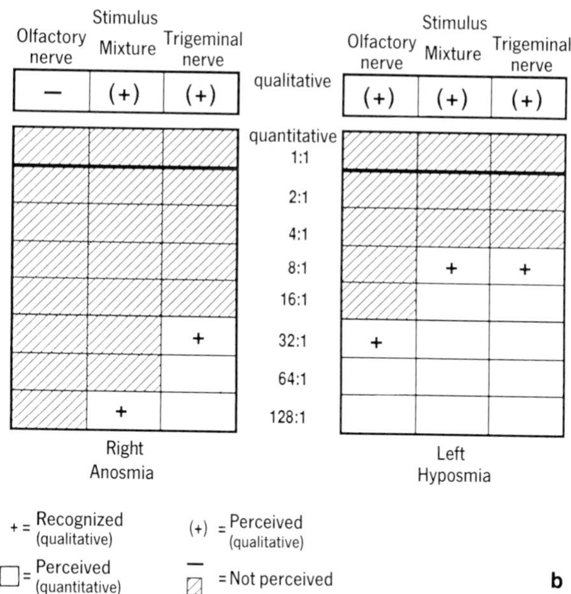

Figure 3.**10** Olfactogram of semiquantitative testing for smell using the Elsberg series of flasks of olfactory substances. The recognition of natural substances is recorded qualitatively and that of synthetic stimuli is graded quantitively. **a** Normal findings. **b** Hyposmia.

Further Investigations

Allergy testing of patients with chronic hyperplastic sinusitis is reasonable, even if the yield of desensitization of appropriate cases has so far been low. The demonstration and elimination of allergens can be a useful supplement to surgery.

The value of allergy testing can be assessed from the history and local findings. Patients with chronically thickened sinus mucosa should be investigated *before* surgery especially for the effect of perennial allergens. If the skin tests, intranasal provocation and *in-vitro* investigations identify the allergen, the patient should be treated conservatively by avoidance of the allergen, systemic medication or desensitization. In addition, anatomical obstructions of the upper airway should be corrected surgically.

However, allergic diagnosis and treatment are disappointing for patients with true polyposis of the sinus mucosa which can be combined with endogenous bronchial asthma and sensitivity to analgesics (the aspirin triad). In these cases *surgical* clearance is the treatment of choice, and allergic management is a useful supplement.

Dental examination should never be omitted in chronic maxillary sinusitis. A panorex view of the upper jaw is a useful screening test, and suspect cases should always be assessed by a dentist. Dental causes are said to account for 10%–20% of cases, but in the author's personal series dental granulomas requiring treatment are unusual. Nevertheless, exclusion of a potential focus is necessary to create optimal conditions for healing of the maxillary mucosa. Conversely an extensive dental infection does not exclude the affected sinus from consideration for intranasal surgery. The best treatment may be dental treatment of the root combined with intranasal endoscopic treatment of the antrum.

Pulmonary function tests are essential for medical advice of the patient with asthma or bronchitis, and allow the anesthetist to recognize peri- and postoperative risks and to arrange prophylactic breathing exercises. A test for non-specific bronchial hyperreactivity also helps the surgeon to identify patients with a subclinical asthma. Whereas about 25% of asthmatics suffer chronic hyperplastic sinusitis, this proportion rises to 40% of those who also have analgesic sensitivity. This sensitivity is often unrecognized, but can be uncovered by pulmonary function tests after an oral dose of aspirin. Patients sensitive to analgesics have a worse prospect of healing of their sinus mucosa. The individual patient should have a peak flowmeter to demonstrate exogenous bronchial asthma, and to optimize long-term medication.

Supplementary investigations by other specialities are often needed especially in:

- children with sinusitis, particularly those with mucoviscidosis, by the pediatrician;
- patients with unexplained pain or disturbances of sensation, by the neurologist;
- women with unexplained swelling of the skin and mucosa or pregnancy, by the gynecologist;
- patients with stridor and other systemic disorders, by the internist.

The interdependence of disease of the respiratory mucosa with other systems is close, and demands a familiarity with neighboring specialties.

The treatment decision is based on evaluation of the history, endoscopic findings and imaging. The latter also decides the type of procedure, its extent and the choice of anesthesia.

Naturally the surgeon should not fall into the trap of regarding every opacity or thickening as indicating tissue hyperplasia requiring surgery. Collections of fluid (blood, secretion or pus) foreign bodies and fungus infections are impressive, but can usually be recognized from the typical convex fluid level or dense opacity. A much more difficult question to answer is the reversibility of visible mucosal swellings if a decision must be made between conservative or surgical treatment. In this case the length of the history, the failure of serious attempts at treatment, etc., are often more helpful than imaging. Lesions in children, and post-traumatic mucosal thickening are both capable of remarkable remission.

The demonstration of mucosal lesions by radiography or CT scan is also an important indication of the prognosis. For example, loss of bony outlines and massive scarring preventing the maintenance of patency of hollow spaces casts doubt upon the prospects for a revision operation. This applies also to patients with immunological diseases, a systemic disorder such as mucoviscidosis or sensitivity to analgesics. Therefore complete investigation demands additional functional tests: the results may not affect the therapeutic decision, but can indicate that it must be supplemented by further measures.

4. Instrumentarium

The Surgical Endoscope

Intracavity surgery demands a well illuminated, sharp and, at times, magnified field of vision with no blindspots. The operating microscope is very useful when used through a wide portal in the upper part of the oral vestibule, and for transnasal surgery of the posterior ethmoid and sphenoid cavities, but it is unsuitable as soon as the surgeon wishes to see around corners into niches, recesses or ducts. Angled telescopes are therefore indispensible, especially for intranasal surgery of the anterior ethmoids and the sphenoid cavity, particularly with access via the middle meatus.

Rigid tubes with high luminous intensity and Lumina eyepieces (Wolf) or Hopkins rods (Storz) are preferred, with 25° (quasi straight), 70° and 110° direction of view (Figure 4.**1**). They are almost all wide angled.

Cold-light illumination is always used, provided by a powerful light source and conducted by a glass-fiber bundle. In this way illumination strengths up to 15,000 lx (standard light source) are achieved. The viewing angle runs from −40° to +120°, and the depth of focus extends from 10 to 80 mm. The surgeon must first accustom himself to the rapidly changing magnification of his target. For example reducing the working distance from 30 to 10 mm produces a magnification of 1.5 fold (Figure 4.**2 a, b**).

Flexible endoscopes provide poorer illumination and the image is less sharp. They are seldom used for surgery, but are preferred for diagnostic endoscopy of the nasal ducts and the nasopharynx, and also can be used for follow-up after antral or sphenoid sinusotomy (Figure 4.**3 a, b**).

Transendoscopic dissection is too inflexible, and paraendoscopic instrumentation has therefore been developed instead: the instruments have a relatively narrow shaft, they can be introduced under optical control and can be moved freely (Chapter 6).

The versatility of paranasal sinus endoscopes has been considerably extended by the incorporation of a suction-irrigation handpiece with interchangeable aspiration and irrigation on the end of the endoscope (Figure 4.**4**). Freeing the lens of blood, secretion and misting by irrigation keeps the field of vision clear, whereas the usual telescopes must be continuously removed from the nose to allow them to be cleaned and demisted. However, effective irrigation of the operative field with a powerful jet of water has to be developed: the current irrigation apparatus on the point of the endoscope is so far inefficient for this purpose. The prototype of a new suction-jet irrigation handpiece has already proved valuable.

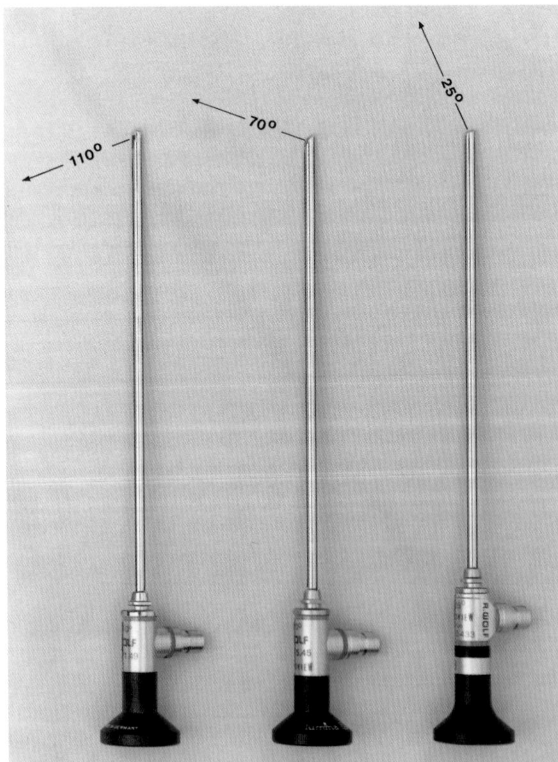

Figure 4.1 Angled suction-irrigation telescopes for endoscopic sinus surgery. The most usual viewing angles are 25°, 70° and 110°. High-illumination wide-angle objectives are usually preferred.

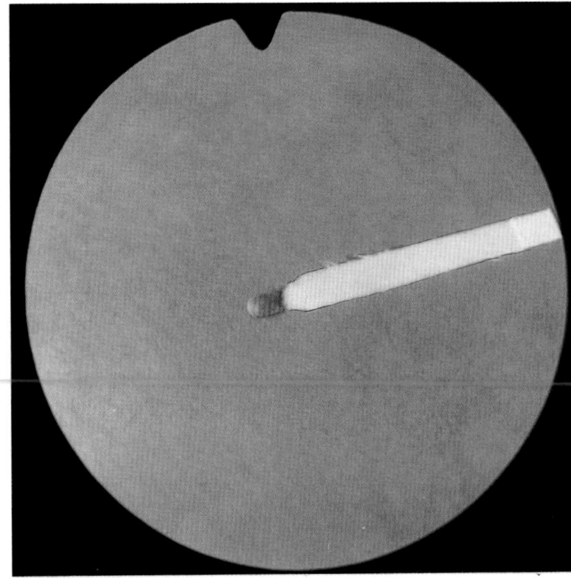

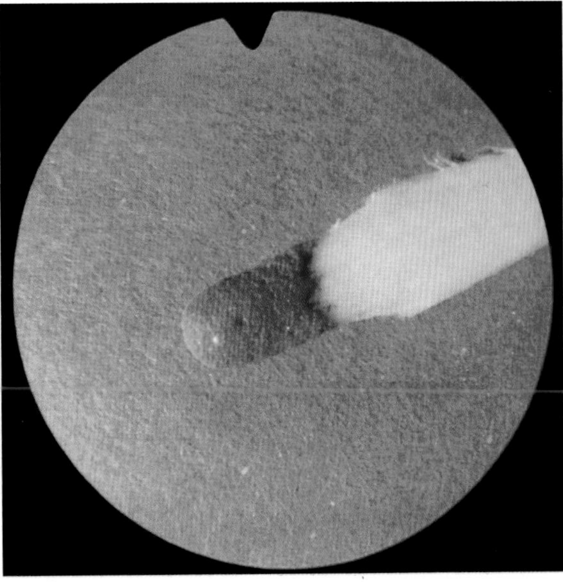

Figure 4.**2** Change of magnification produced by changing the working distance. **a** 4 cm working distance.

b 1 cm working distance (25° Panoview Plus telescope, Wolf, Knittlingen).

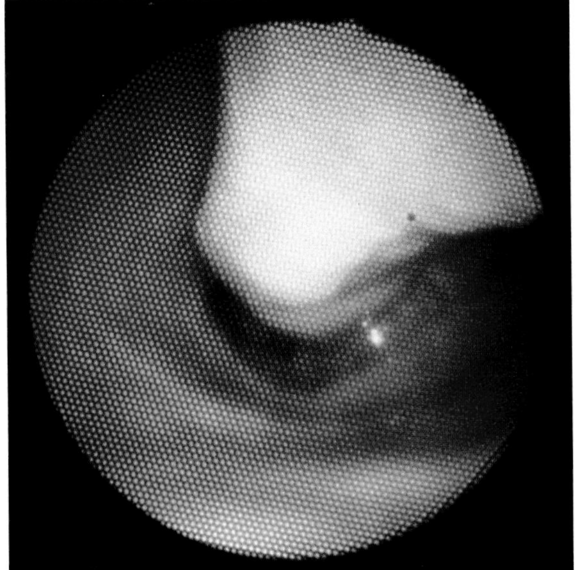

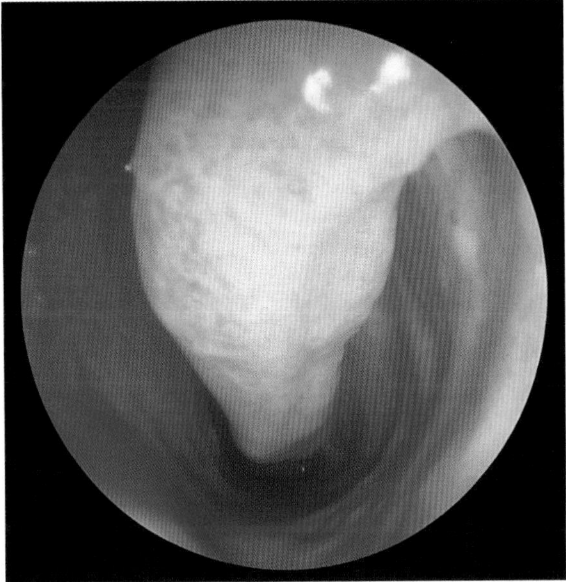

Figure 4.**3** View of the left inferior meatus.
a with a flexible endoscope,

b with a 25° rigid telescope.

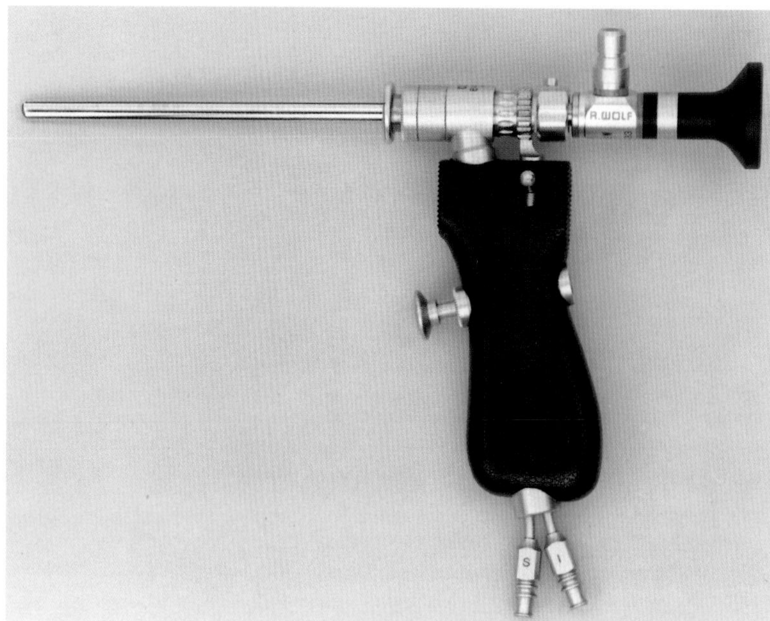

Figure 4.**4** Suction-irrigation handpiece for fitting to various angled telescopes. The author's surgical endoscope for sinus surgery (1981).

Instruments

A wide range of instruments is available for transnasal surgery including fine, slender scalpels, fissure knives, sickle knives, perforators, rasps and punches with varying angles of jaws and shaft (Figure 4.**5**).

Punches and forceps with various curves of the handle are suitable for resection of bony walls. New sharp cutting punches are still being developed to allow removal of tissue with preservation of neighboring viable mucosa. The diamond burr and sharp curettes should be used for removing bone, for example to widen a narrow frontal duct (Figure 4.**6**).

High-frequency diathermy (Figure 4.**7**) has proved suitable for making a bloodless incision through the mucosa and scar tissue. The argon laser (Figure 4.**8**, 4.**9**) is also used because it allows conduction of energy through flexible glass fibers, providing better cutting and coagulation (Wigand 1981). Bipolar coagulation forceps are used to coagulate small arteries and veins.

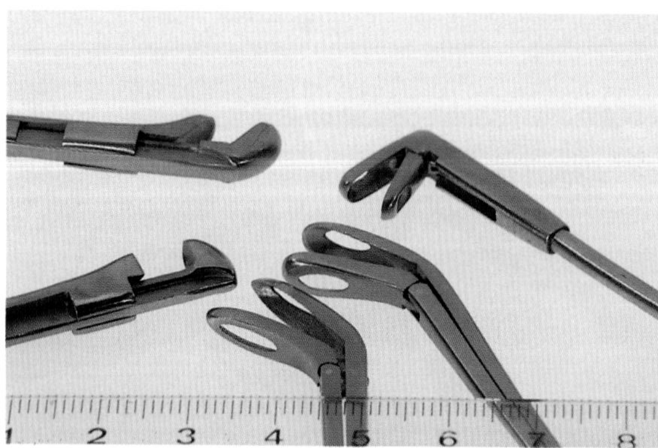

Figure 4.**5** Instruments for endoscopic sinus surgery, showing the jaws of various forceps and punches. From left to right: 45° punch, 90° pointed punch with long jaws, 45° upward-cutting ethmoid forceps, blunt 45° upward-cutting ethmoid forceps, blunt 90° angled ethmoid forceps.

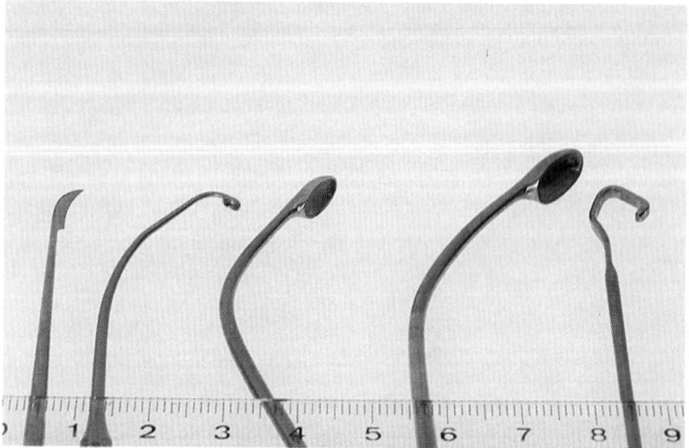

Figure 4.**6** Instruments for endoscopic sinus surgery, from left to right: the sickle knife, curved sharp curettes in several sizes, and on the right a bone hook for removing bony fragments during inferior meatal antrostomy.

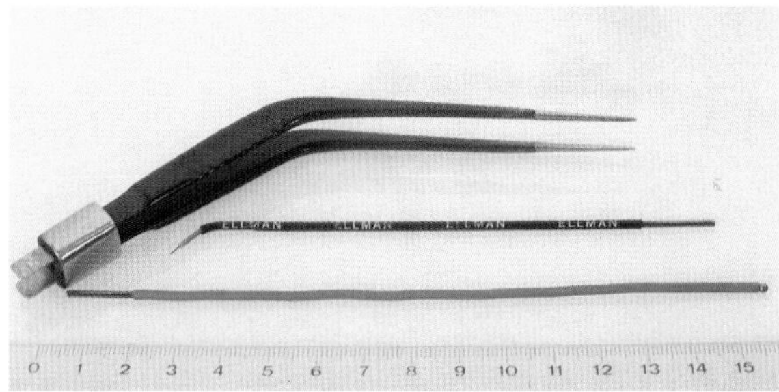

Figure 4.**7** Instruments for endoscopic sinus surgery, from above downwards: forceps with offset handle for intranasal bipolar coagulation, semi-rigid electrode for high-frequency cutting diathermy, and semi-rigid coagulation probes (Ellman, Frankfurt).

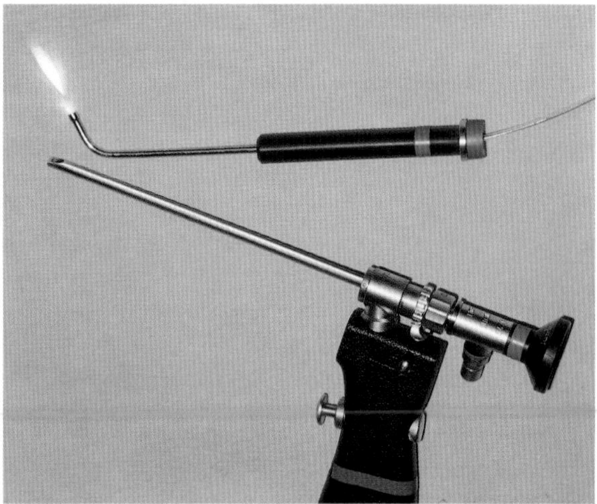

Figure 4.**8** Principle of paraendoscopic argon laser surgery in the sinuses. A flexible cable in a curved tube is shown above, and below the suction-irrigation endoscope for optical monitoring.

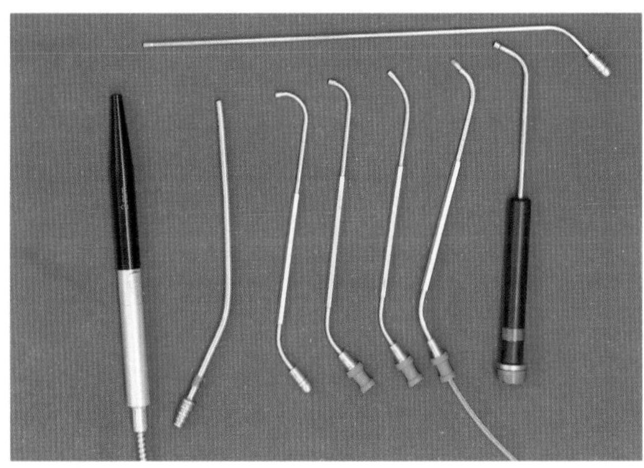

Figure 4.**9** Various curved introduction tubes for attaching flexible fibers for the use of the argon laser in sinus surgery. A straight handpiece is shown on the left, and various straight and hollow probes on the right and above.

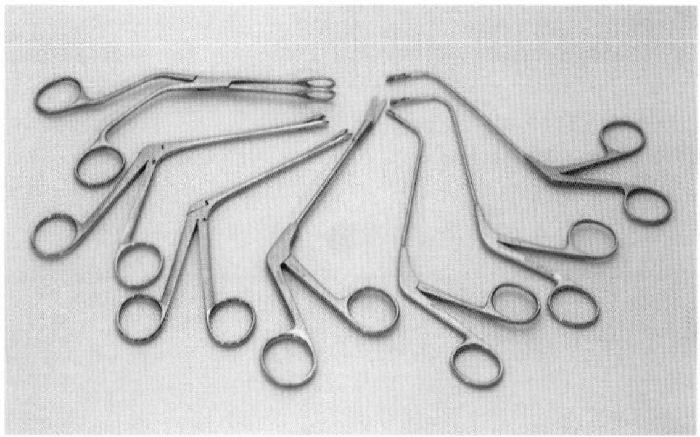

Figure 4.**10** Instruments for endoscopic sinus surgery. From left to right: ring-shaped septal forceps for removing the perpendicular lamina, No. 1 and No. 2 straight Blakesley's ethmoid punch, strong ethmoid scissors with serrated cutting edge, small curved double forceps with perpendicular jaws, small highly curved double forceps with horizontal jaws, curved double forceps with horizontal jaws.

Angled gripping instruments with which one can pack, cut, palpate or displace particular areas of the sinus system are still being developed. The set of instruments shown in Figure 4.**10** is suitable, but does not represent the ideal, final solution. The experienced surgeon will be satisfied with a few slender instruments which lie easily in the hand, and which allow all necessary dissection with continuous practice.

Other Auxiliary Techniques

Other technical accessories can facilitate the course of the operation and the treatment after operation.

The intraoperative control of mucosal bleeding by pledgets soaked in 1/1000 adrenalin solution has proved useful. The appropriate safety measures to prevent side effects must be observed. Superficial oozing from the bone can be controlled by surgical cellulose which is also suitable as a spacer in a narrow gutter.

Silastic sheet is used to splint the nasal septum after septoplasty if pieces of cartilage or bone have been replaced. It is particularly useful in the narrow gap between the middle turbinate and the septum to prevent adhesions in the olfactory cleft, especially after revision surgery. The sheet is stitched on both sides of the septum with two through-and-through sutures (Figure 4.**11**). Larger sheets reaching higher have been inserted into the middle nasal meatus lateral to the middle turbinate to avoid its lateral adherence.

An unsolved problem is the maintenance of patency of narrow connecting passages, for example the frontonasal duct, after the loss of mucosa. The race between epithelialization from the surrounding edges of the mucosa, and the granulation tissue sprouting from the floor of the defect often ends in scar tissue obliteration of the narrow area. Resorbable or non-resorbable plastic tubes as spacers have often proved disappointing: restenosis is frequent even if the tube is left in place for from 6 to 10 weeks.

Biological tissue glue, such as the two-component glue with a fibrin basis (Tissucol), has proved particularly useful for fixing mucosal flaps, for example a rotation flap of the olfactory mucosa used in reconstruction of the olfactory cleft. Also it can be used to prevent oozing.

Commercially available vaseline gauze strips 1 or 2 cm wide are useful for packing the nasal cavity, in layers adapted to the conditions within it. Other authors prefer inflatable tubes or foam. Expansile packing (e. g. Merocel) is attractive to use but can be difficult to remove once it has been in place for more than 2 days. Patients particularly appreciate the introduction of breathing tubes through the nasal packing. These are self made from plastic tubing, for example a feeding tube suitably cut and bent (Figure 4.**12**). It is very important to moisten the tube internally with a silicone spray to prevent blockage by blood clot.

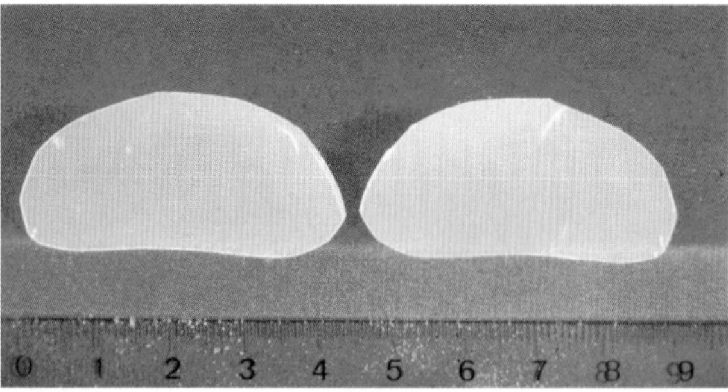

Figure 4.**11** Sheets of X-ray film for splinting both sides of the anterior part of the septum.

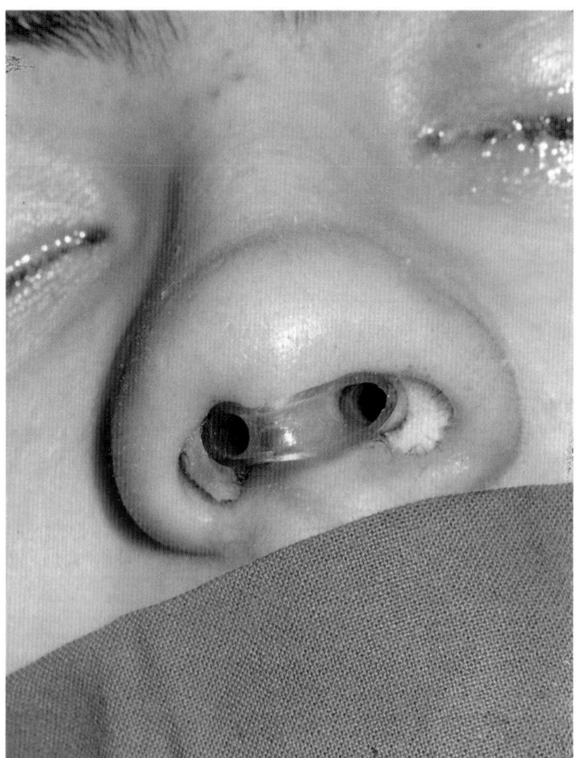

Figure 4.**12** Respiration tubes for introduction through the nasal packing. These are made from a feeding tube, and each side is about 8 cm long.

5. Anesthesia and Position of the Patient

Present-day anesthesiology provides excellent conditions for operations on the paranasal sinuses, either under general or local anesthesia. The techniques available do not obstruct the operative procedure: indeed they facilitate it or even make it possible in the first place. The decision between local or general anesthesia depends on many factors and is discussed with the patient, weighing all the advantages and risks. The author prefers general anesthesia for almost all operations, particularly on account of the necessity to teach in a University clinic, but is also convinced that effective dissection can be carried out under local anesthesia with appropriate precautions. For more extensive procedures on the ethmoid and on the base of the skull, general anesthesia is almost always recommended to spare the patient anxiety, and to prevent swallowing of blood and fluid by the use of a pharyngeal pack.

Local Anesthesia

A suitable anesthetic for *septal correction* is diffuse infiltration of the entire septum with a 1% xylocaine solution with adrenalin 1/200,000: from 5 to 10 ml should suffice. The columella and the mucosa of the premaxilla should be infiltrated to allow the placing of a hemitransfixion stitch and dissection of the base of the septum. Many surgeons are afraid of the possible trauma to the delicate septal mucosa by the pressure of infiltration, and therefore prefer a nerve block (Figure 5.**1**). Infiltration of the lateral wall of the inferior meatus, and submucosal infiltration of the canine fossa suffice for simple *antral operations*.

Additional anesthesia for operations within the antral cavity is achieved by a depot of anesthetic at the lateral edge of the posterior choana directed towards the pterygopalatine fossa (Figure 5.**2**).

Localized operations on the ethmoids such as hiatotomy, infundibulotomy and partial anterior or posterior ethmoidectomy can be done successfully under local anesthesia. Topical anesthesia is suitable using cotton wool carriers or small gauze strips soaked in 1–4% xylocaine or lidocaine placed in the middle and upper meatus after a preliminary spray with a suitable topical anesthetic. Many rhinologists insist on the topical use of cocaine solution.

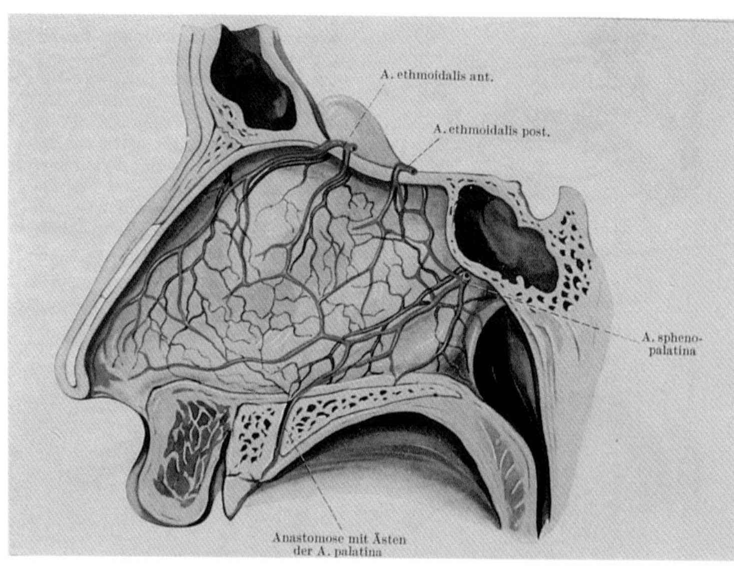

Figure 5.**1** Vascular supply of the nasal septum. The corresponding sensory nerves run with main branches. The posterior septal nerve runs with the septal branch of the sphenopalatine artery (Deneker, H. J., R. Meyer: Plastische Operationen an Kopf und Hals, Springer, Berlin 1964).

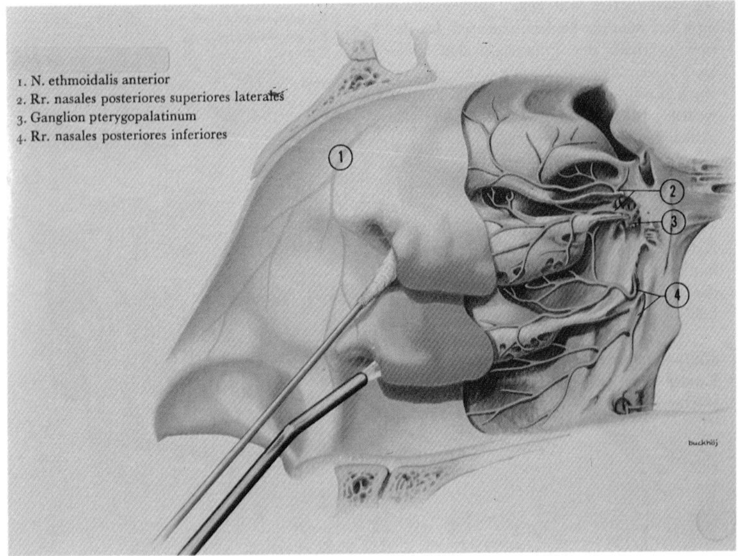

Figure 5.**2** The sensory nerve supply of the lateral nasal wall (Eriksson, E.: Atlas der Lokalanaesthesie, Springer, Berlin 1980).

Additional infiltration with 1% xylocaine plus adrenalin at the pterygopalatine foramen and in the medial canthus at the point of entry of the ethmoidal arteries into their canals to block the anterior and posterior ethmoidal nerves generally provides satisfactory anesthesia of the ethmoid area.

In recent years neuroleptanalgesia has been introduced for operations on the nasal skeleton. It permits any form of exposure, resection, etc., with minimal disturbance to the respiration and circulation, and also allows infiltration or topical application of a local anesthetic containing adrenalin to induce an optimal bloodless field. The current standard procedure in our clinic is as follows:

Anesthesia for Ethmoid Operations using Endotracheal Intubation Anesthesia

M. Brandl

The anesthetic of choice for ethmoid operations is a modified neuroleptanalgesia with fentanyl as an analgesic, and benzodiazepine. If it is likely that the operation will last a long time flunitrazepam is used, whereas for operations forecast to last between 2 and 3 hours midazolam is preferred because of its shorter half-life.

Since correction of the position of the tube during the operation is very difficult, it must be fixed with particular care. Modern tubes made of silicone and rubber with a spiral wire and a high-volume, low-pressure cuff should be used to prevent narrowing due to kinking.

The oropharynx is packed with a moist gauze roll to prevent postoperative vomiting caused by flow of blood into the stomach. In many clinics a nasogastric tube is placed for the same reasons. Since many patients vomit after operation despite this prophylactic measure, the intraoperative sedation with benzodiazapine can be supplemented by butyrophenone derivatives, preferably using 2.5–5 mg dehydrobenzperidol. The moderate alpha-blocking activity of DHBP is furthermore very suitable for preventing hypertonic circulatory response. The incorporation of the above mild dosage does not affect the recovery phase adversely.

If a hypertensive crisis occurs during the operation despite satisfactory analgesia, due either to the high pain intensity during ethmoid operations or to topical hemostasis using pledgets soaked in adrenalin, the first measure is to attempt to compensate the rise of blood pressure by increased concentration of the inhaled anesthetic. Simultaneous tachycardia can be treated by beta-adrenoceptor blockade; hydralazine preparations or urapidil are indicated for hypertension with a normal pulse rate. Hypertensive crises cannot always be prevented by calcium antagonists in high doses, nor by prophylactic calcium antagonists.

Controlled hypotension with nitroglycerine or sodium nitroprusside is only needed in unusual cases. Furthermore, the use of vasodilators does not necessarily achieve a bloodless field (the high-pressure, low-flow technique). Controlled hypotension with marked reduction of the mean arterial blood pressure is not carried out in most patients because of the attendant risks, particularly for geriatric or pregnant patients. It is usually satisfactory to maintain the blood pressure at the lower limit of normal (controlled normotension).

Ethmoid operations last a relatively short time in competent surgical hands, and occasionally can end earlier than expected. Since the anesthetist cannot recognize and assess the stage of the operation, the surgeon should advise him repeatedly of the likely duration of the procedure. This is the only way of guaranteeing extubation in the operating room at the end of the operation without losing time, and without risk to the patient.

Position of the Patient

The author prefers the normal prone position for all operations on the nasal sinuses without particular elevation or lowering of the head. In this way the gaze can alternate rapidly between the roof or floor of the nose, and all instruments can be manipulated by their handgrips without obstruction by the oral endotracheal tube. Elevating the head causes the handgrip to impinge on the anesthetic tube or the chest: conversely, extension of the head impedes vision of the floor of the nose or antrum. Operations with the patient sitting are unsuitable for general anesthesia, but can certainly be considered for relatively brief procedures.

The surgeon stands on the right-hand side of the patient, with the instrument table on the left-hand side of the operating table and the endoscopic accessories to the left of the surgeon, at the head of the table (Figure 5.**3a, b**). This arrangement allows the

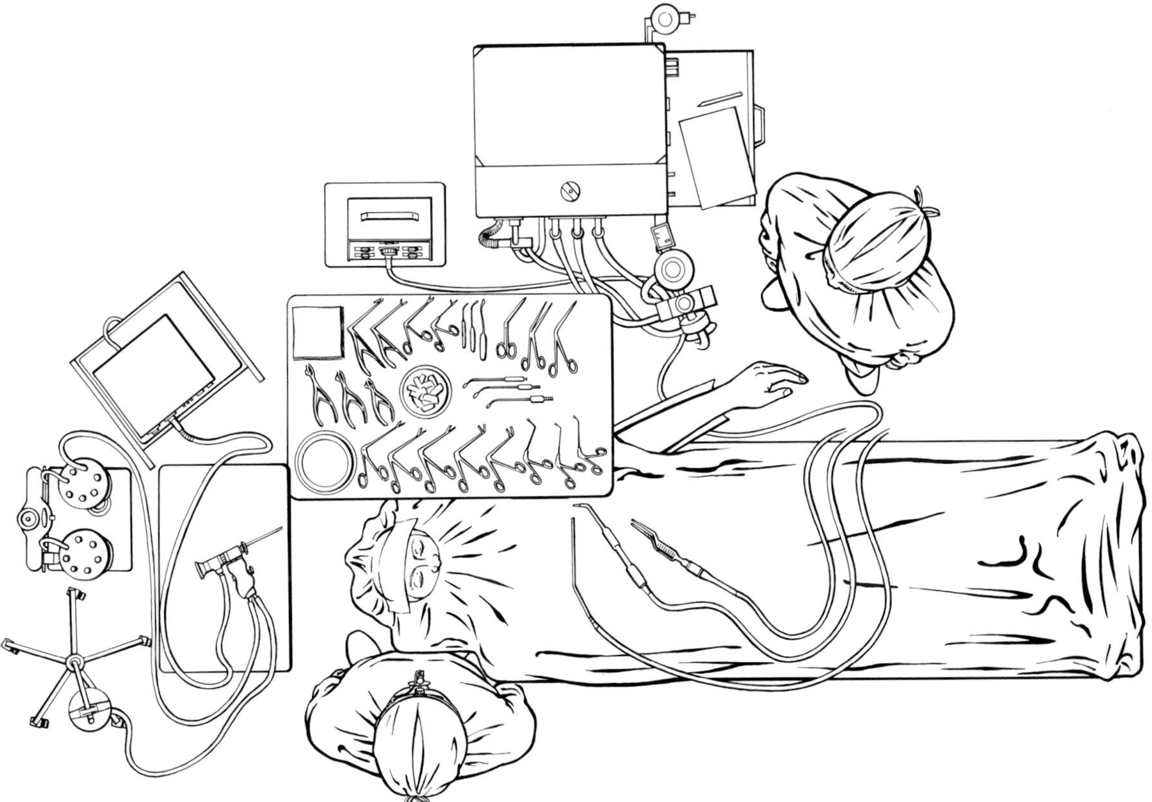

Figure 5.**3** Position of the patient for endoscopic sinus surgery. **a** Plan.

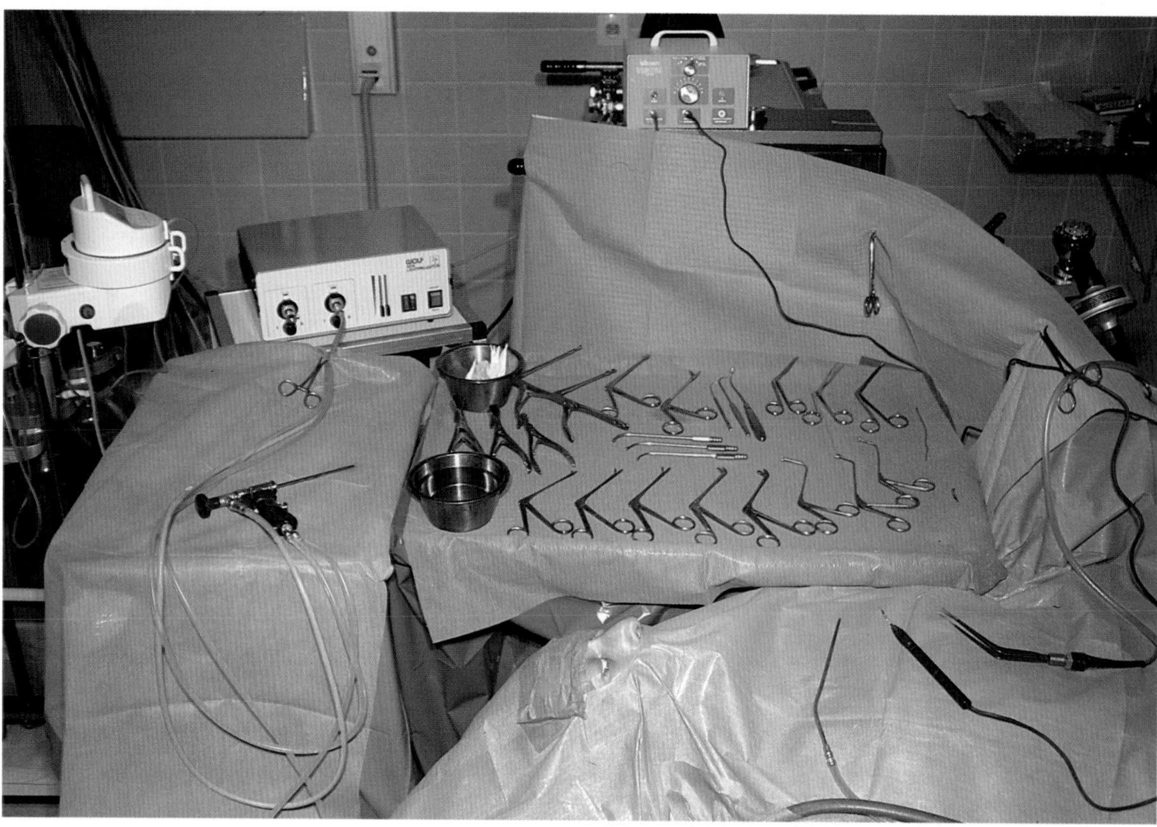

b Instruments arranged facing the surgeon:

suction with a straight nasal sucker;
fine electrocoagulation;
bipolar electrocoagulation forceps;
metal bowl with saline;
metal bowl with adrenalin-soaked pledgets;
nasal specula in three different sizes;
two nasal punches, a backward-cutting punch (Ostrom), scissors,
three different sizes of curved sharp curettes, two turbinectomy scissors and one packing forceps;
three antral suction tubes in different sizes;
five Blakesley's forceps in different sizes;
three various curved double forceps (thin);
irrigation-suction endoscope;
infusion stand with warming apparatus attached and a saline bottle;
suction;
coldlight source;
fine electrocoagulation;
anesthetic apparatus.

surgeon to choose an instrument quickly, and dispenses with the need for a scrub nurse. She can be replaced by a visitor or assistant who stands on the right-hand side of the surgeon, and can then follow the operation and participate in the endoscopy. This position of the patient and the instrument table requires the cooperation of the anesthetist who must understand the special working conditions of the rhinologist, and the need to lead the anesthetic tubing to the foot of the patient rather than place it in the usual position.

6. Operations

Operations in the Nasal Cavity

Septoplasty

In many cases correction of the nasal septum is a prerequisite for good exposure, for safe operating conditions, and for the creation of an ideal shape for the nasal cavity. Furthermore, it is often indicated on its own merits to improve ventilation of the chronically inflamed mucosa. The treatment plan should therefore include mobilization and straightening of the septum.

Septal resection as described by Killian with destruction of cartilage should be abandoned because it robs the septum quite unnecessarily of its support, and does not improve the function of the upper segment that is so important in the physiology of the airstream. It has been replaced by the cartilage-sparing technique originally described by Cottle. The method can naturally be modified in the individual case, and the following personal method is only one of many variations (Wigand 1978).

Firstly, a hemitransfixion incision is made along the edge of the septal cartilage in the left or right nasal vestibule at the mucocutaneous junction (Figure 6.**1**). Cutting diathermy is particularly suitable for this incision. The perichondrium is completely elevated through this incision down to the floor of the nose on both sides using a semi-sharp elevator. This dissection is continued under vision posteriorly and inferiorly over the junction of cartilage and bone. Tunneling is unnecessary if the surgeon has learned to release the inrolled edge of the quadrilateral cartilage from the premaxilla by sharp dissection (Figure 6.**2**), and to free it completely from the base of the septum posteriorly over the vomer (an area described by Masing as the septal pouch) (Figure 6.**3**).

The anterior edge of the bony perpendicular plate of the ethmoid is now demonstrated by dividing the junction of bone and cartilage. After exposing the perpendicular plate on both sides it is divided above and below with a sagittal chisel cut (Figure 6.**4**), elevated from the sphenoid and the vomer using a special punch with large blades, and removed in one piece (Figure 6.**5**). It is then straightened, narrowed if necessary, and preserved until the end of the operation in saline solution.

The perpendicular plate is only replaced after straightening of the septum, partial resection of the triangular block of the vomer (Figure 6.**6**), removal of projecting pieces of cartilage and chiseling off the obstructing ridge projecting laterally from the premaxilla and the palatal ridge. It is wedged, glued or stabilized by splints of silastic sheeting. Good end-to-end adaptation to the posterior edge of the quadrilateral cartilage should be achieved. The last step of septal correction should be left until the endoscopic

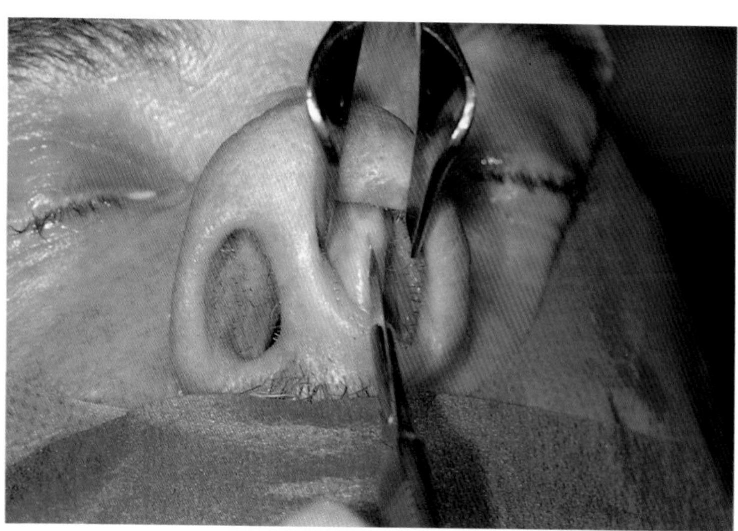

Figure 6.**1** Hemitransfixion incision in the left nasal vestibule over the entire length of the inferior edge of the septum.

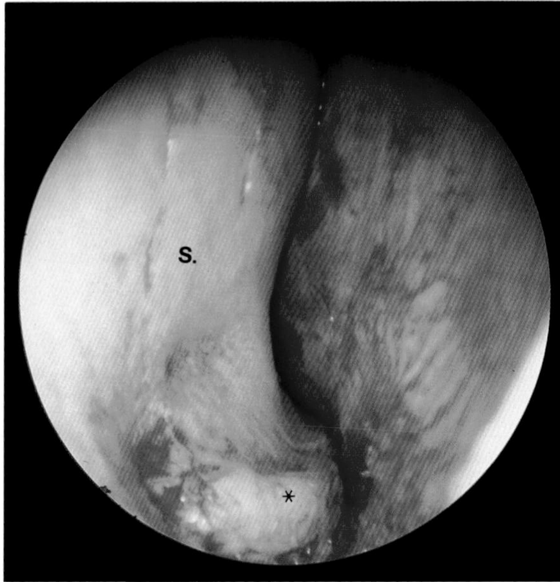

Figure 6.**2** Dissection of the bone-cartilage junction over the premaxilla after complete exposure of the septum. The septal mucosa with the perichondrium can be seen from inside on the right. Excess cartilage forms a spur on the floor (*).

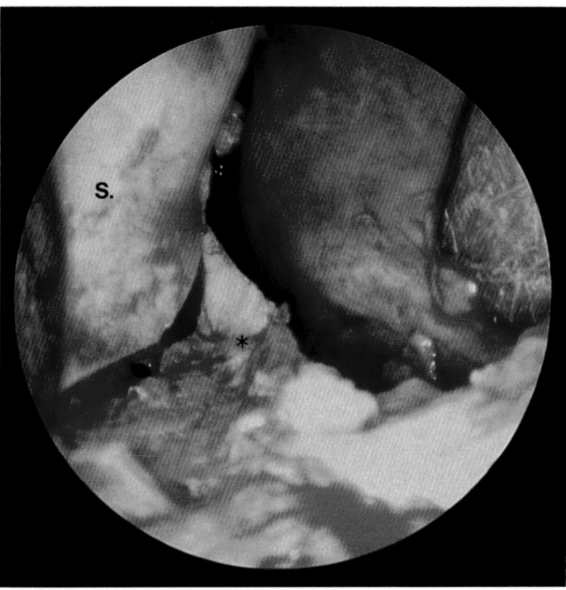

Figure 6.**3** The premaxilla (*) seen from above before it is narrowed. The septal mucosa is freed on both sides form the edges of the bone down to the floor of the nose. Excess cartilage is resected.

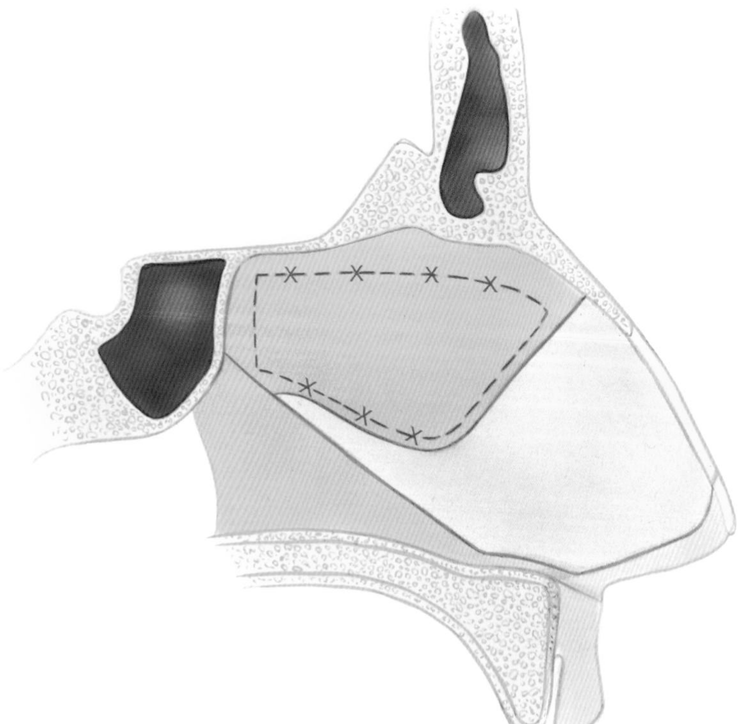

Figure 6.**4** Diagram of freeing of the perpendicular plate. The upper and lower chisel cuts (x–x) are shown that allow the plate to be removed in one piece. View from right.

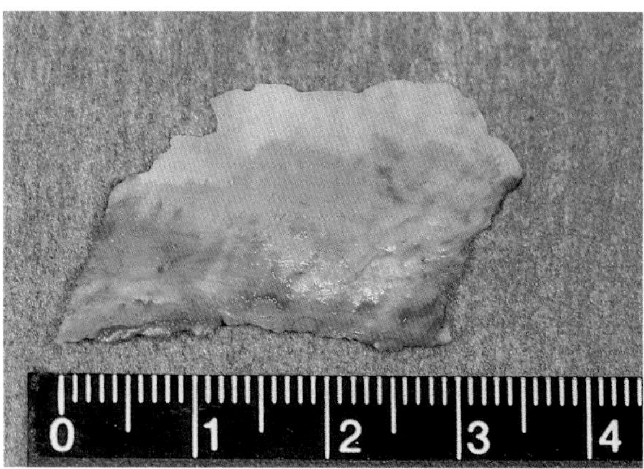

Figure 6.5 A piece of the perpendicular plate of the septum that has been removed. It is reimplanted after being straightened at the end of the operation.

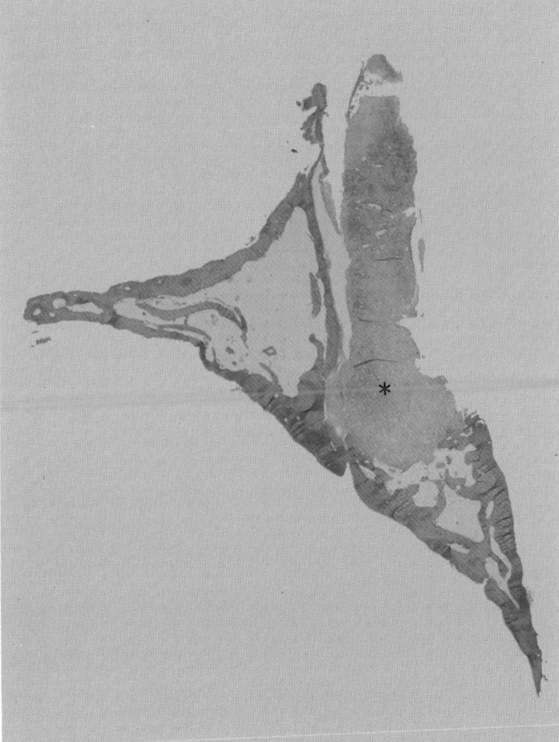

Figure 6.6 Histological transverse section of the triangular block of vomer with the inferior edge of the quadrilateral cartilage (*) inserting into it (elastic-van Gieson 4×).

sinus procedure is finished to take full advantage of the septal mobility.

The last step of the septal procedure is the vestibular stitch, a special stitch (Figure 6.**7**) that not only adapts the wound edges but also rotates the quadrilateral cartilage in an anterosuperior direction. The cartilaginous septum thus regains its previous tension with respect to the nasal dorsum which it often loses after removal ot the perpendicular plate. The cartilage is held in its original position by the rotation suture, and sinking of the weak triangle is prevented. Posterior rotation of the quadrilateral cartilage is much more often the cause of saddling of the nasal dorsum than resection of cartilage at the lower border. In addition to the cartilaginous rotation suture, two further deep interrupted sutures are placed through the wound edges to close the hemitransfixion incision securely. Additional use of fibrin glue may be helpful both in the case of damage to the mucosa and for replantation of bone or cartilage. An adhesive is not usually needed.

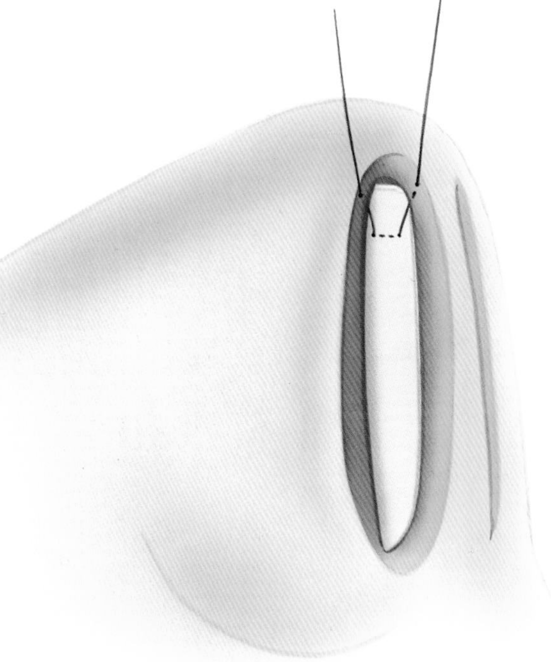

Figure 6.7 Diagram of a cartilaginous rotation suture for closure of a right side hemitransfixion incision. A firm knot rotates the loosened quadrilateral plate superiorly into its original position in the nasal columella.

Turbinectomy

The various indications and techniques for narrowing the nasal turbinates, particularly the inferior, do not need to be considered here. However, many ethmoid operations demand reduction of the inferior or middle turbinate, particularly if the nasal airway must be improved, or the surgical field must be extended to give a good view and allow instrumentation for the treatment of sinusitis.

The best procedure for reduction of the inferior turbinate is submucosal resection of the length of the turbinate bone using Legler's method after using a cutting snare to remove a hyperplastic posterior end of the turbinate. This technique preserves the mucosa and can be individually modified. However, it is often essential to resect the excessively hypertrophic turbinate itself. In these cases longitudinal resection with cutting diathermy could be considered. In the author's experience a strip turbinectomy with the long nasal scissors applied along the free lobular edge of the inferior turbinate has proved useful, although crusting and bleeding from the wound edges in the initial postoperative phase, and pain during postoperative treatment, are quite common. The open wound edge can be treated with caustic or fibrin glue.

The middle turbinate may also require limited resection if its anterior end is polypoid and blocking access to the middle nasal meatus or the olfactory cleft (Figure 6.**8**). In this case conservative removal of the excess tissue with the curved nasal scissors, or diathermy is indicated. The tissue removed must be subjected to histology to show whether the lesion was a polyp rich in glands (Figure 6.**9**), a papilloma or some other tumor. If a voluminous bullous turbinate obstructs the middle meatus, thinning by longitudinal splitting is suitable (see Figure 6.**58**).

Posterior partial resection of the middle turbinate is often necessary during complete ethmoidectomy because the body of the middle turbinate blocks access to the posterosuperior ethmoid cells. This can easily be dealt with by a curved scissors (see

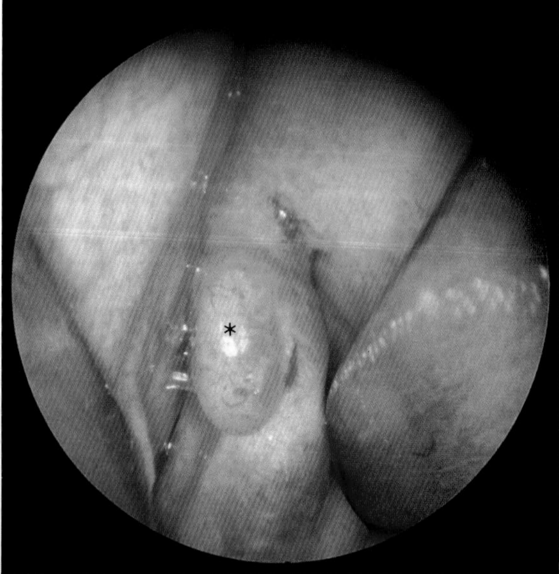

Figure 6.**8** Soft polyp hanging from the head of the middle turbinate.

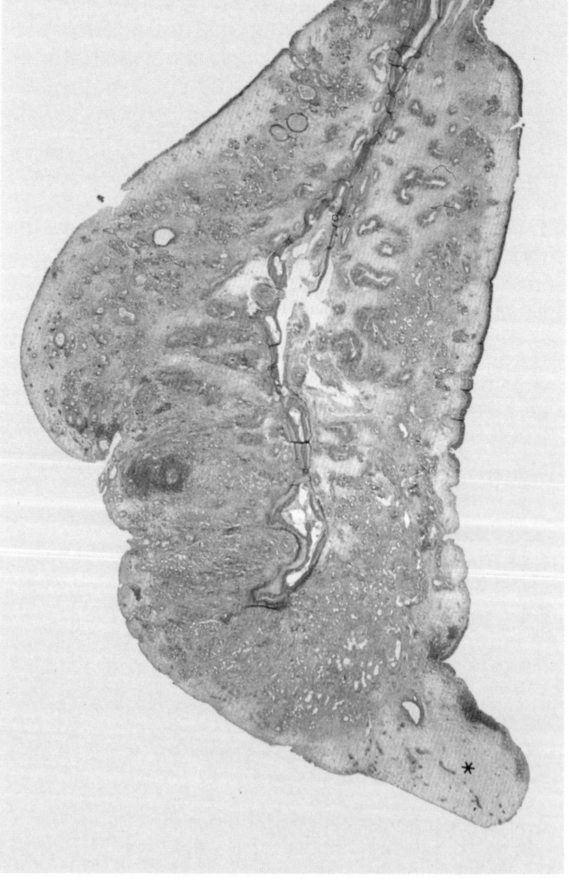

Figure 6.**9** Histology of the soft polyp (*) shown in Figure 6.**8** showing pseudo-erectile tissue rich in glands and vessels (elastic-van Gieson 3×).

Figure 6.**48**); the mobilized part of the turbinate is removed with a forceps or punch. For many years the place of partial or sub-total resection of the middle turbinate has been controversial, but wide experience has shown that these operations carry no ill effects, in particular ozena due to drying of the nasal mucosa by excessive volume of air. However, no more of the turbinate should be removed than is necessary because superiorly it carries olfactory fibers, and its medial lamina contributes decisively to the structure of the olfactory cleft.

Biopsy and Tumor Removal

Biopsies can be taken for histology, and localized areas of tissue can be removed very precisely using the endoscope. A self-retaining speculum and the operating microscope may be useful for dissection in the nasal introitus and the anterior third of the nose, for example, for precise excision of papillomas from the nasal vestibule. However, the surgical endoscope comes into its own for manipulations in the posterior third of the nasal cavity. The endoscope is also a great help in transnasal biopsy of the nasopharynx. In most cases, local anesthesia suffices, but general anesthesia with packing of the pharynx may be more comfortable for both patient and surgeon if severe bleeding is to be expected, for example after a punch biopsy of a nasopharyngeal angiofibroma or if anatomical narrowing makes access for the biopsy forceps difficult. The high-frequency diathermy needle with a slender grip and interchangeable hooks, loops, etc. (see Figure 4.**7**), has proved invaluable for bloodless removal of tissue specimens, and for dividing adhesions.

Intranasal endoscopic surgery for tumors may be successful, depending on the site, extent and pathology of the lesion, and it may also be used as a palliative partial resection or for complete excision with a healthy margin. Lesions with a narrow base or those confined to one turbinate are particularly suitable for complete removal. The endoscopic findings must be supplemented by tomography in most cases, to exclude extension beyond the nasal cavity, and invasion of the skull base. Preferably the tumor should have been shown to be benign by previous biopsy. The technique is determined by circumstances: lesions with a soft pedicle can be removed with the cutting snare, but broad-based sessile lesions require excision, possibly with division of their bony base by the chisel, and if necessary resection of the turbinate. Bulky benign lesions can be removed piecemeal by the punch forceps under endoscopic control. The base should be removed by drilling the underlying bone with a diamond burr. This method is particularly suitable for the treatment of circumscribed inverted papillomas, as personal experience extending over many years has shown.

Intranasal excision of a malignant tumor confined to the nasal cavity, under endoscopic control, can be practiced with success, after preoperative CT scan for careful assessment of the extent of the lesion (Figure 6.**10**). However, this procedure is only justified for very small lesions whose complete extent is within the vision of the endoscope. The treatment plan must include histological assessment of specimens taken from the apparently healthy margin of the wound, vigourous drilling of the underlying bone and continuous close endoscopic follow-up. Under these circumstances, intranasal surgery for small malignant tumors may be justified for frail patients who are unwilling to undergo an operation producing a scar on the face, or for patients in poor condition.

Endoscopic Use of the Laser

Division of a choanal atresia in the newborn and infants using the operating microscope and a carbon dioxide laser has proven to be very valuable. It is simple, but application of the beam to the correct point can be obstructed by the turbinates or septal spurs. The nasopharynx should be protected before beginning coagulation. The technique and the aftercare will not be discussed at this point.

The carbon dioxide laser can be controlled carefully under the operating microscope but can be directed upon only part of the nasal mucosa because the beam is directed forwards. For this reason the argon or the Nd:YAG laser are useful in the angular nasal cavity. In the latter case the laser beam can be conducted around corners by a flexible cable (see Figure 4.**8**) directly to the target using special curved hollow probes, and its action monitored by the irrigating-suction endoscope. The laser is the treatment of choice for coagulation of bleeding lesions, such as hereditary telangiectasia, and for the localized cautery of a hypertrophic inferior or middle turbinate.

If the laser is used for coagulation or excision of tissue with a cartilaginous framework such as the septum or the nasal ala the inevitable spread of heat can lead to chondronecrosis.

Removal of Foreign Bodies

Small foreign bodies such as pieces of paper, parts of plastic toys or pellets, may impact in the nasal airways and be difficult to remove without injuring the mucosa, turbinates or septum. The exact position of the foreign body, and the precise application of the instruments can be monitored endoscopically. Endoscopy is of particular value for removal of foreign bodies and particles of ointment from the antral cavity after antrostomy, and has proved particularly useful for identifying and removing remnants of foam or gauze packing hidden in a newly created antrostomy.

Operations on the Maxillary Antrum

Indications

- recurrent acute inflammations and empyema of the maxillary sinus,
- chronic maxillary sinusitis,
- as one of the procedures for pansinusitis,
- complications of inflammatory disease,
- foreign bodies and trauma,
- biopsy and drainage of tumors.

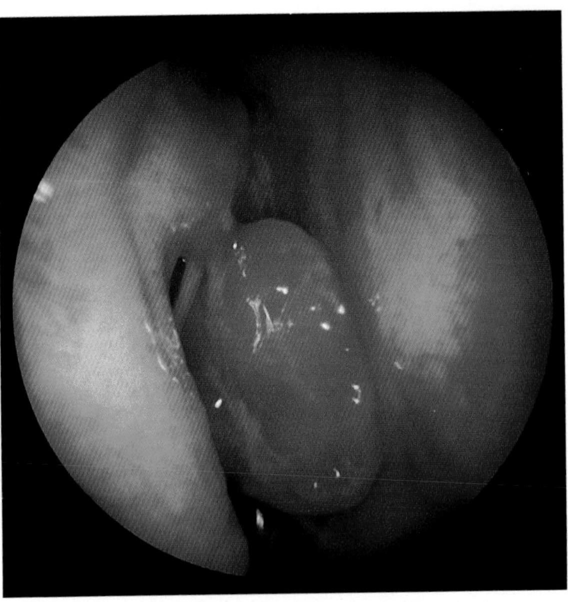

Figure 6.**10** Circumscribed hemangiopericytoma of the head of the middle turbinate. The histological diagnosis was provided by the Pathological Institute of the University of Erlangen-Nuremberg.

Principles

The purpose of the operation is to create a unilocular antral cavity, lined by mucosa, with secure ventilation and drainage through a permanent outflow to the middle and/or the inferior meatus. Mucosa should be preserved as much as possible to encourage mucosal regeneration, and to prevent the formation of scar tissue, so that only gross disease should be removed. A middle meatal antrostomy is preferred to an inferior meatal antrostomy. Correct manipulation of the instruments prevents perforation of the orbit. Endoscopic control with an angled telescope is mandatory, and care should be exercised during curettage because of the danger of injury to the tooth buds and to the infraorbital nerve.

Operative Technique

Intranasal antral procedures can be divided into two phases: (1) antrostomy, (2) intracavitary manipulation. Often the latter is unnecessary, and antrostomy is then the sole purpose of the procedure. Revision operations after a previous intranasal or transoral (Caldwell-Luc) operation are more difficult, demanding a partly intranasal and a partly transoral procedure via the canine fossa.

Inferior Meatal Antrostomy

Topical anesthesia with 4% xylocaine, infiltration with xylocaine 1%, and vasoconstriction of the mucosa of the inferior meatus using pledgets soaked in 1/1000 adrenalin are all worthwhile. The inferior meatus is brought into view by elevating the constricted inferior turbinate and displacing it medially using Killian's speculum (Figure 6.**11a, b**). The medial wall of the antrum is perforated with a semi-sharp elevator or chisel at the point where the bony wall is thinnest, about 8 mm behind the anterior insertion of the inferior turbinate and about 5 mm above the floor of the nose (Figure 6.**12**). The thin bone behind the perforation is pushed into the meatus by medially directed pressure. The posterior half of the antrostomy is punched out using Blakesley's semi-sharp nasal punch (size 2 or 3) or a conchotome (Figure 6.**13**), using the sharpest cut possible to prevent laceration of both the nasal and antral mucosa. Blunt avulsion of fragments of bone often strips the neighboring mucosa from the bone, leading to necrosis and abnormal ciliary transport. The anterior part of the antrostomy is now created using acute-angled forceps or punches such as Ostrom's

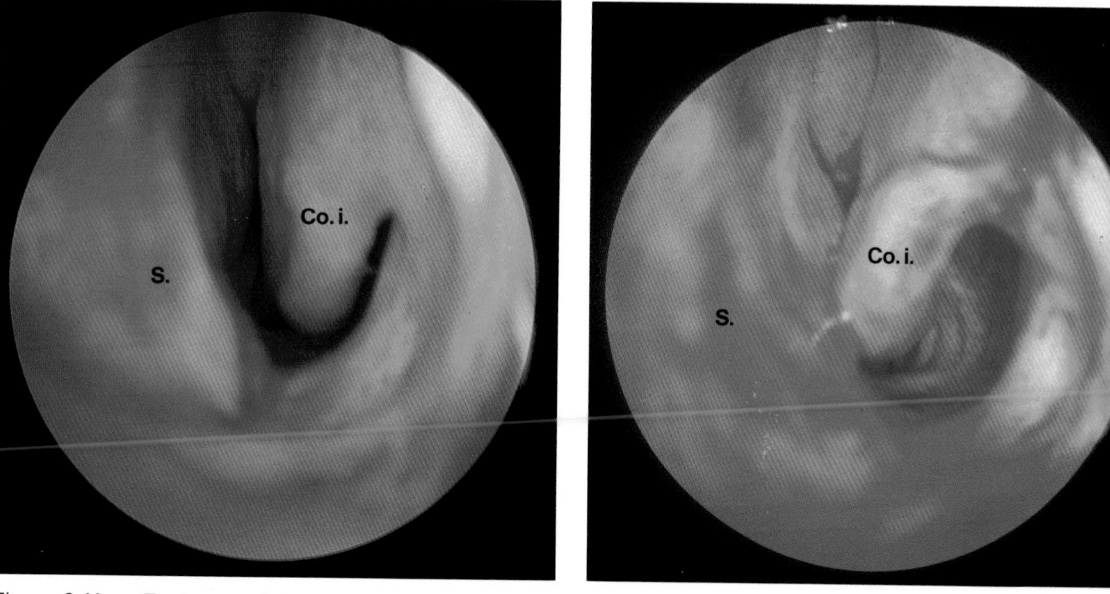

Figure 6.**11** **a** Exposure of the left inferior meatus originally covered by the left inferior turbinate. **b** A good view after medial displacement of the inferior turbinate.

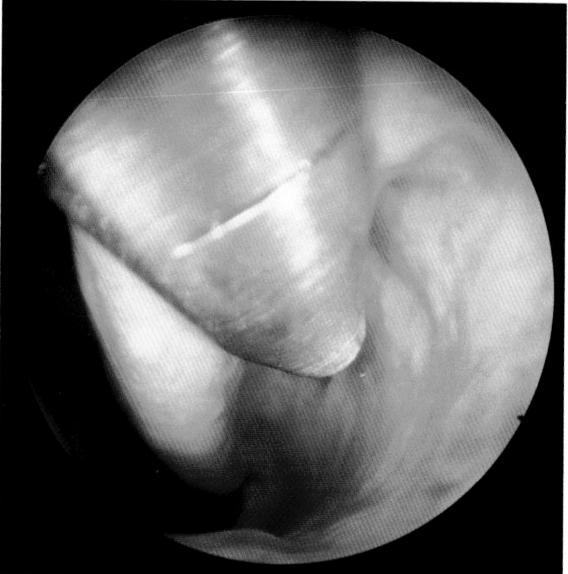

Figure 6.**12** Inferior meatal antrostomy on the left side. The elevator marks the point of perforation. The slit formed by the ostium of the lacrimal duct in front and above can be well seen. Care must be exercised when using the punch in this direction.

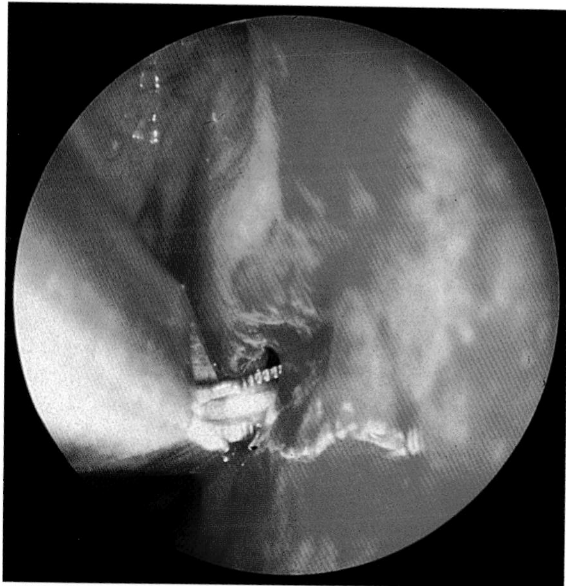

Figure 6.**13** Inferior meatal antrostomy on the left side. A small window is formed by breaking through the posterior edge of the perforation which is then enlarged by a punch (25° telescope).

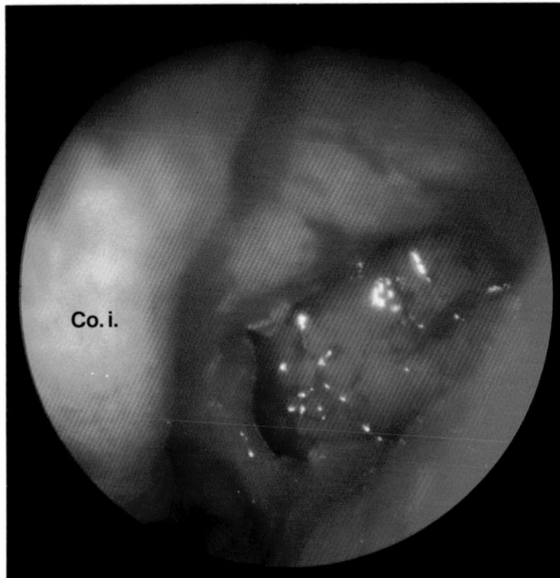

Figure 6.**14** Inferior meatal antrostomy extended posteriorly and anteriorly (25° telescope).

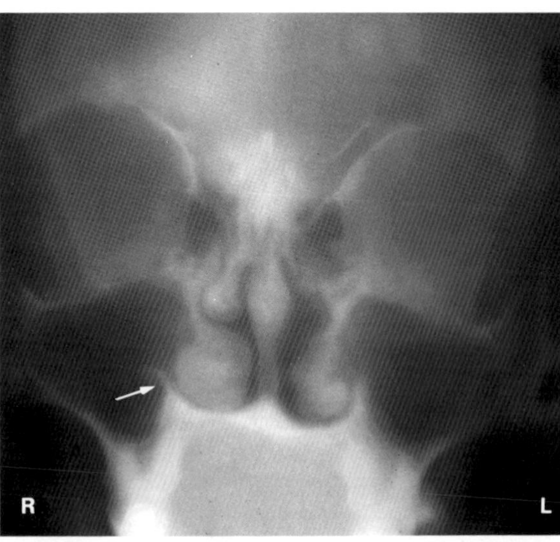

Figure 6.**15** Incorrect inferior meatal antrostomy on the right side causing postoperative pain over the maxilla. A plate of bone marked with an arrow projects into the antrum, and the lower edge of the antrostomy is too high.

(Figures 6.**13** and 6.**14**). A specially curved bone hook is available for levering out pieces of bone which have been pushed into the cavity (see instrumentation in Chapter 4). Pieces of bone displaced into the antrum may cause neuralgia and continuing secretion, probably due to disturbance of the mucociliary self-cleaning mechanism (Figure 6.**15**).

The antrostomy should have vertical and horizontal diameters of at least 8 × 10 mm, since it has a marked tendency to contract or even become obliterated, and its edges should be smooth. Lining of the antrostomy by eversed antral mucosa is recommendable. Removal of the covering bone, three radial incisions of the adjacent mucosa, and eversion of the latter into the nasal meatus are the steps necessary in this technique. The upper edge of the new window should not reach as far as the insertion of the inferior turbinate, otherwise scar tissue retraction pulls the inferior turbinate into the antrostomy, particularly if a turbinectomy is performed at the same time. The lacrimal canal must not be damaged during punching out of the anterior edge of the antrostomy because scar tissue can obstruct the duct, leading to permanent epiphora. Spacers, for example that described by Bumm, may be useful for maintaining the patency of the antrostomy.

Middle Meatal Antrostomy

An antrostomy should preferably be created at the point where nature has decreed that the short canal from the antral cavity opens, where secondary ostia are more often found, and where the physiological transport pathways draining the antral mucosa end.

The simplest procedure is to enlarge the natural ostium, particularly the secondary ostium in the fontanelle (Buiter's fontanellotomy). A very limited resection of the medial antral wall can be done beneath the semilunar hiatus under endoscopic control (Figure 6.**16**).

However, the need to manipulate instruments within the antral cavity usually demands the creation of a larger window. Personal experience with several hundred middle meatal antrostomies, and Hosemann's photographic studies (1985), show that even large defects of the centre of the antral wall above the inferior turbinate do not interfere with the drainage of the secretions and particles. Depending on the presence of polyps, or on the need for freedom of movement for instruments within the antral cavity, the author creates a modest sized (8–10 mm) or sub-total window in the middle meatus. The details of endoscopic anatomy determine which structures are sacrificed, but the window should be made as small as possible to avoid unnecessary disturbance of the natural transport pathways. Whether the creation of a window at any site other than the natural ostium can be challenged on basic principles, as indicated by Hilding's experiments, has so far not been

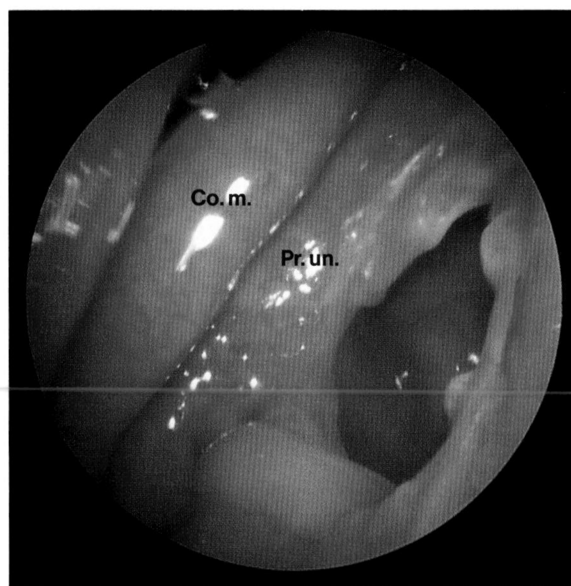

Figure 6.**16** Small middle meatal antrostomy beneath the uncinate process 4 weeks after operation. A stream of mucus draining from the antral cavity, and marginal granulations can be seen.

determined scientifically. The 45° upward-cutting pointed ethmoid punch is suitable for opening the antral cavity: the author has designed his own model with prolonged jaws. Correct control of the instruments is vital to ensure the security of the contents of the orbit: the closed pointed punch (or the half-open punch in the hands of an experienced surgeon) is placed on the dorsum of the middle turbinate about halfway along its long axis. This is followed by a controlled forward thrust, directed in a strictly horizontal plane (Figure 6.**17a, b**). As the frontal sections in Chapter 2 show, the orbital wall can never be perforated in this direction of thrust. If perforation can be achieved under endoscopic vision, then the opening is usually created through the posterior fontanelle (Buiter and Straatman 1981) at the point where the semilunar hiatus expands between the edge of the bulla and the uncinate process, and where the medial antral wall is membranous.

If the half-opened punch has been used, closure of the forceps achieves the first limited resection (Figure 6.**18**), and the antral cavity can be inspected

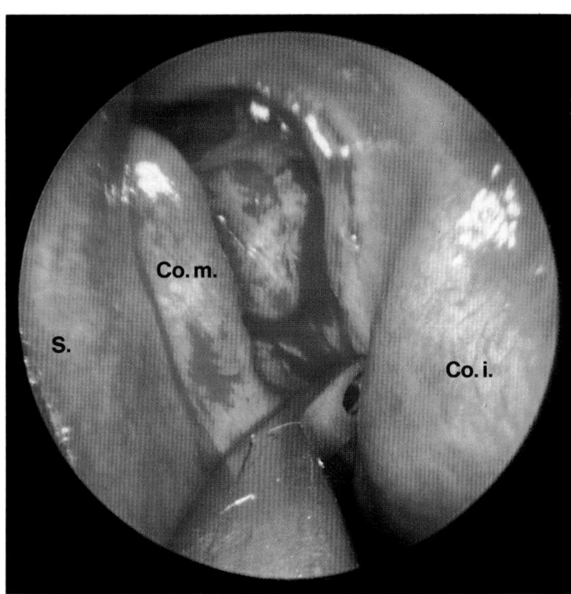

Figure 6.**17** Middle meatal antrostomy. **a** A 45° angled ethmoidal forceps is applied immediately above the inferior turbinate. The jaws must penetrate in a horizontal direction. Blood appears from the middle meatus after the removal of polyps (25° telescope).

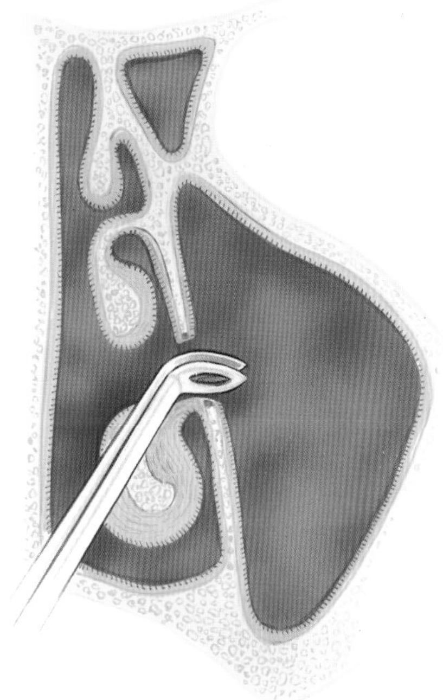

b Diagram of safe middle meatal antrostomy.

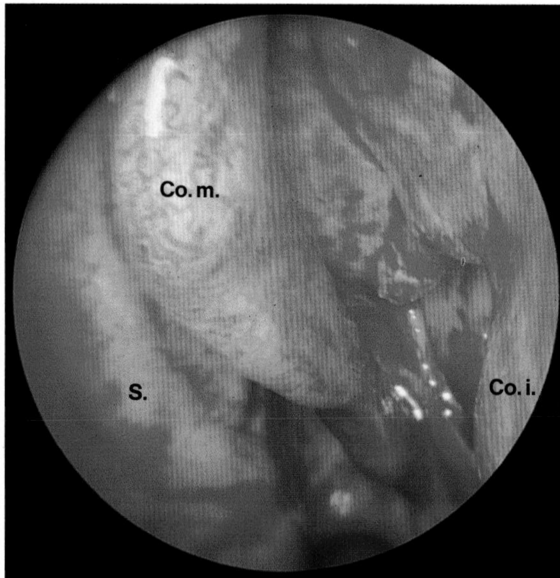

Figure 6.**18** Newly created, still small supraturbinal nasoantrostomy. The view is limited by the inferior and middle turbinate (25° telescope).

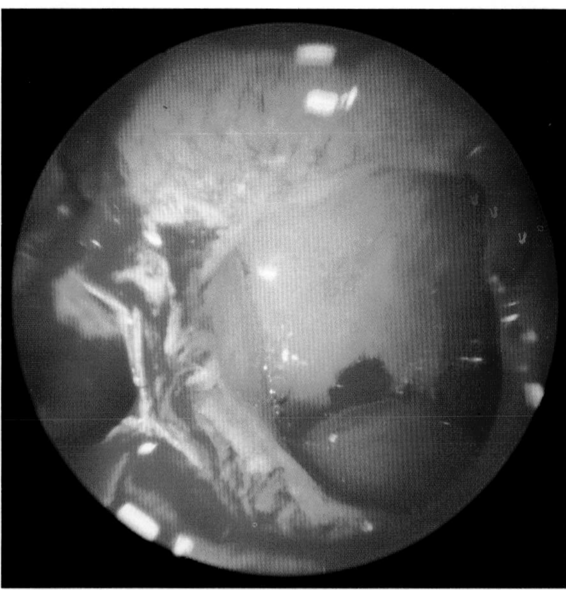

Figure 6.**19** Fresh, large, middle meatal antrostomy with a view of an inferior cyst (70° telescope).

through this opening using an angled telescope. Generous resection of the medial antral wall to create a defect 8 mm high and 10 mm wide is needed for extensive intracavitary manipulations, and to create a permanently open window (Figure 6.**19**). Ostrom's backward-cutting punch is particularly valuable for this step.

If the lower edge of the antrostomy lies far inferiorly on account of individual circumstances such as polyps or the necessity to manipulate instruments, the inferior meatus can easily be opened lateral to the body of the turbinate, but this does not usually have any ill effects. Posteriorly and above, the party wall is best removed with a cutting conchotome or the straight Blakesley's forceps, and in complete antro-ethmoidal operations this can be continued to its upper edge (see below). Endoscopic checking and smoothing of the rim of the antrostomy is important after every procedure. Brisk bleeding from the posterior edge of the window can be controlled by bipolar coagulation or compression with pledgets soaked in adrenalin.

The author has recently stopped simple excision of a large antrostomy but tries to dissect the lateral nasal wall: while the nasal mucosa and the underlying bone are removed, the antral mucosa is radially incised and eversed into the middle nasal meatus (eversion technique). This maneuver is to enhance mucociliary transport into the nose.

Operations within the Maxillary Cavity

Whereas an intranasal antrostomy can be carried out at least partially under direct vision, manipulations within the antrum itself must always be performed using an angled telescope. Blind operations do not achieve the goal of the operation, endanger important structures and must be avoided. Almost all procedures can be undertaken either through an inferior or a middle meatal antrostomy. If the field of vision is inadequate a better view can be gained by using an endoscope introduced through an anterior, canine fossa, antrostomy. All experienced surgeons agree that the degree of freedom when using small gripping instruments passed through the endoscope is very limited, whereas all situations can be tackled with instruments, suction, laser, etc., passed *alongside* the endoscope (para-endoscopic surgery) (Figure 6.**20**).

Figures 6.**21** and 6.**22** show examples of the removal of polyps and cysts under endoscopic control. Orientation in space and accurate identification of the target always have precedence. Only grossly abnormal lesions which appear to be irreversible should be removed, whereas hyperplasia, edematous swellings, etc. (Figure 6.**23**), which are capable of resolution should be given the chance to do so. Sadly there are no macro- or even microscopic mucosal characteristics on which to base the decision, so that mucosa should be preserved as far as possible. It is very easy to elevate or tear healthy mucosa with unsuitable instruments, leading to worsening of the situa-

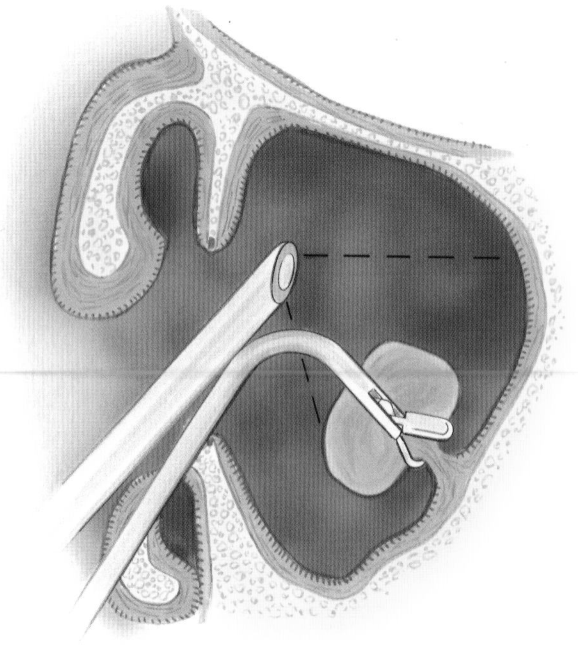

Figure 6.**20** Diagram of the principle of para-endoscopic instrumentation in the antral cavity.

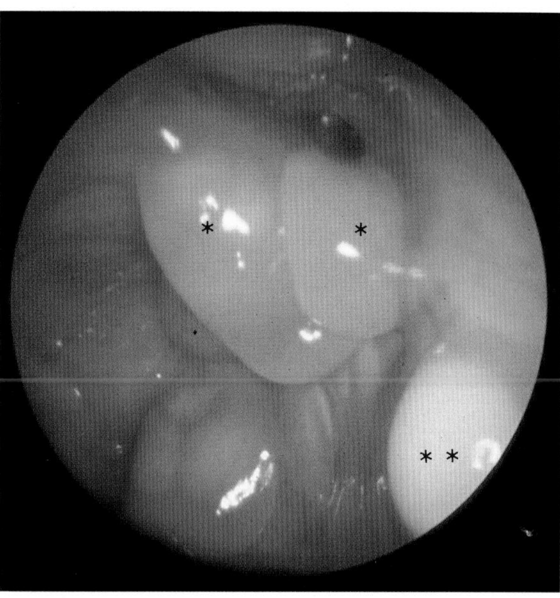

Figure 6.**21** Polyp (*) and retention cyst (**) in the left antral cavity seen through a middle meatal antrostomy, looking towards the zygomatic recess (70° telescope).

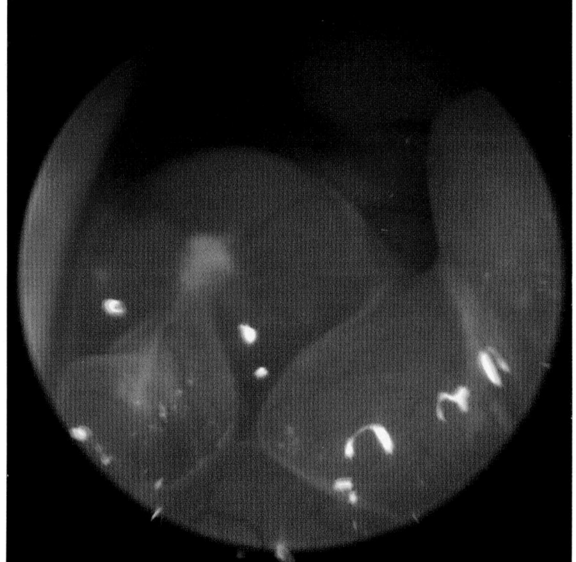

Figure 6.**22** Large edematous polyp of the left antrum after middle meatal antrostomy (70° telescope).

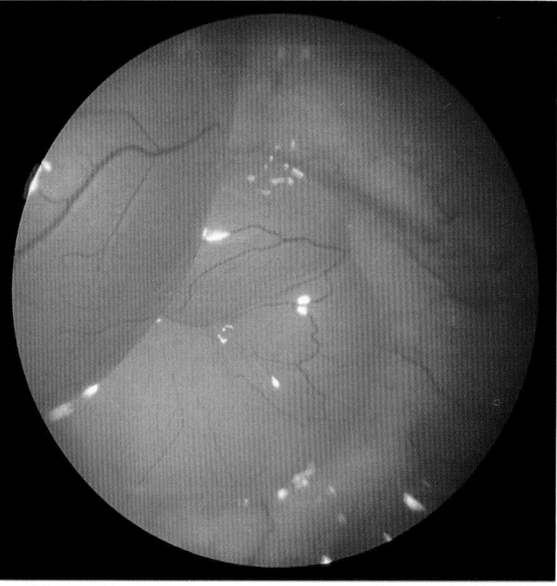

Figure 6.**23** Edematous mucosa on the posterior and anterior wall of an antrum not requiring removal (middle meatal antrostomy, 70° telescope).

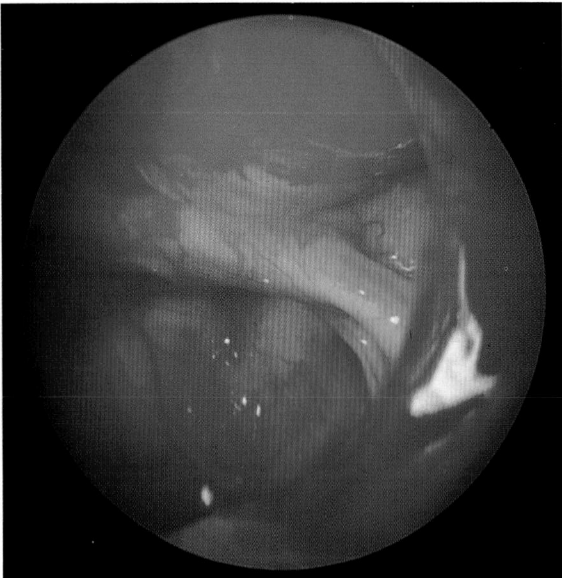

Figure 6.**24** Infraorbital nerve hanging from the roof of the left antrum. It is particularly in danger shortly before its entry into the anterior wall of the antrum (70° telescope).

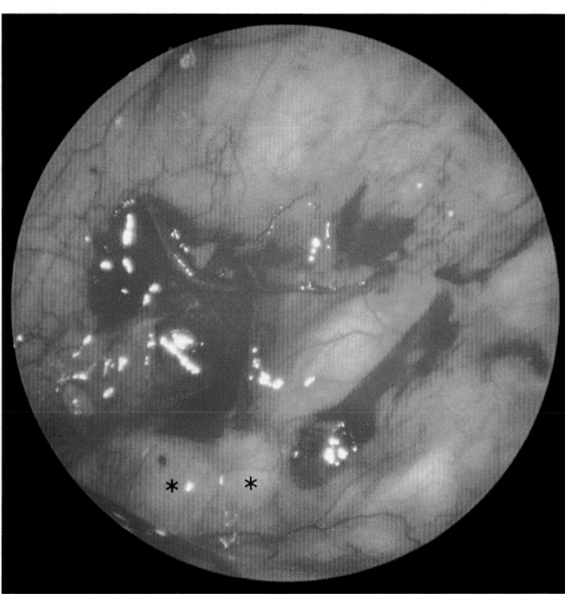

Figure 6.**25** Projecting paper-thin bony sockets of the molar teeth (*) in the floor of the alveolar recess of the right antrum. Middle meatal antrostomy (70° telescope).

tion. At the moment, it is not clear whether non-touch laser surgery or electrocautery will be of a greater help in this area. Mucosa which has been stripped from bone by forceps or suction should be replaced immediately, but sadly does not always heal.

The infraorbital nerve is sometimes exposed in the roof of the antrum (Figure 6.**24**); it must never be damaged. Also, roots of the teeth lying in the antral cavity must be respected. They are yellow in colour and can be confused with retention cysts, and the beginner may be tempted to use the obsolete technique of curettage (Figure 6.**25**). On the other hand, inferior recesses must be opened completely otherwise scar tissue can form loculi in which a concealed empyema can develop. The author has found concealed purulent foci using the endoscope in an unsuspected maxillary cavity at reoperation after a previous Caldwell-Luc antrostomy. These loculi had obviously been overlooked at the first operation, and only came to light after an energetic search stimulated by an abnormal CT scan.

It may be necessary to create a second window in the inferior meatus if suitable instruments are not available to grasp a lesion, such as a cyst, lying in an unfavorable position, and which cannot be reached from the middle meatus. The author has seen no particular postoperative problems from the creation of a second window, but avoids it if possible.

The last step of the operation is hemostasis using bipolar coagulation or pledgets soaked in adrenalin. Once the lumen appears to be free, the edges of the antrostomy are inspected with the endoscope, and freed of mucosal tags or bone spicules. It is usually not necessary to pack the antral cavity: indeed, packing induces a foreign body mucosal reaction, as does blood clot. Loose packing for 24 hours with strips of gauze impregnated with ointment, or plastic foam in a finger cot, usually suffices but can often be dispensed with.

The above brief remarks establish the central role of the endoscope and angled telescope in antral surgery. There is a widespread but false view that endoscopic maxillary surgery is limited to carrying out a simple antrostomy. However, the comprehensive endoscopic treatment of the antrum demands greater knowledge of topographic anatomy, better instruments and is technically more difficult than the transoral Caldwell-Luc operation.

Revision Surgery

Second operations, particularly after a previous radical antrostomy, are much more difficult because the scar tissue lining and changes in the bony framework of the maxilla make orientation much more difficult, and obstruct access or even make it impossible. The CT scan (Figure 6.**26**) is a necessary part of the work-up and may cast doubt on the place of an intranasal procedure if a transoral revision appears to be inevitable. However, a transoral revision can often be avoided, although the patient's consent should always be obtained for this procedure should it become necessary.

The principles of the procedure are identical to those of the first operation. The creation of an adequate antrostomy is the first priority, and it often exposes the disease. If a small antral cavity is found in the inferior meatus (Figure 6.**27**) and another cavity is found beyond the remaining antrostomy in the middle meatus (Figure 6.**28**) with an intervening plate of scar tissue demonstrated by a CT scan, it is worth attempting to cut out this plate using a perforator, curved forceps and punches. On the other hand if a CT scan has demonstrated a low-lying orbit, which is frequent after a Caldwell-Luc operation, posterior retraction of the facial soft tissues or an abnormal double cavity with a thick dividing wall (Figure 6.**29a, b**), an intranasal endoscopic procedure would probably be too difficult, and a thorough transoral revision is indicated.

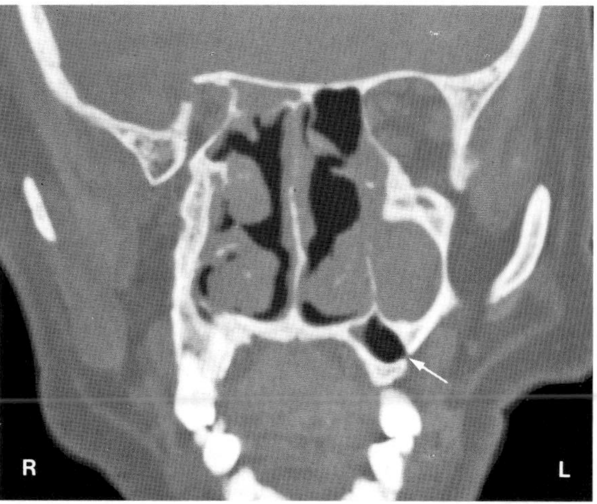

Figure 6.**26** Concealed alveolar recess with retention of mucus after a previous Caldwell-Luc procedure. The main symptom was maxillary pain. CT scan shows erosion of the left antral cavity with scar tissue, and a partially air-containing alveolar recess (marked with an arrow). Both ethmoid sinuses had been partially resected by the transmaxillary route. An intranasal revision procedure is still possible.

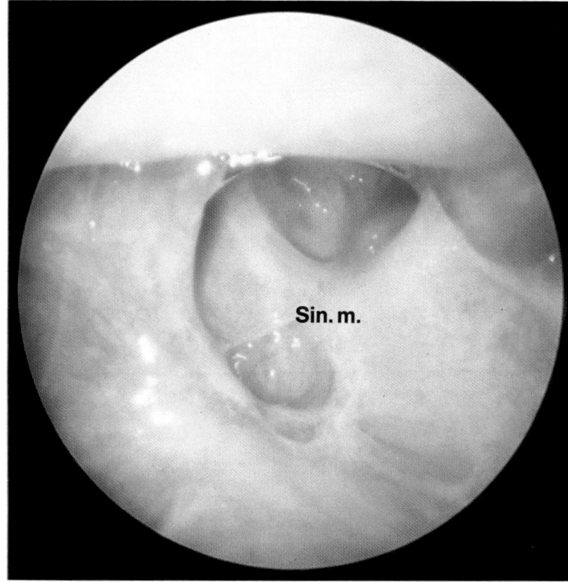

Figure 6.**27** Small left residual antrum after Caldwell-Luc operation. Inferior meatal antrostomy (70° telescope).

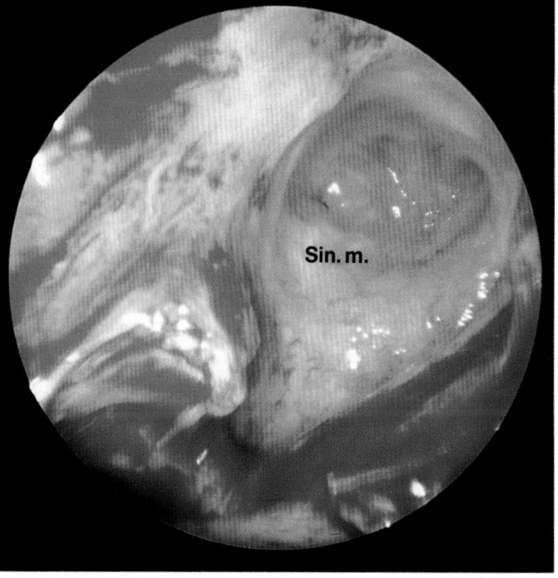

Figure 6.**28** Small isolated antral cavity on the left side after Caldwell-Luc operation combined with a transmaxillary ethmoidectomy. Left middle meatal antrostomy (70° telescope).

The previous operation may have included a transmaxillary ethmoidectomy, leading to scar tissue obliteration of the connections between the cells or recesses and the nasal cavity, causing loculated inflammation. Patients with this type of loculated disease may suffer bronchitis or neuralgia. Endoscopy or radiographs are often misleading, indicating that the antral cavity is open and free of disease, so that many of these patients are for a long time misdiagnosed as suffering from psychological overlay or depression, before a CT scan reveals the hidden focus.

Applications

Chronic Maxillary Sinusitis

Chronic antral mucositis with its intermediate forms from mucosal hyperplasia, via polypoid mucosal hypertrophy to an empyema resistant to treatment, provide the bulk of the indications for operation. Removal of cysts and polyps from the wall of the maxillary antrum will be used as examples of the operative procedure (see Figures 6.**21** and 6.**22**). The ideal procedure is the endoscopic removal of isolated cysts or polyps from an otherwise healthy antrum (Figure 6.**30**). These lesions do not always cause symptoms, but can contribute to bronchitis, pharyngitis, laryngitis, or even may constitute a focus with distant effects. Complete removal of these large cysts is not always simple. The double forceps often tears the thin wall, allowing the serous contents to gush out, so that the pedicle of the polyp or the lining of the cyst are not easy to find and remove without tearing the healthy mucosa lying on the wall of the antrum. Eradication using the diathermy loop or the argon laser has proved valuable. Pseudocysts often recur.

Operative treatment of diffuse polypoid pansinusitis demands attention to the antrum. It is remarkable that the antral cavity often shows only a smooth mucosal thickening whereas marked polypoid formation is present in the ethmoid (Figure 6.**31**), indicating primary disease of the ethmoidal mucosa with secondary affection of the antrum. The prospects of recovery of the antrum are good if the diseased ethmoid mucosa is treated, whereas an operation on the antrum alone is illogical.

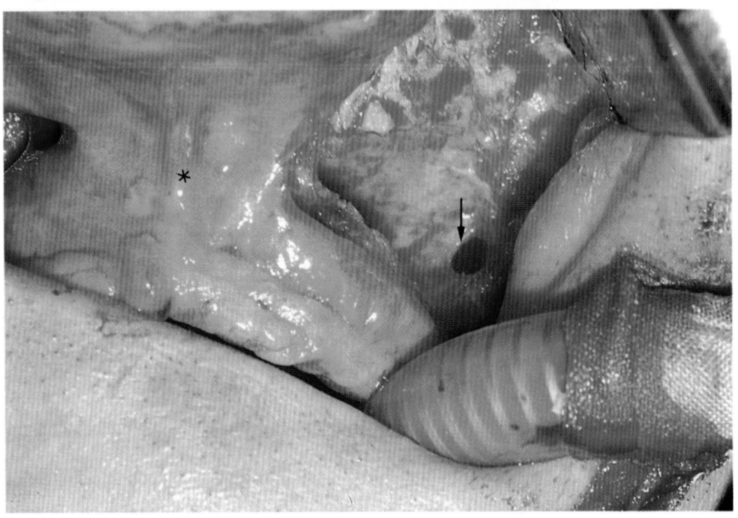

Figure 6.**29** Radiograph of a mucosal cavity (marked by an arrow) closed off by scar tissue lying in the zygomatic recess of the left antrum after previous Caldwell-Luc antrostomy. **a** Massive fibrosis with lateral retraction of the inferior turbinate. The ethmoid has been inadequately treated. The patient complained of maxillary pain and had the symptoms of chronic sinusitis and bronchitis.

b Exposure of the lateral antral recess (marked by an arrow) occluded by scar tissue at transoral revision. Frenulum (*).

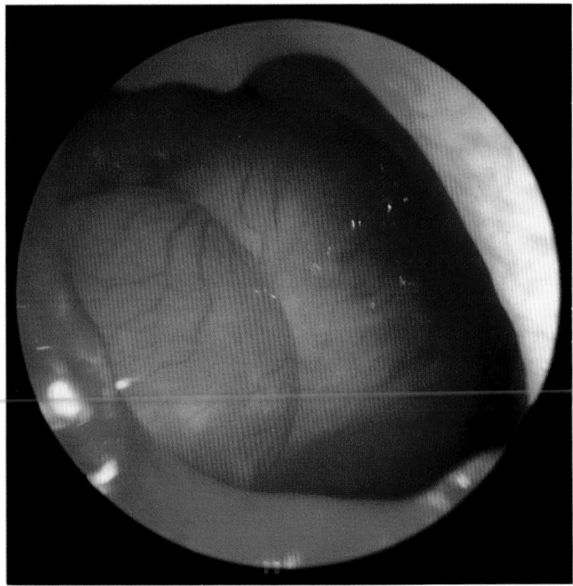

Figure 6.**30** Large middle meatal antrostomy for the removal of two edematous polyps from the left antrum (70° telescope).

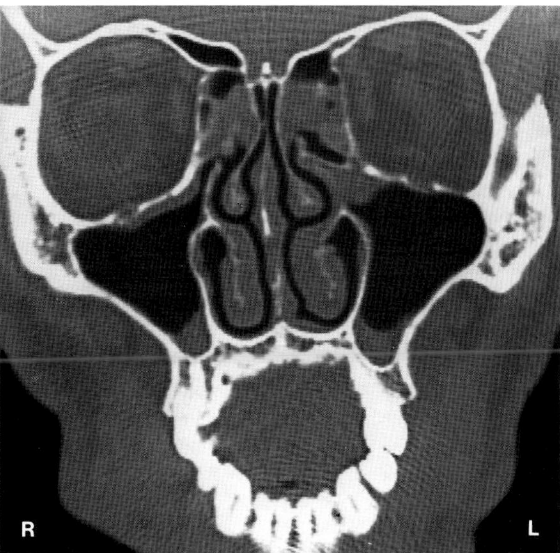

Figure 6.**31** Coronal CT scan showing massive ethmoidal polyposis with discrete hyperplasia of the antral mucosa.

In other cases inflammation of the antral mucosa is pronounced, whereas the ethmoid is relatively healthy. However, the ethmoids are never completely healthy, since an antral inflammation of nasal origin always spreads via the ostiomeatal unit of the middle meatus which belongs to the anterior ethmoid sinuses. A pathologically important, circumscribed, anterior ethmoiditis must be sought: it may not be visible on plain views but can be demonstrated before operation by a precise tomogram (Figure 6.**32a, b**). From this it follows that it is necessary in chronic disease to plan a middle meatal antrostomy and demonstrate the drainage channel for the anterior ethmoid, that is the semilunar hiatus and the ethmoid infundibulum.

The best results are obtained if the antral mucosa is retained and the window is modest in size. However, if a pronounced polyposis is present in both regions, removal of the bony edge of the window should be considered so that no narrow ethmoid recesses remain. The upper wall of the antrum must then merge into the soft curve of the lateral ethmoid wall without any step. Otherwise recurrent polyps can easily develop in the narrow area (Figure 6.**33**).

Moderately severe inflammatory hyperplasia of the antral mucosa causing uniform mucosal thickening on radiographs resolves after simple opening of the nonfunctioning ethmoid infundibulum from the semilunar hiatus without creating an antrostomy, although the results are unpredictable and the patient should be warned of the possibility of a second procedure. However, infundibulotomy alone cannot guarantee healing of the antrum for long-standing severe polyposis of both the ethmoids and the antral cavity. A new antral window must then be created to allow access to the maxillary polyposis.

Maxillary Sinusitis of Dental Origin

Inflammation of the dental roots or an antro-alveolar fistula do not automatically demand transoral exposure of the antrum by the Caldwell-Luc technique. Endoscopic treatment of the antral cavity at the same time as, or after, treatment of the dental disease or closure of the fistula suffices to achieve healing of the antral cavity.

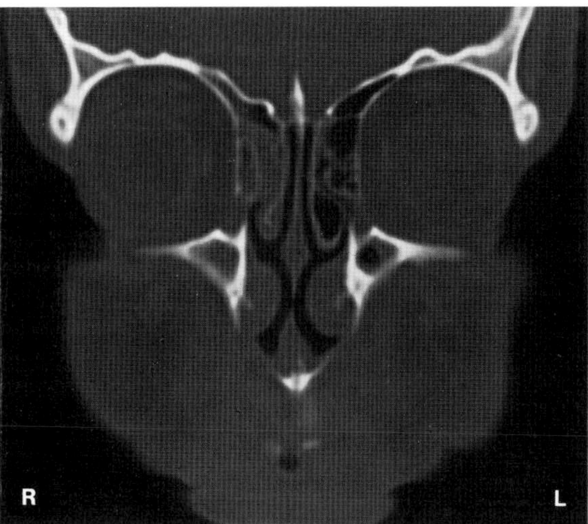

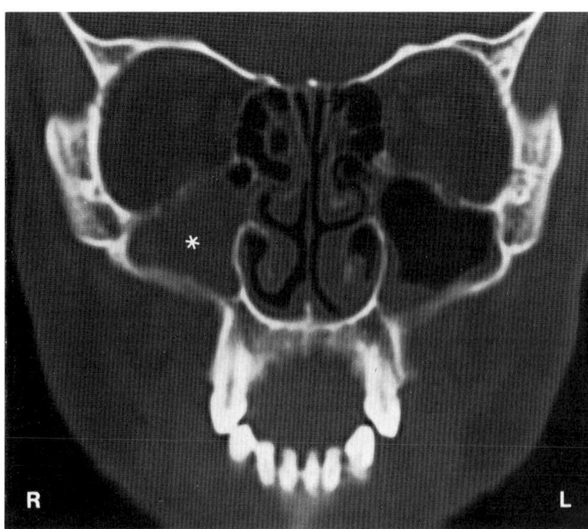

Figure 6.**32** CT scan showing anterior ethmoiditis with extensive chronic maxillary sinusitis on the right side (*).
a Coronal section through the anterior ethmoid.

b The posterior ethmoid cells are still aerated.

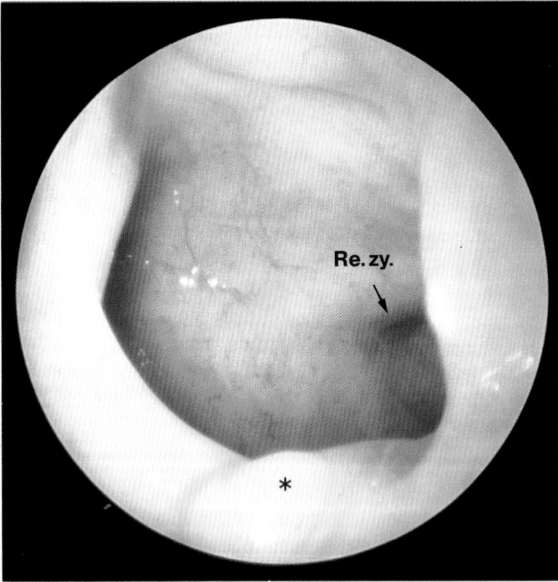

Figure 6.**33** Middle meatal antrostomy on the left side with a marked superior extension 6 years after operation. Mucosal streams (*) demonstrates the mucosal pathway at the lower edge of the window. Good recovery of a severe polypoid-hyperplastic mucosa (70° telescope).

Complications of Inflammatory Disease

A radical procedure via the transoral approach is obsolete even for the treatment of inflammatory complications. In many cases, drainage of the suppuration by the intranasal route coupled with high doses of appropriate antibiotics suffices to control the osteitis, periostitis and inflammation of the facial soft tissues arising from the antral cavity. Similar satisfactory results can be obtained for early orbital complications, but in these cases the antral operation is usually combined with an ethmoidectomy.

Also an antral mucopyocele can be managed satisfactorily by marsupialization through a wide intranasal antrostomy. Figure 6.**66** shows such a pseudotumor with caries of the bony floor of the orbit and facial swelling, one of the main symptoms being boring facial pain with double vision. A generous antrostomy brought the acute symptoms under control within hours.

Antrostomy in Children

Antrostomy is rarely indicated in infants because ethmoiditis is the commonest form of sinusitis at this age. However, if antrostomy is necessary, two disadvantages must be borne in mind: (1) the septal correction which is so often necessary may be refused at this age, (2) the patient cannot be expected to tolerate the necessary intranasal aftercare, including suction, installation of drugs and endoscopy.

However, operation cannot be avoided in all cases. The decision is easier in children older than 10 years. In children of school age ethmoiditis probably

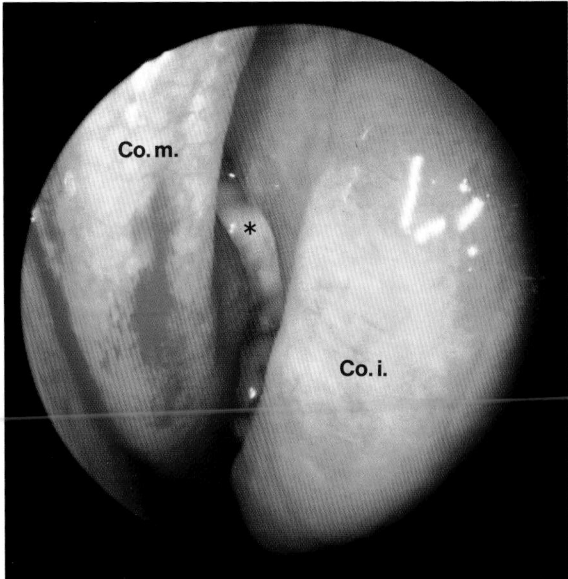

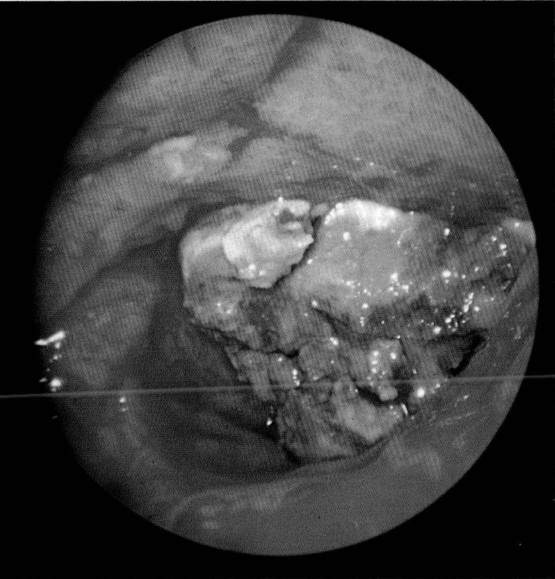

Figure 6.**34** Antral mycosis. **a** Fungal mycelia (*) in the left middle meatus (25° telescope).

b Inspissated fungal mass. View with a 70° telescope through a large spontaneous middle meatal window due to erosion.

precedes maxillary sinsuitis so that antrostomy alone does not tackle the basic pathology. Nevertheless, an ethmoidectomy is undesirable at this age, and it may be necessary to carry out an antrostomy alone as a compromise; experience shows that this often leads to resolution of the ethmoiditis presumably because resolution of the inflammation in the maxillary cavity has a favorable retrograde effect on the drainage through the ethmoid infundibulum. In childhood the good results of Thornwald's drainage and irrigation of the antrum via a retained catheter is probably explained in the same way.

The technique of antral surgery in children is the same as that in adults. It is possible to create a middle meatal antrostomy, preferably using smaller forceps and punches than usual, but an inferior meatal antrostomy alone is usually not sufficient treatment for chronic sinusitis. If lasting resolution of the mucosal disease demands supplementary procedures such as adenoidectomy or adenotonsillectomy, an inferior meatal antrostomy can contribute to healing. The window often closes spontaneously, but by then aeration and drainage are achieved through the recovered ostium in the middle meatus.

Foreign Bodies and Trauma

Once the surgeon has become familiar with the techniques for intranasal operations on the antrum he is ready to proceed to the para-endoscopic removal of foreign bodies, and the treatment of trauma. It is easy to remove inspissated masses remaining after treatment by irrigation, yeast concretions (Figure 6.**34 a, b**), dental root fillings or bullets (Figure 6.**35**) via a middle or inferior meatal antrostomy after careful radiological localization of the foreign body.

Debridement of the antral cavity after fractures of the middle third of the face, removal of bony splinters which may cause neuralgia and organized hematomas which can form a cholesterol granuloma can be carried out under favorable circumstances via the transnasal route. Penetration of the floor of the orbit with reduction of mobility of the bulb and impaction of the muscles and orbital fat is better dealt with by an external (infra-orbital) approach with

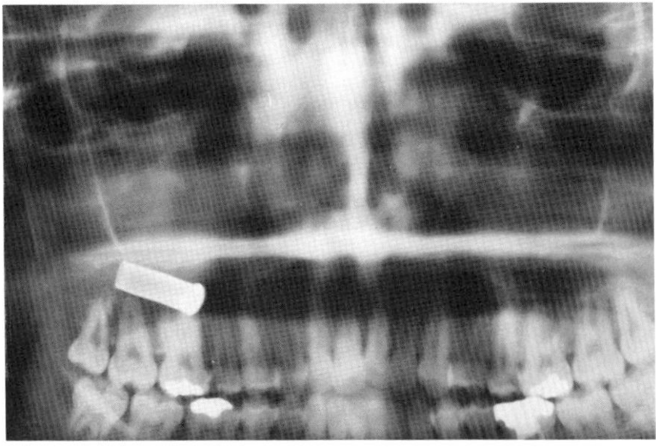

Figure 6.**35** Bullet in the right antrum which had entered through the face. It was removed endoscopically by the infraturbinal route. Panorex X-ray before operation.

splinting, but in suitable cases intranasal endoscopic assessment and temporary support of the orbital floor often succeed.

Antral Tumors

Benign tumors of the antrum are rare, so that endoscopic removal of such tumors is rarely indicated. Inverted papillomas may be controlled by an endonasal approach. Malignant tumors cause no symptoms when they are small, so that an approach through the inferior meatus is restricted to taking tissue for histology, creating drainage for necrotic material during radiotherapy, and for endoscopic follow-up. On the other hand an endoscope with an angled telescope can be used to supplement wide transfacial or transfrontal exposure of a tumor affecting several levels.

Operations on the Ethmoid Sinus

Indications

- chronic recurrent maxillary sinusitis,
- chronic hyperplastic polypoid sinusitis of the ethmoid and the maxillo-ethmoidal junctional zone,
- complications of inflammation,
- foreign bodies and trauma of the ethmoid and of the anterior skull base,
- tumors of the ethmoid and neighboring areas,
- transnasal access to the frontal and sphenoid sinuses, and to the orbit and lacrimal duct.

Principles

The operation should be tailored to the individual patient and the extent of the chronic sinusitis, but the goal must always be restitution of free aeration and drainage of the ethmoid compartment. The middle turbinate with its attachment at the roof of the ethmoids is a key landmark ensuring the security of the procedure. It may be partially or completely removed depending on the extent of the disease, but the value of preserving or reconstructing the olfactory cleft must be stressed.

The middle meatus is the gateway to the ethmoids. The functional pathway from the semilunar hiatus to the ethmoid infundibulum and then to the frontal sinus, the anterior ethmoid cells and the antral cavity via the primary maxillary ostium should be exploited surgically. The posterior ethmoids are more clearly seen after a posterior partial resection of the middle turbinate. Ethmoid operations are usually combined with correction of the upper part of the nasal septum. The correct choice and direction of the instruments minimizes the danger of injury to the orbit and the anterior skull base, but a CSF fistula due to tearing of olfactory fibers may occur, and should be repaired immediately. Partial resections may be more difficult and more dangerous than complete clearance if the surgeon has not acquired sufficient experience with complete ethmoidectomy.

Operative Technique

Opening of the Semilunar Hiatus (Hiatotomy) and the Ethmoid Infundibulum (Infundibulotomy)

The functional ostiomeatal unit consisting of the middle meatus and the semilunar hiatus (Naumann 1977) plays a pivotal role in mucosal disease of the sinuses, because most inflammations of the maxillary, frontal and ethmoid sinuses arise from this point (Messerklinger). In particular, swelling and hyperplasia of the mucosa in the ethmoid infundibulum obstruct aeration and drainage of the antrum, the anterior ethmoids and the frontal sinus leading to the development of sinusitis. Widening of the infun-

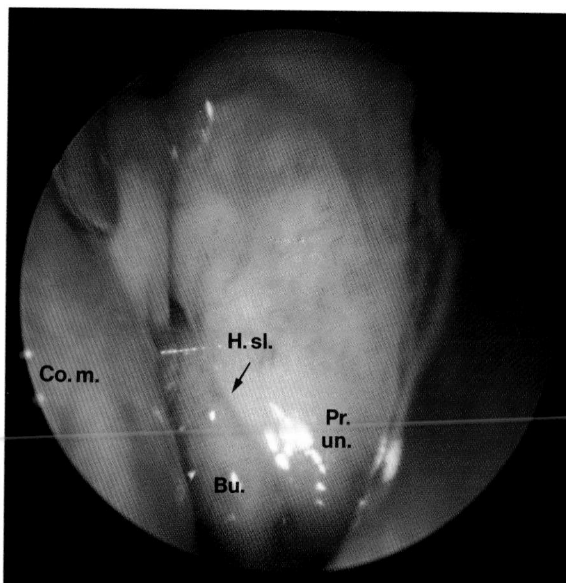

Figure 6.**36** Left middle turbinate with the complex of the middle turbinate, the bulla and the uncinate process. On the left and above can be seen the point of the elevator for retraction of the middle turbinate. The semilunar hiatus is visible as a thin upward curved line (25° telescope).

dibulum alone therefore often leads to recovery of severe hyperplasia of the sinus mucosa (Messerklinger 1979). This principle of treatment has been less used as a routine in many clinics than ethmoid aeration via intranasal or transmaxillary access. Because of the individual variation in shape of the middle meatus surgical exposure of the infundibulum under endoscopic vision must be adapted to the type and extend of the resection of bone and mucosa (Figure 6.**36**).

The middle meatus can be well seen with the 25° telescope: The characteristic protrusion of the ethmoid bulla and the marked groove of the semilunar hiatus are easily located. A secondary antral ostium is often to be found close to its posterior end, but it may be concealed, covered by swollen mucosa or be absent. The ethmoid infundibulum is an anterior prolongation of the semilunar hiatus, lying between the ethmoid bulla and the uncinate process.

The ethmoid infundibulum can be exposed by opening the semilunar hiatus (hiatotomy) by careful removal of its walls, in particular the upper edge of the uncinate process. Polyps projecting from its gutter (Figure 6.**37 a, b**) must often be removed first with a delicate grasping forceps. A strip of mucosa and bone is then removed from the uncinate process using a sickle knife carried forwards parallel to the upper edge on the hiatus (Figure 6.**38 a, b**). A fine cutting forceps is placed in the existing gutter and used to remove tissue from the uncinate process until

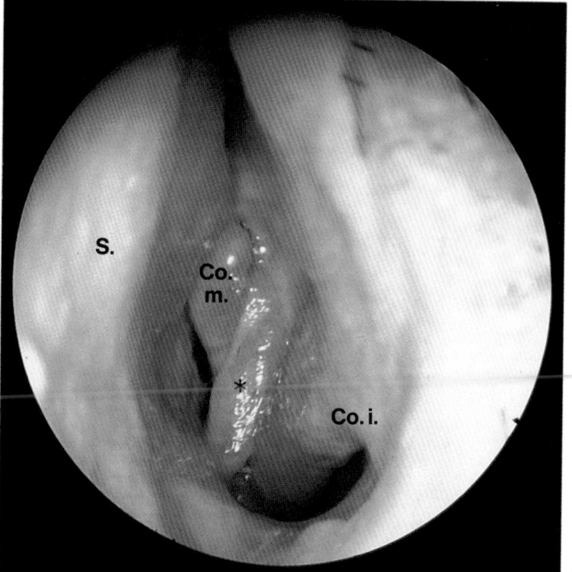

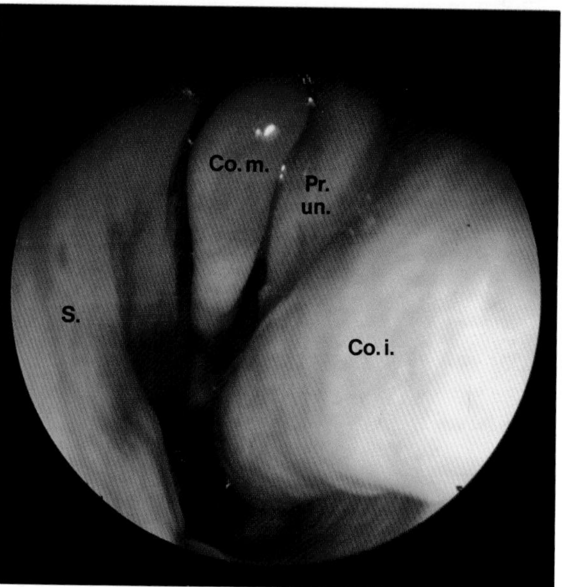

Figure 6.**37** Occlusion of the middle nasal meatus by polyps (*) protruding between an atrophic middle turbinate and reaching as far as the flat gutter of the floor of the nose (**a**). **b** Nasal cavity after extraction of the polyp.

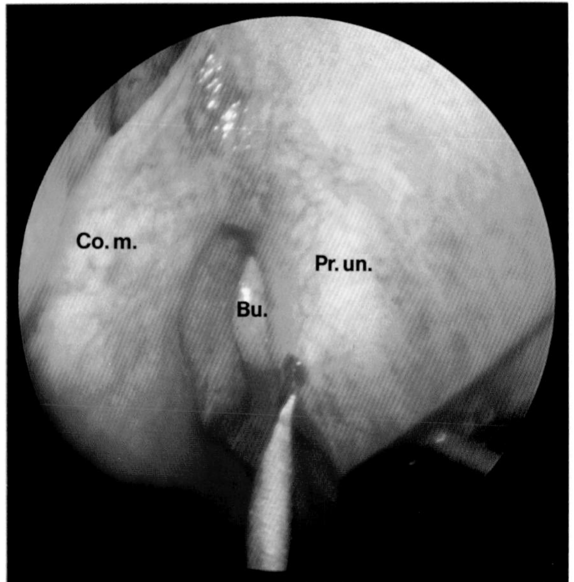

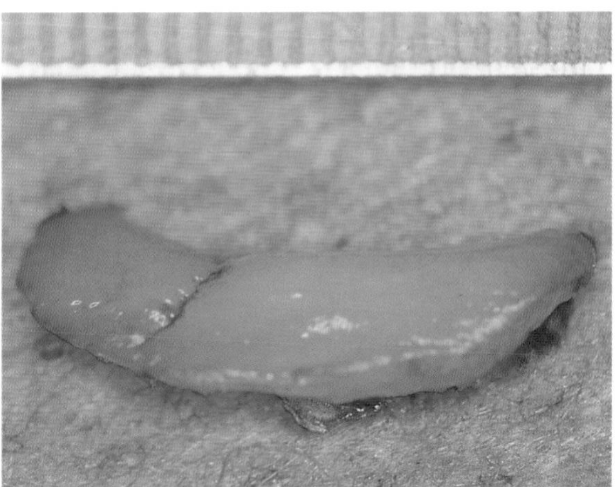

Figure 6.**38** Resection of the uncinate process to expose the ethmoidal infundibulum. **a** Sickle knife at the start of the resection line (25° telescope).

b Resected segment with a millimeter mark above.

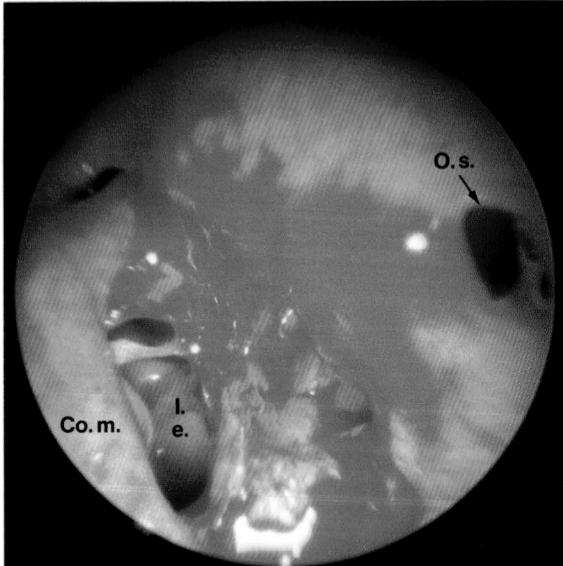

Figure 6.**39** The opening of the anterior ethmoid cells after resection of the left uncinate process. The ethmoid infundibulum is thus exposed. A small polyp lies centrally, and on the right there is a secondary maxillary ostium in the anterior fontanelle (70° telescope).

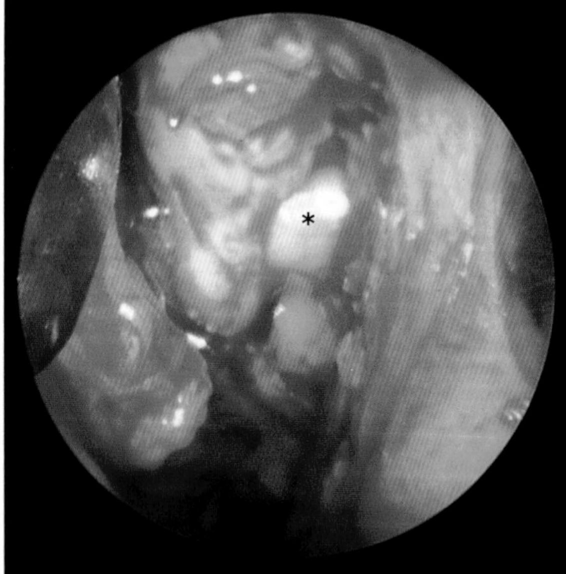

Figure 6.**40** Infundibulotomy and partial resection of the bulla. A white polyp (*) obstructs the view into the terminal recess anteriorly. On the left side can be seen a speculum beneath the middle turbinate (left side, 25° telescope).

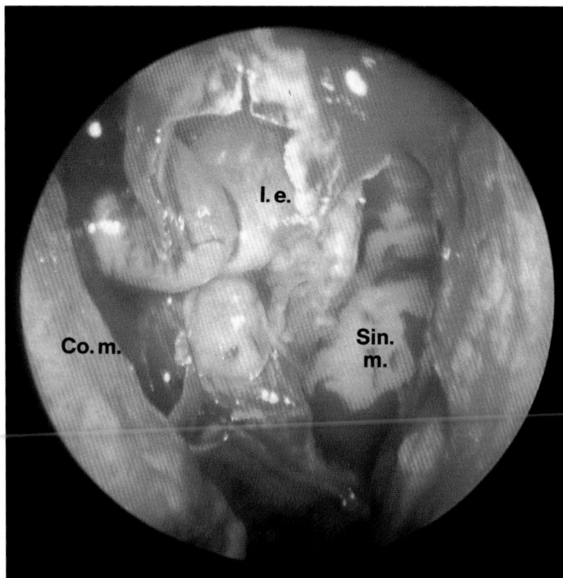

Figure 6.**41** Anterior partial ethmoidectomy. Several small polyps have been removed after exposure of the infundibulum and the cells are opened. On the right side can be seen the opening of a newly created middle meatal antrostomy (70° telescope) (same patient as in Figure 6.**40**).

the primary antral ostium, several anterior ethmoid cells and the frontonasal duct are visible in the now open infundibulum, allowing free drainage (Figure 6.**39**). If inflammatory hyperplasia is found in the cells of the bulla, the cells can be carefully opened from the hiatus, checked and if necessary removed (Figures 6.**40**, 6.**41**). The procedure ends with minor procedures such as removal of polyps or minimal extension of the window at the maxillary ostium.

Strictly speaking simple enlargement of the semilunar hiatus by resection of the upper edge of the uncinate process should be termed a *hiatotomy* whereas *infundibulotomy* indicates wide opening of the ethmoid infundibulum including removal of cells and septa of the ethmoid bulla in most cases. The surgeon learns how much tissue to remove determined by the individual pathology and anatomy, and a strict division into two types of operation is not always practical.

Anterior Ethmoidectomy

Often chronic hyperplastic mucosal inflammation affects only the cells bordering the middle meatus, as can be well shown by CT scans (see Figure 3.**5**). Circumscribed posterior ethmoiditis is less common. Clearance of different regions of the ethmoid may therefore be indicated.

The goal of *anterior ethmoidectomy* is complete exposure of the anterior ethmoid. The use of an operating endoscope with angled telescope is absolutely essential since residual cells walled off by scar tissue cause foci of recurrent ethmoiditis. Therefore it is also advisable to secure free drainage for the frontal sinus. Blind resection without optic control is dangerous because perforation of the orbit or the anterior cranial fossa and tearing of the olfactory fibers leading to a CSF leak can happen more easily in the anterior than in the posterior ethmoid.

Strictly speaking, anterior ethmoidectomy can be carried out in two ways; neither one nor the other should be preferred, but the one appropriate to the extent of the disease, or a combination of the procedures, should be chosen.

An initial middle meatal antrostomy has proven to be a particularly safe procedure; an antrostomy is often indicated per se because the antral cavity is frequently involved. The antrostomy is created by resection of the posterior fontanelle, and possibly of the lower edge of the uncinate process beneath the semilunar hiatus (see Chapter 6). The neighboring anterosuperior and medial bone can now be punched out from the opening thus created, with the orbital wall under direct vision, until the ethmoid infundibulum is exposed entirely (Figure 6.**42 a, b**). The remaining cells of the bulla and the anterior ethmoid cells can be opened a cell at a time using the angled telescope until the anterior ethmoid compartment is reduced to one common cavity covered by mucosa. Its borders – the lamina papyracea, the skull base and the boundary with the frontal sinus – are reached relatively safely in this way. In the author's clinic, injury to the orbital periosteum has now become extremely rare, even if the bony dividing wall is absent.

In order to achieve better exposure of the anterior ethmoid cells it is often necessary to remove bone around the *agger nasi* with a punch, since it overhangs and obstructs the view. If the frontal duct is still not visible after exposure of the most anterior cells under the agger, its position is determined by carefull probing and its lumen exposed by removal of overlying polyps (Figure 6.**43 a, b**). Dissection should never be carried in front of the small mound of bone where the anterior end of the middle turbinate meets the agger nasi (Figure 6.**44**), since the olfactory cleft and the base of the skull begin above or in front of this point.

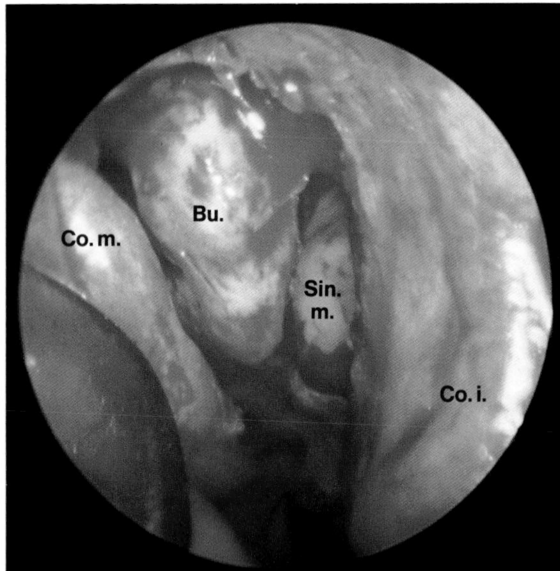

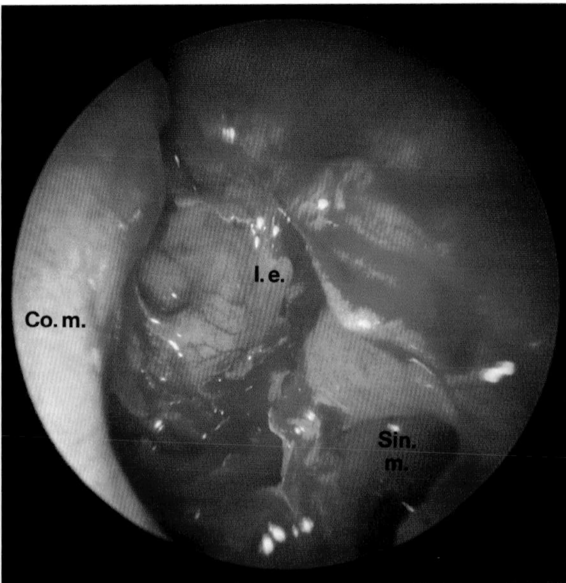

Figure 6.**42** Resection of the bulla after middle meatal antrostomy and infundibulotomy.
a Exposure of the left ethmoid bulla.

b The view after removal of the bulla and its cells. The anterior ethmoid cells are still intact (70° telescope).

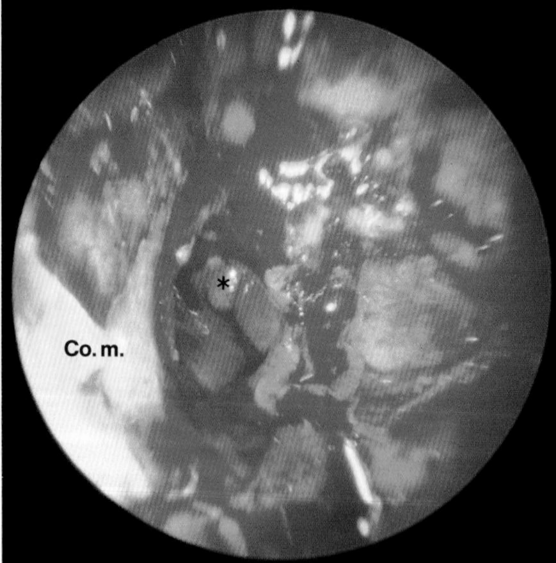

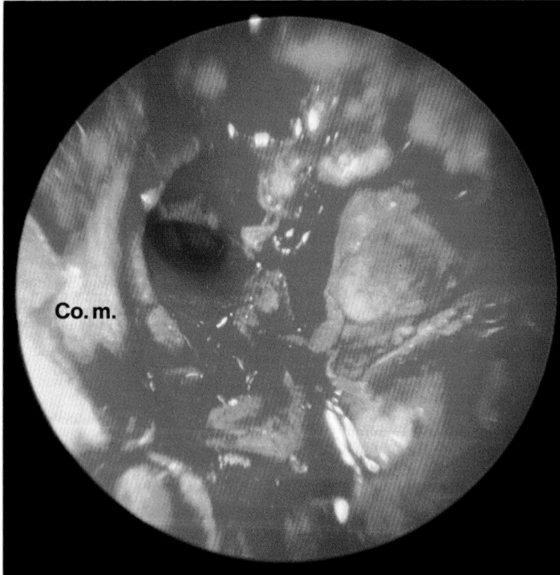

Figure 6.**43** Exposure of the nasofrontal duct.
a A small polyp (*) obstructs the view into the nasofrontal duct after exposure of the anterior ethmoid cells.

b A free view of the frontal duct is only obtained after endoscopic removal of the polyp (70° telescope).

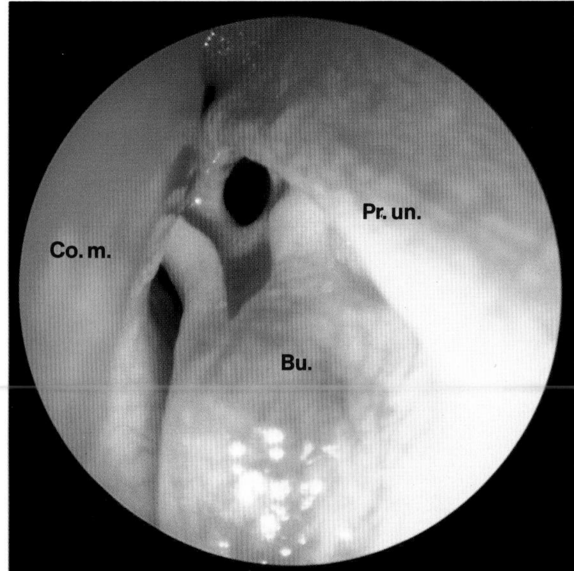

Figure 6.**44** Anterior end of the semilunar hiatus. A small bridge of bone lies at the junction of the anterior limit of the uncinate process and the bulla. A similar one runs upwards from the process to the middle turbinate, and in this case is limiting the nasofrontal duct from in front. A third bony bridge which is very well developed in this case runs between the turbinate and the bulla. At the upper edge of the picture lies the scarcely visible junction of the agger nasi and the middle turbinate (70° telescope).

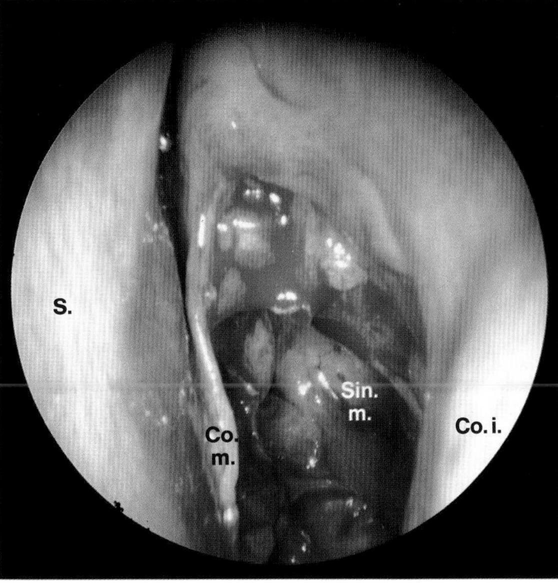

Figure 6.**45** Opening of the left antrum into the middle meatus by anterior ethmoidectomy. The medial lamella of the atrophic middle turbinate has been preserved. The anterior ethmoid cells filled with polyps lie under the agger nasi (70° telescope).

The middle turbinate may be left entirely intact at infundibulotomy or anterior ethmoidectomy for circumscribed ethmoiditis. Although disease of individual cells may require the cells to be opened and the lateral part of the turbinate to be removed, its medial surface should be completely preserved.

The second method of anterior ethmoidectomy is based on that originally described by Halle (1915), and later developed into an endoscopic procedure by Messerklinger (1987) and Stammberger (1985), in which the anterior ethmoid is entered through the semilunar hiatus and the ethmoid bulla. After exposing the semilunar hiatus and the ethmoid infundibulum, and opening the bulla widely the ethmoid system is opened cell-by-cell without fenestrating the antral cavity anew. This method conforms to physiological and pathological principles. In practice the end result in hyperplastic ethmoiditis requiring surgery is often the same as in the above resection technique because the boundary with the antral cavity beneath the uncinate process is also opened by systematic removal of cells (Figure 6.**45**).

The second approach via the ethmoid infundibulum is more dangerous than the first, because the orbital wall often runs only 2–3 mm from the infundibulum, and can thus be damaged by careless blind dissection using a sharp sickle knife or similar instrument, whereas the primary middle meatal antrostomy exposes the antral roof and thus the orbital wall immediately, so that they are constantly under vision and are therefore safe during removal of the uncinate process and the neighboring ethmoid cells with the punch.

Posterior Ethmoidectomy

A partial *posterior ethmoidectomy* is seldom indicated for chronic ethmoiditis because this disease spreads via the middle meatus, mainly affects the anterior ethmoids and is seldom limited to the posterior compartment. However, this operation is often indicated to expose the sphenoid sinus. There are no disadvantages arising from a wide upper nasal cavity after posterior extension of the ethmoidectomy. Septal correction is advisable to improve the view.

The operation begins with a hiatotomy to allow the cells to be opened systematically rather than randomly. After resection of the posterior half of the upper edge of the uncinate process and opening of the posterior bulla cell, the basal lamella of the middle turbinate is usually encountered dividing the an-

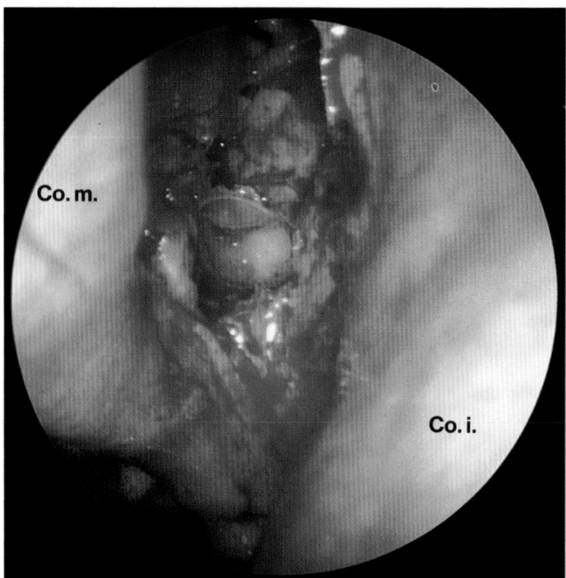

Figure 6.**46** A view of the posterior ethmoid cells after perforation of the basal lamella of the left middle turbinate (25° telescope).

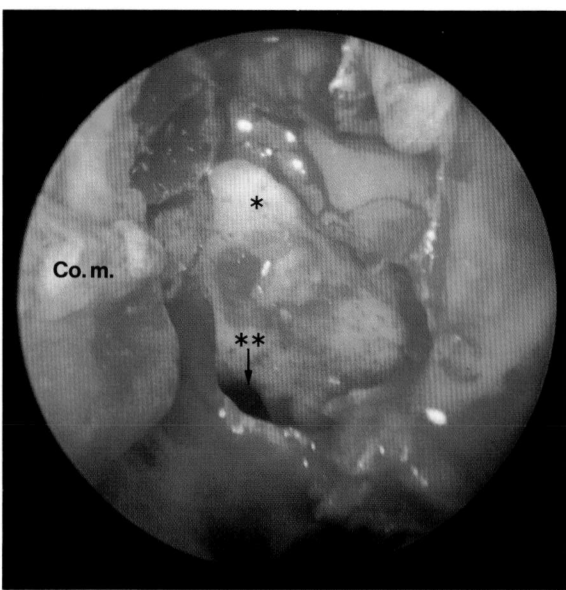

Figure 6.**47** After removal of the posterior ethmoid cells the anterior wall of the left sphenoid sinus and its ostium come into view (70° telescope). It remains partially covered by the posterior attachment of the middle turbinate (* equals ethmoid roof, ** equals sphenoid ostium).

terior from the posterior ethmoid compartment. It is perforated carefully (Figure 6.**46**), the posterior ethmoid cells removed stepwise, and the anterior wall of the sphenoid sinus and its ostium exposed (Figure 6.**47**). If dissection is continued on the anterior wall of the sphenoid sinus through the ethmoid cells, the insertion of the superior turbinate to the anterior wall of the sphenoid cavity often obstructs a free view of the sphenoid ostium. Mosher (1929) pointed out that the insertion of the superior turbinate to the anterior wall of the sphenoid sinus normally divides the wall into a medial part opening into the superior nasal meatus and a lateral part bordering the ethmoid in a ratio of 1:2. The above dissection of the posterior ethmoids can usually be carried out without difficulty, with total preservation of the middle turbinate provided that the ethmoid has not been destroyed by polyposis or undergone necrosis and provided that the ethmoid does not extend far laterally at its posterior end. In these circumstances the following variation is recommended:

The view into the posterior ethmoids is greatly facilitated and the security of the operation considerably improved by resection of the posterior third of the *middle turbinate,* by a cut curving backwards and upwards using the curved turbinectomy scissors, a counter incision at the end of the turbinate and removal of the divided end of the turbinate (Figure 6.**48**). The posterior insertion of the middle turbinate is then clearly exposed, forming a landmark leading to the sphenoid ostium. At the same time the posterior ethmoid cells are also exposed; they are removed by breaking down the party walls with ethmoid forceps, or with a forward-cutting punch directed carefully towards the anterior wall of the sphenoid sinus, until the latter is freely exposed (Figure 6.**49**).

Simultaneous opening of the *sphenoid sinus* is achieved by pushing a slender closed ethmoid forceps into the sphenoid ostium, and the widening the defect of the anterior wall by opening up the forceps. If the ostium cannot be found the anterior wall is carefully perforated after determining the correct point from the appropriate landmarks (see Chapter 2 on Endoscopic Anatomy). This initial opening can then be extended using a 45° or 90° punch until the anterior wall of the sphenoid sinus is completely removed (Figure 6.**49 a–c**). Bleeding from the branches of the sphenopalatine artery can be controlled by the curved bipolar coagulation (Figure 6.**50**). The roof and lateral wall of the sphenoid sinus are now exposed as landmarks to allow a posterior ethmoidectomy to be carried out safely: prolongation of the sphenoid roof anteriorly meets the ethmoid roof at the same level, and with only slight curvature of the surface. The removal of all cells can now be checked exactly and safely using a bone punch with a blunt head without danger to the base of the skull.

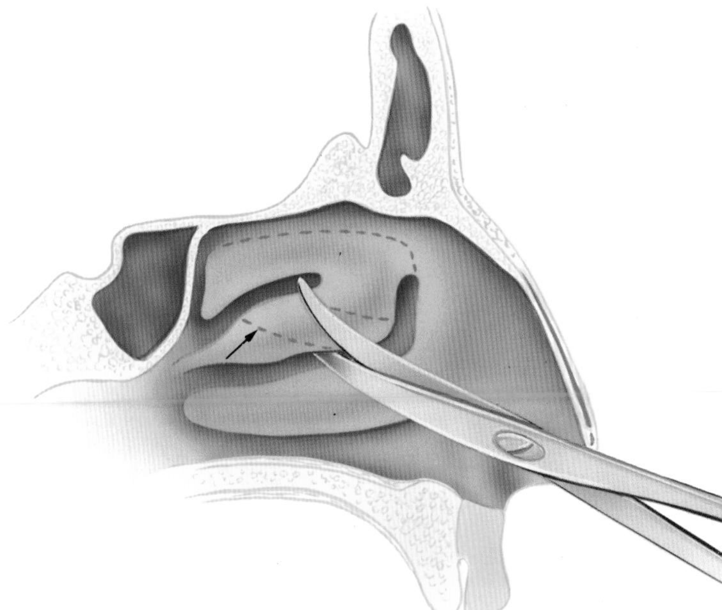

Figure 6.**48** Resection lines for partial removal of the middle turbinate. At the very top lies the incision for subtotal resection. A second line below marks the incision for a 50% resection with preservation of its olfactory mucosa. The third line (marked with an arrow) defines an incision which per se releases the middle turbinate from its lateral position. This incision may otherwise initiate a resection of the posterior third.

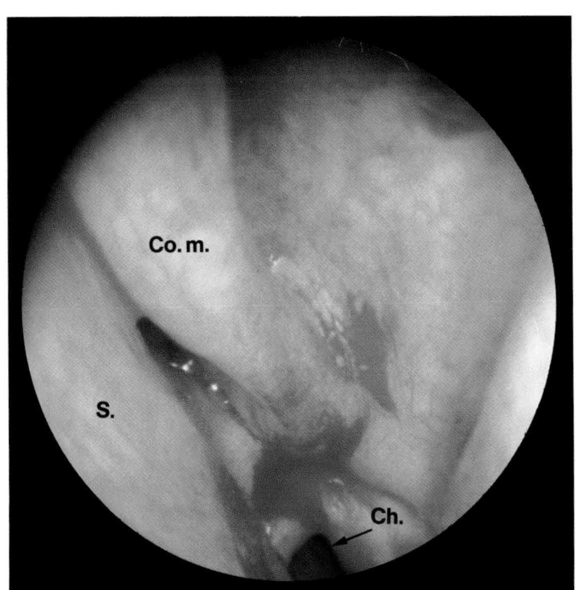

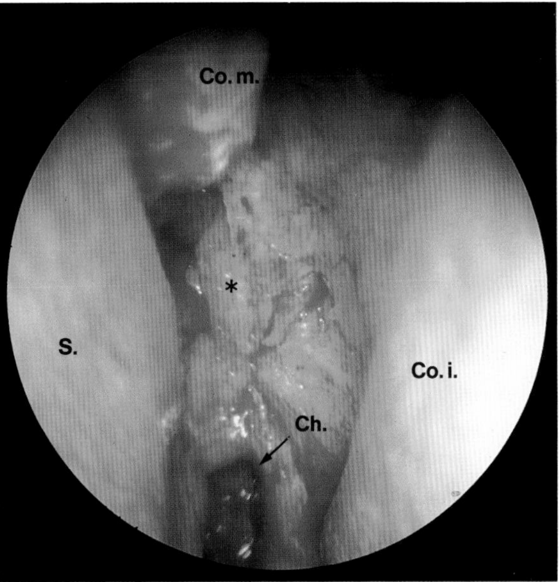

Figure 6.**49** Anterior wall of the sphenoid sinus. **a** Covered by the posterior attachment of the middle turbinate. **b** Exposed (*) by resection of its posterior third. The left choana lies below.

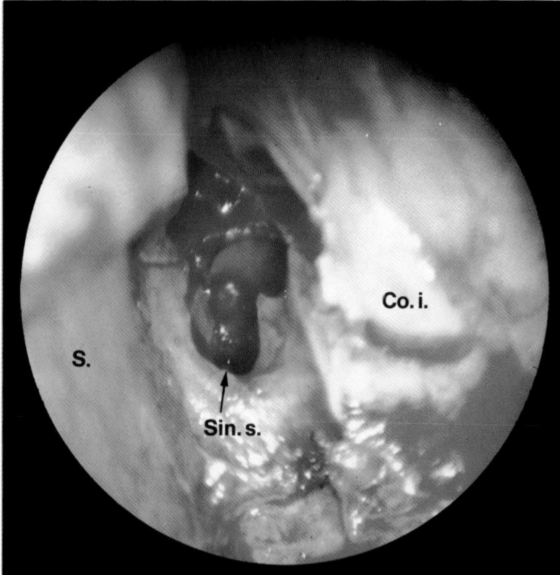

c Fenestration of the anterior sphenoid wall (25° telescope).

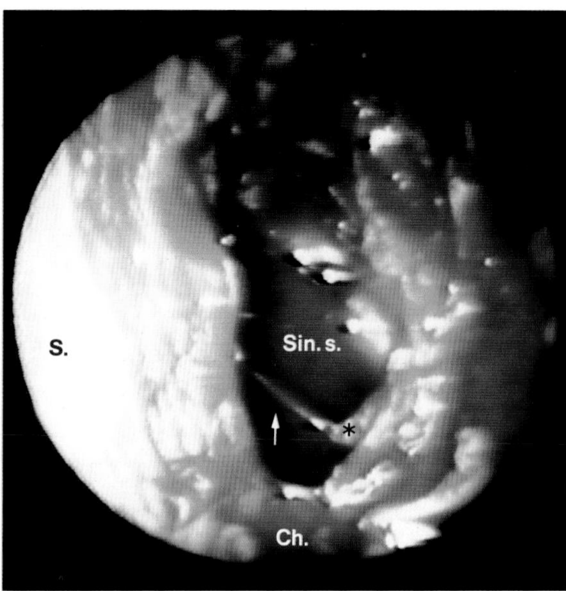

Figure 6.**50** Bleeding sphenopalatine artery during opening of the sphenoid (the arrow shows a small stream of blood). The stump of the vessel (*) is dealt with by the bipolar coagulation forceps under direct vision (25° telescope; extract from a video).

The lateral wall of the sphenoid sinus also marks very accurately the contour of the lateral wall of the ethmoid compartment, as the series of CT scans shows, running forwards in a smooth gentle curve towards the orbit (see Chapter 2 on Endoscopic Anatomy). It is relatively thick unlike the thin party walls of the ethmoid cells, so that careful dissection precludes injury to the orbit or the optic nerve.

The canal for the optic nerve may lie almost free in the lateral part of the sphenoid cavity (Figure 6.**51**) but the author has always found it to have a bony cover. Passage of the optic nerve through an ethmoid cell running very far laterally and superiorly is rare, but should be mentioned.

The anterior extent of removal of the posterior ethmoids for posterior ethmoiditis depends on individual findings. If the middle ethmoid cells are also affected, an infundibulotomy is recommended to secure drainage from the remaining anterior cells.

Posterior ethmoidectomy is seldom carried out in isolation, but is usually combined with anterior ethmoidectomy to allow removal to diseased *posterior ethmoid cells.* It begins with penetration of the basal lamella which has previously been exposed through the bulla, and proceeds from in front backwards.

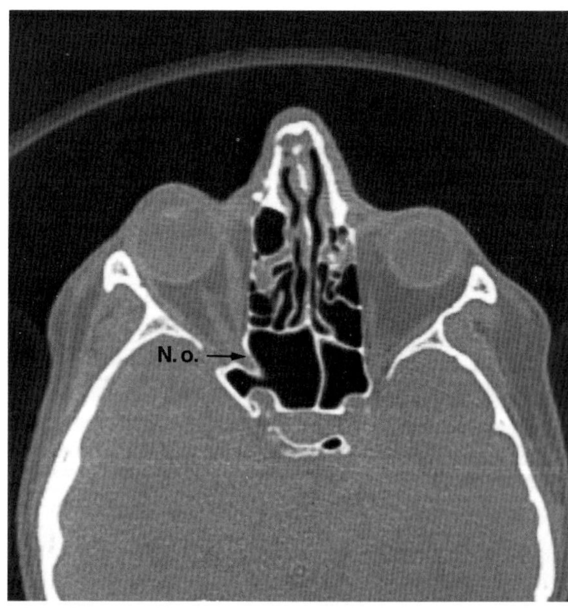

Figure 6.**51** Passage of optic nerve through a large left sphenoid cavity. High-resolution CT scan.

Complete Ethmoidectomy with Opening of the Sphenoid, Frontal and Antral Cavities

Complete ethmoidectomy is supposed to be one of the most dangerous operations in this area. The literature and discussions at conferences show that various techniques are used for reasons of safety. Radical removal of all the mucosa is said to be better carried out through an external facial incision, but if complete clearance is not indicated many surgeons prefer transmaxillary access after an incision in the oral vestibule. Finally it appears that most authors only choose a strictly intranasal procedure if limited cell clearance is desired. These differences apply more or less to the present day (for example Naumann 1987). On the other hand the purpose of surgery with preservation of mucosa, independent of the route of access, is the creation of a unilocular ethmoid cavity with no party walls from which mucosal polyps can be removed with preservation of the mucosal surfaces of the external walls.

Anteroposterior Exposure

This exposure can be achieved with an intranasal technique, either using a classical transbulla procedure described by Halle, or the method beginning in the infundibulum described by Messerklinger and Stammberger. An infundibulotomy is then followed by clearance of the bulla and the anterior ethmoid cells. Next, the posterior ethmoids are opened from the basal lamella, and cleared cell-by-cell in an anteroposterior direction. Stammberger (1985) does not insist on the obligatory opening of the sphenoid and frontal cavities, and he also rejects resection of the middle turbinate.

Posteroanterior Exposure

A description of the technique of intranasal complete ethmoidectomy developed since 1975 in the author's clinic now follows. Unlike previous methods it is based on retrograde exposure of the ethmoids, beginning at the sphenoid sinus and working in a posteroanterior direction along the base of the skull. This has been developed into a standard technique giving a clear exposure which is therefore free of complications, and which also give reliable results. It is indicated for severe diffuse polyposis of the ethmoids: it is usually combined with septoplasty and opening of the sphenoid, frontal and antral cavities (pansinus operation).

The main prerequisite for the safety of the procedure is an optimal view of the surgical field. It is true that a large part of the procedure can be carried out under direct vision through the nostril using a long nasal speculum, but for the deeper regions optical magnification is necessary, using the operating microscope where forward vision suffices, and the angled telescope to see around corners. The author usually uses a 70° angled telescope with an irrigation-suction handpiece.

The second principle is complete opening of the cells to guarantee healing of the chronic polypoid mucosal inflammation. Remaining cells are often the point of origin of persistent disease. These two aspects therefore led us to develop complete ethmoidectomy, in which an entirely visible ethmoid compartment is created with no remaining narrow areas and no remaining cells. The resulting wide upper nose was a new and surprising experience, that did *not* lead to drying of the regenerating mucosa nor to the development of ozena. Thus the middle turbinate can be removed partially or sub-totally with no ill effects.

Polyps filling the nasal cavity (Figure 6.**52**) are removed with forceps or snares after intensive decongestion of the mucosa with adrenalin-soaked pledgets, providing a reliable view of the shape and position of the often markedly atrophic or polypoid middle turbinate (Figure 6.**53**).

Opening of the sphenoids begins with a posterior *partial resection of the middle turbinate*. An incision curved concavely upwards is made with the turbinectomy scissors curved on the flat (see Figure 6.**48**) so that the posterior part of the turbinate inserting into the ethmoid is reduced in size. The loose posterior turbinate stump can be removed with a No. 3 ethmoid forceps through the curved incision and through a counter incision at the end of the turbinate. The incision curving obliquely downwards generally straddles the lateral ethmoid and encompasses about one-third to one-quarter of the free body of the turbinate. Bleeding from the sphenopalatine artery is controlled by bipolar coagulation and compression with a pledget.

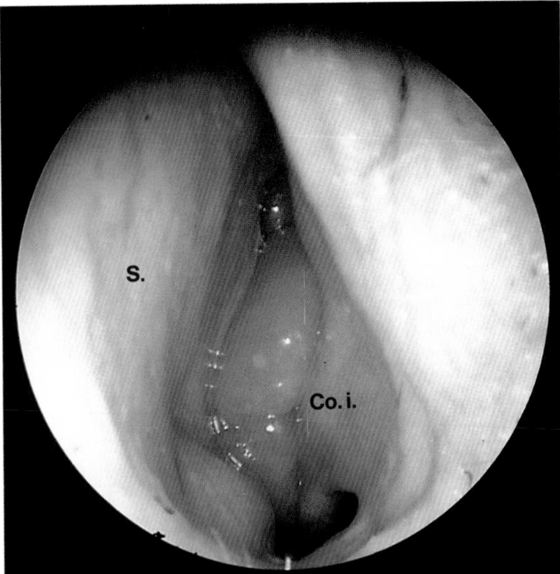

Figure 6.**52** Massive nasal polyposis obstructing the view of the left middle turbinate (25° telescope).

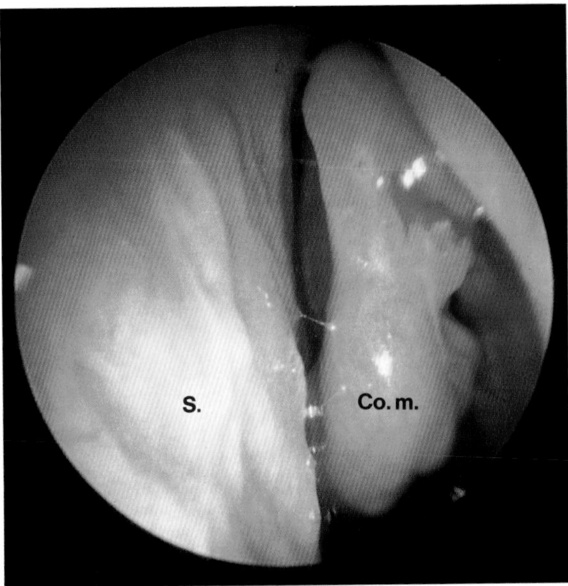

Figure 6.**53** After careful removal of the polyps the left middle turbinate and the middle meatus come into view. Mucosal defects and partial opening of the ethmoidal cells can make orientation difficult (25° telescope).

The posterior ethmoid labyrinth is opened by posterior, limited removal of the free body of the middle turbinate. Figure 6.**54** shows some cells with their party walls. Polypoid mucosal edema, tenacious mucus or pus often ooze out in cases of polypoid ethmoiditis. The tangle of cell walls and polyps is removed carefully using a large Blakesley No. 3 forceps; the instrument must always be directed posteriorly.

At a point from 1 to 2 cm above the upper edge of the posterior nasal choana there is no danger of perforation of the base of the skull because the surgeon encounters the thick anterior wall of the sphenoid sinus or the rigid plate of the sphenoid plane if he goes too high.

The lateral boundary of the posterior ethmoid demands care: occasionally the canal of the optic nerve may form a visible bulge or can even be surrounded by an extensive Onodi cell so that it lies almost completely within this cell. However, the optic nerve is safe from injury if the forceps are not directed laterally during this first phase of removal of the posterior ethmoid cells, but are introduced towards the anterior wall of the sphenoid sinus in the midline, parallel to the septum.

It is advisable not to expose the posterior ethmoid cells as far as the ethmoid roof directly at this point, but firstly to expose and remove the *anterior wall of the sphenoid sinus,* to avoid dissection towards the base of the skull (Figures 6.**55,** 6.**56**). The

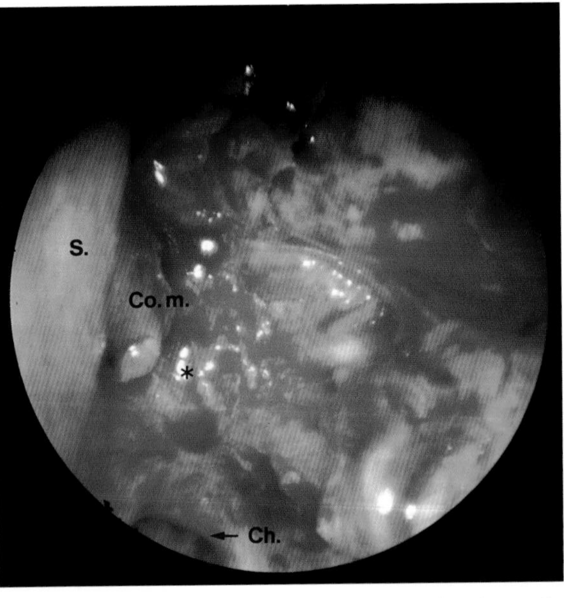

Figure 6.**54** Beginning of a posteroanterior ethmoidectomy for polypoidal pansinusitis. The anterior wall of the sphenoid is exposed (*) by resection of the posterior third of the left middle turbinate and removal of the posterior ethmoid cells. The upper edge of the choana lies at the lower edge of the picture (70° telescope).

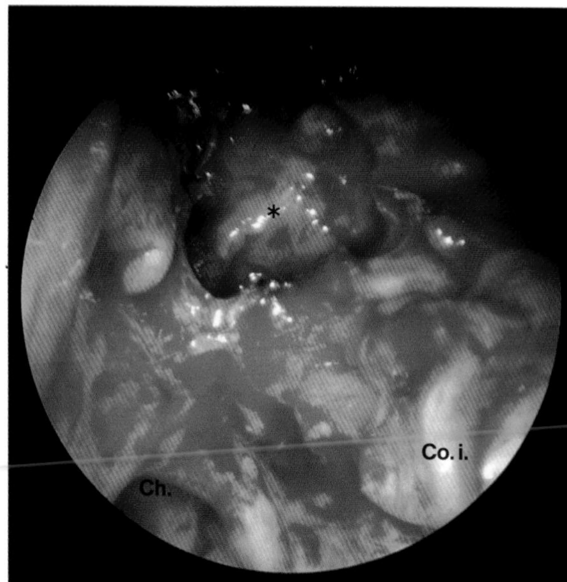

Figure 6.**55** The anterior wall of the left sphenoid sinus has been opened and a view of the roof of the cavity above (*) is shown. The base of the skull is reached in this manner (70° telescope).

level of the roof of the ethmoid sinuses can be deduced from the direction of the easily visible roof of the sphenoid so that resection of the posterior ethmoid cells with a punch can now proceed safely in a posteroanterior direction (Figure 6.**57**). The blunt end of the punch cannot perforate the anterior cranial fossa even if excess pressure is exercised.

First of all, however, some remarks must be made about exposure of the sphenoid cavity behind an unusually well developed ethmoid. The surgeon who is familiar with the anatomical landmarks can open the sphenoid cavity without difficulty once the presence and shape of the cavity have been confirmed by radiography, preferably CT scans.

The anterior wall of the sphenoid sinus is easily exposed by careful removal of the posterior ethmoid cells after resection of the posterior end of the middle turbinate. It is easy to find a thin point using a suction tube, and to break into the sphenoid at this point using gentle pressure.

In other cases the closed pointed Blakesley's (No. 1 or 2) forceps can be used to find the ostium

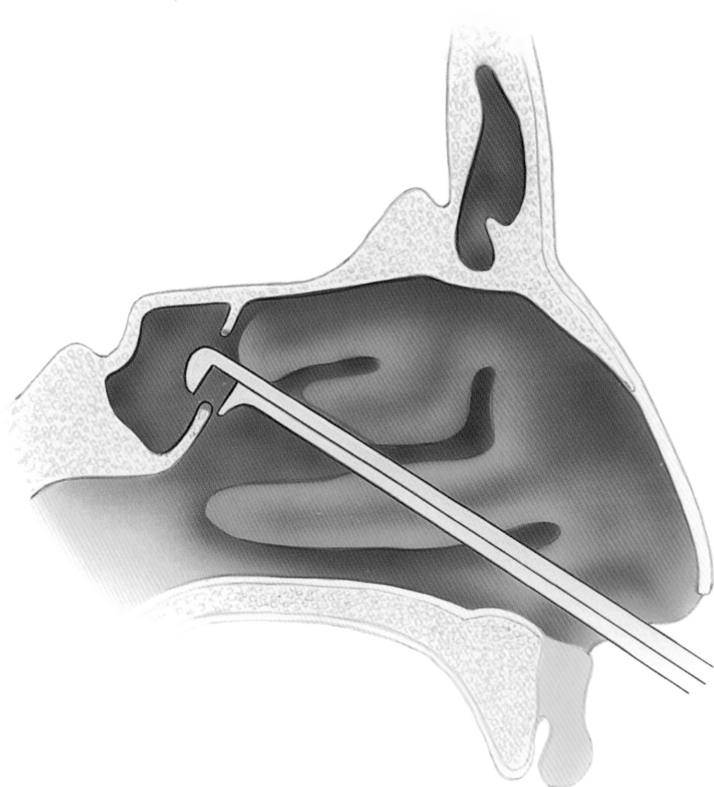

Figure 6.**56** Removal of the anterior wall of the sphenoid sinus by a punch. There is no danger to the optic nerve and the carotid artery, but brisk bleeding from the sphenopalatine artery is frequent.

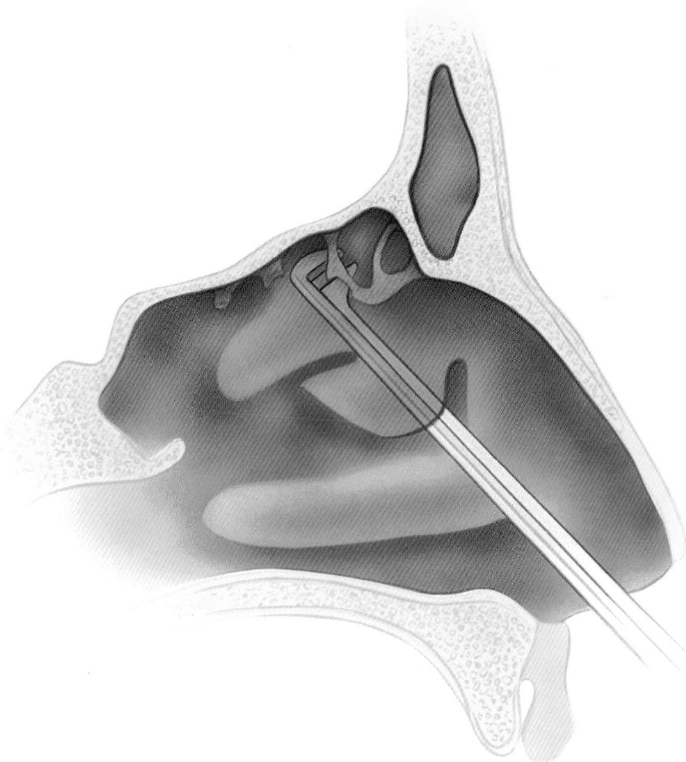

Figure 6.**57** Removal of the ethmoid cell walls in a posteroanterior direction by the punch in complete ethmoidectomy.

and to enlarge it by opening the blades. The position of the sphenoid ostium can be deduced from the relation between the posterior insertion of the middle turbinate and the choana. A point about 5 mm above and 3 mm medial to the attachment of the inferior turbinate usually lies in front of the sphenoid cavity, and at this point the ostium or a semi-transparent bony area can be found marking the underlying cavity (see Figure 6.**54**). Another easy method of finding the point of opening is to introduce a suction tube 10–12 mm above the apex of the choana, then to pass it slowly in a medial direction and finally to push gently in the midline. The wall gives suddenly, and the suction tube then lies within the sphenoid cavity. The Blakesley's forceps is now introduced closed and pulled out again in the open position, producing an opening of sufficient width through which the 45° or 90° forceps can be introduced for *complete removal of the anterior wall of the sphenoid sinus.* Arterial bleeding from the edge of the resection, usually inferolaterally, is dealt with by coagulation or packing.

The patient's eyes and his circulation deserve special attention during all procedures in the posterior part of the ethmoids and the sphenoid cavity. The pupil should be repeatedly inspected to ensure that it is constricted and reacts to light. A reflex mydriasis indicates a functional lesion of vision that resolves spontaneously. The operation should be suspended and an opthalmologist asked to inspect the optic fundi to exclude ischemia of the central artery, indicating thrombosis or even a lesion of the optic nerve. Also an exploratory transethmoid opening of the orbital cavity by resection of the lamina papyracea and longitudinal incision of the orbital periosteum may be indicated in the search for a hematoma either outside or inside the orbital periosteum due to damage to an ethmoid artery which then retracts into the orbit. In the worst cases a transfacial or transfrontal orbitotomy must be carried out. The author has seen reflex transitory mydriasis on two occasions during ethmoid operations; they both resolved without seqeulae within 30 minutes.

Reflex increase in pulse rate and blood pressure during resection of bone in the posterior ethmoid and sphenoid sinus region is quite common. They are harmless but in high-risk patients require attention from the anesthesiologist.

Complete *exposure of the posterior ethmoids* is not always simple. The cell septa are punched out, beginning on the roof of the cavity of the sphenoid sinus and remaining in the same level along the base of the skull in a posteroanterior direction. They are removed with their abnormal contents such as polyps, cysts or pus. Great attention must be paid to complete removal of bony spurs and party walls which encourage the retention of secretions. This removal of the posterior ethmoid cells can often be carried out under direct vision. However, all the cells of the posterior ethmoid, including any lateral processes must be removed so that optical control using an angled telescope is necessary. Others prefer routine use of the operating microscope (Teatini 1982, Draf 1980). The bony party walls should be removed, using sharp punch or forceps, and the cell contents cleared, but the outer wall of the ethmoids should remain covered by mucosa. Unfortunately the mucosa covering the roof and the lateral wall of the ethmoid is often not completely preserved because it is torn by blunt instruments.

Once the posterior ethmoid is opened and hemostasis has been achieved with pledgets soaked in adrenalin, an outstanding view is obtained, facilitating removal of the anterior ethmoid. Before undertaking the next step the topography should be checked again by looking for the upper end of the curved incision through the posterior part of the middle turbinate. This point marks the anterior point of removal of the resected end of the turbinate, and also the posterior point of the main part of the middle turbinate still attached to the base of the skull. The posterior end of the attachement of the medial lamella of the turbinate to the base of the skull is an important landmark indicating the posterior edge of the cribriform plate. The mucosa extending up to this point in the gutter between the nasal septum and the middle turbinate forms the olfactory region and must be preserved at all costs. Olfactory fibers run rostral to this landmark and also within the medial surface of the turbinate; if they are torn, the dural sheaths are split causing a CSF leak.

In contrast, the ethmoid cells behind the insertion of the middle turbinate into the roof of the ethmoid, are roofed by the firm bone of the sphenoid plane, excluding inadvertent perforation with the forceps or punch.

Management of the Middle Turbinate

The middle turbinate is an integral part of the ethmoid cell system forming both a key and an obstruction to complete ethmoidectomy. It may be poorly or well pneumatized, or even expanded due to excessive pneumatization forming a bullous turbinate. If it is affected by polypoid ethmoiditis it must be cleared, producing a cavitation of the turbinate. After scrupulous removal of the cells from the turbinate, sometimes little remains other than a membranous floating medial lamella. In other cases the turbinate is narrow and compact so that it need not be cleared. Often one turbinate obstructs the view of a narrow ethmoid, particularly if the septum is broad. For these reasons, and in the interests of healing and safety, a partial removal of the turbinate should be seriously considered, but sacrifice of tissue should be minimal to prevent unneccessary loss of olfactory mucosa. Objections to resection based on the worsening of the airstream or drying of the nasal mucosa are groundless, even after sub-total resection.

Initially the author carried out a generous resection of the turbinate both for reasons of sefaty and to allow thorough removal of the cells (Wigand 1981), but now practices conservative turbinate resection to preserve the sense of smell. The posterior third is resected to expose the posterior ethmoids in most cases of complete ethmoidectomy for massive polyposis, so that the posterior ethmoids and the sphenoid cavity may be exposed completely, but the main part of the body of the turbinate is preserved. In particular, great care should be exercised to preserve the medial lamella of the turbinate. The extent of anterior partial resection of the turbinate is determined individually by its shape.

If the pneumatization of the turbinate is pronounced (concha bullosa) an initial longitudinal incision with a size 15 scalpel, a fissure knife or bone scissors (Figure 6.**58**) is worthwhile. In this way the medial surface with its fine bony lamella is preserved while the body of the turbinate and its cells can be recognized in steps. If the turbinate is less well pneumatized in its free part but cells are well developed in the upper part then postero-anterior clearance of the middle and anterior ethmoid cells usually suffices.

If the middle turbinate is even better pneumatized with cells extending into its inferior segment close to its edge then all polyps must be removed from the cells of the middle turbinate complex (Figure 6.**59**). Its medial lamella then hangs from a narrow base only, and is even more unstable if the agger nasi is punched out lateral to the anterior area of attachment of the bone to uncover the most anterior ethmoid cells, the agger nasi cells and the frontal duct. In this situation it may be appropriate to cut back as much as fifty percent of the turbinate through a longitudinal curved incision (see Figure

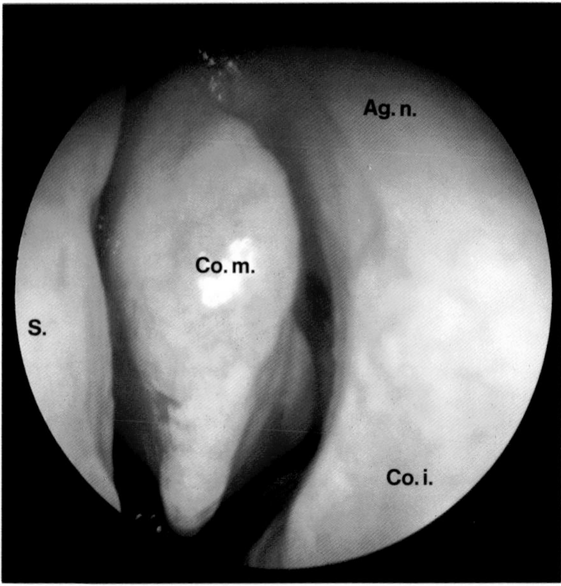

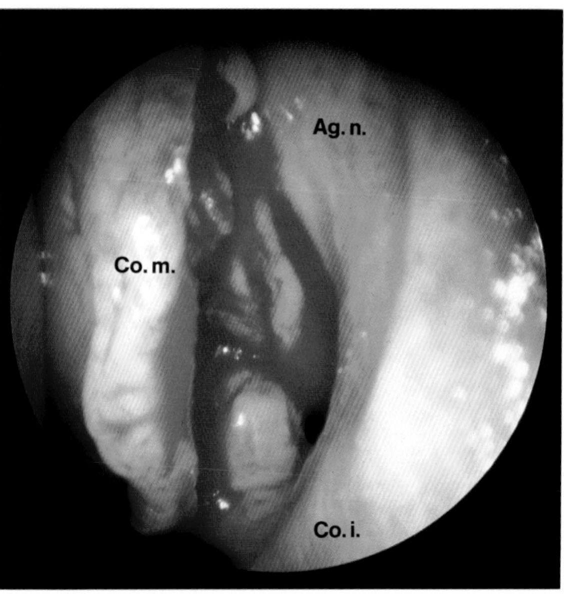

Figure 6.**58** Longitudinal division of the middle turbinate. **a** Dilated head of the anterior end of the turbinate (concha bullosa).

b Preservation of the medial lamella and opening of the polypoid turbinate cells after lateral resection of the turbinate.

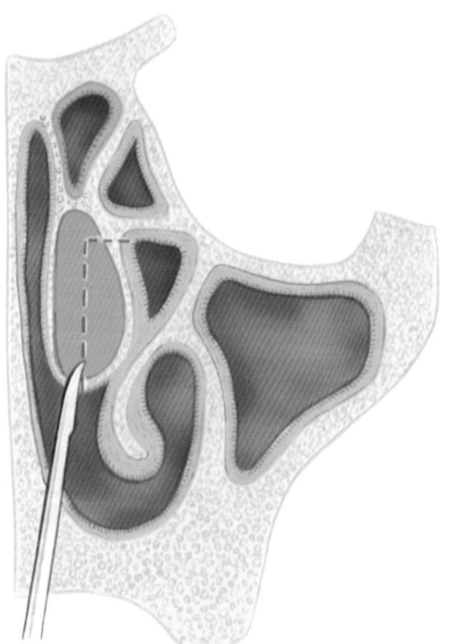

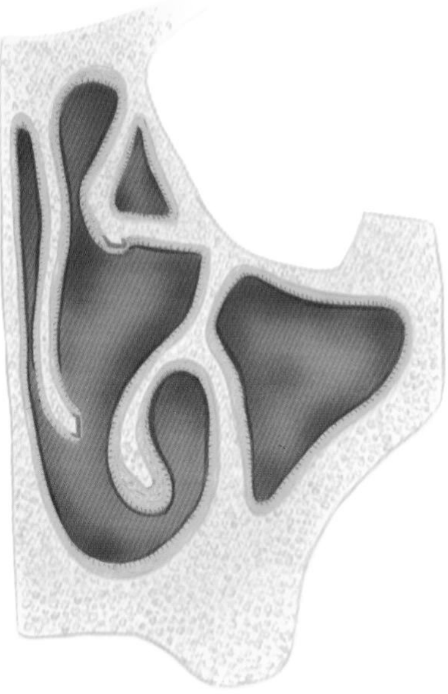

c Resection of the lateral half of a diseased bullous concha. The resection line is shown by a dotted line.

d Status after resection of the lateral part of the diseased bullous concha with restitution of drainage and ventilation.

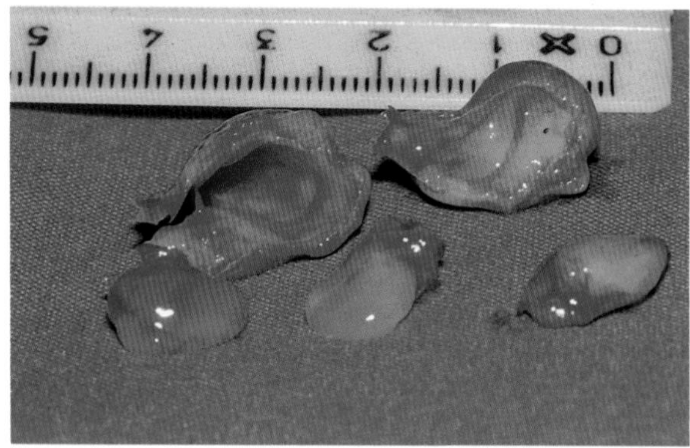

Figure 6.**59** Intraconchal polyps in an inadvertently avulsed middle turbinate.

6.**48**) with no regard for damage to the olfactory function. Personal observations show that normal olfaction is often preserved even if the middle turbinate is lost up to its fixed base. It appears that remnants of the turbinate along with the olfactory area of the septum are able to provide a sense of smell.

A large floating medial lamella of the turbinate can later cause "turbinate flutter" during respiration, and the large wound surface can adhere to the lateral ethmoidal wall. A drop of blood at this narrow point is enough to cause the adhesion. This situation can be managed successfully by folding the floating lamella of the turbinate over to prevent both turbinate flutter and unnecessary loss of valuable olfactory mucosa (Figure 6.**60**). The mucous membrane is folded over to reach the roof of the ethmoid and is fixed with fibrin glue. This type of reconstruction has three advantages: stabilization of the fluttering remnant of the turbinate, patency of the olfactory cleft, and minimizing of the wound surfaces. The frontal duct must not be obstructed by parts of the turbinate.

Dissection of the olfactory cleft requires special attention. One of the main symptoms of chronic sinusitis is loss of the sense of smell, usually due to mechanical obstruction of the olfactory cleft. The sense of smell may return rapidly or gradually after the operation, provided that enough olfactory epithelium remains following restitution of aeration and drainage. It is doubtful whether the olfactory epithelium is capable of regeneration by surface expansion. Therefore great care must be taken, even during minor procedures such as polypectomy, to preserve mucosa on the upper third of the medial lamella of the middle turbinate and on the corresponding surface of the septum, to lacerate as little mucosa as possible and to preserve bone. If ulceration in this region can be prevented, for example by extremely careful diathermy removal of polyps and adhesions under endoscopic control, the prospects of recovery of the sense of smell are good. Unfortunately, repeated extractions of nasal polyps in the doctor's office without correction of the septum and without clear operating conditions often lead to a superficial defect of the turbinate and septum with resulting synechiae of the upper nasal cavity. Many of these patients go through life with no sense of smell.

The middle turbinate may have to be split initially, it may have to be partially resected or it may be left untouched. Which of these is done determines whether dissection of the turbinate follows clearance of the posterior ethmoids or exposure of the middle and anterior ethmoid cells.

Removal of the Middle and Anterior Ethmoid Cells

Then the honeycomb of cells and polyps is removed lateral to the medial lamella of the turbinate preserving the stump of the middle turbinate (which may already have been exposed) or the retained body of the turbinate. The cells are removed with the punch, or opened with a sharp upward-curved forceps and cleared up to the base of the skull. It is useless to plan a previously determined route of removal of named cells tracts. All cells lying between the body of the middle turbinate or its medial lamella and the lateral ethmoid wall (the lamina papyracea) should be broken down gently and removed. The ethmoid gallery is thus cleared between the middle turbinate and the orbital wall as far as the overhang of the agger nasi. An angled telescope must be brought into use at this point for the further rostral part of the procedure. Once again the necessity for care around the point of insertion of the middle turbinate to the skull base is emphasized: a row of olfactory fibers runs through the skull base onto its medial lamella and these can be damaged. Firm resistance during breaking down the party walls of the ethmoid cells or removal of polypoid mucosa may indicate that an olfactory fiber has been grasped in the instrument.

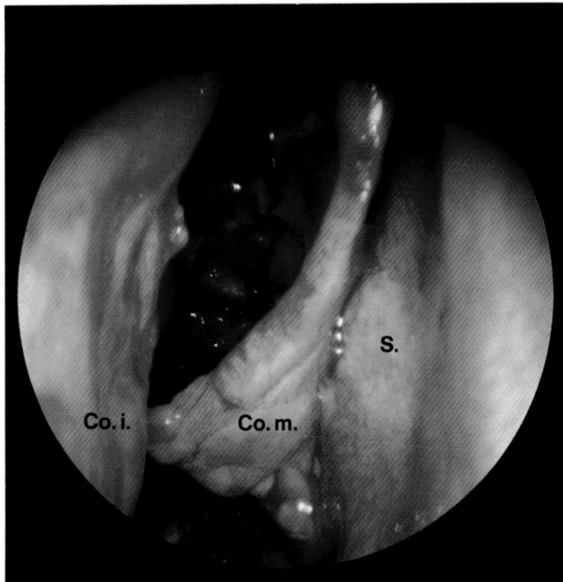

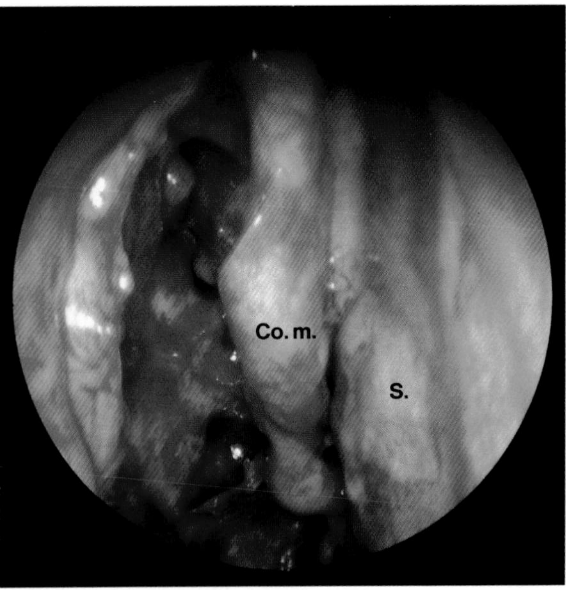

Figure 6.**60** Remodeling of the medial turbinate.
a Only the thin medial lamella remains after clearance of the turbinate cells from the right side of the nasal cavity (70° telescope).

b After careful removal of the medial bony lamella, the mobile mucosal flap developed from the middle turbinate is folded laterally and glued in place. A compact turbinate body is thus attained without loss of the olfactory mucosa, and the olfactory cleft is widened (right nasal cavity 70° telescope).

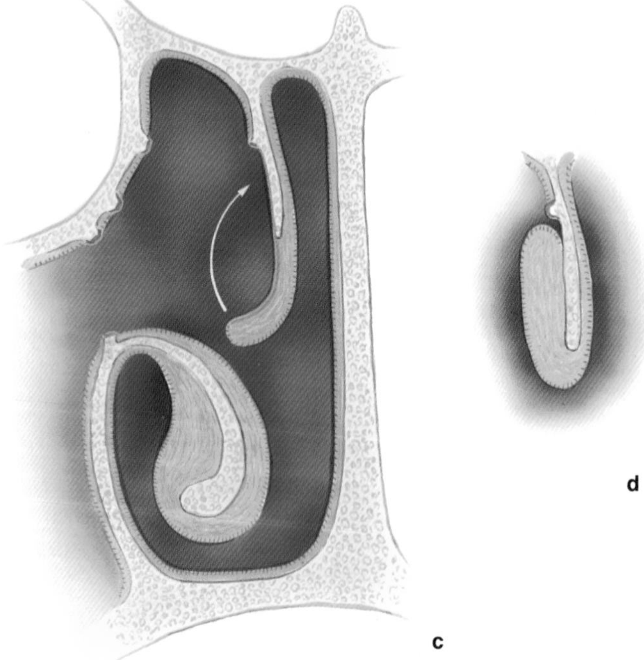

c, d Plastic reconstruction of the middle turbinate.

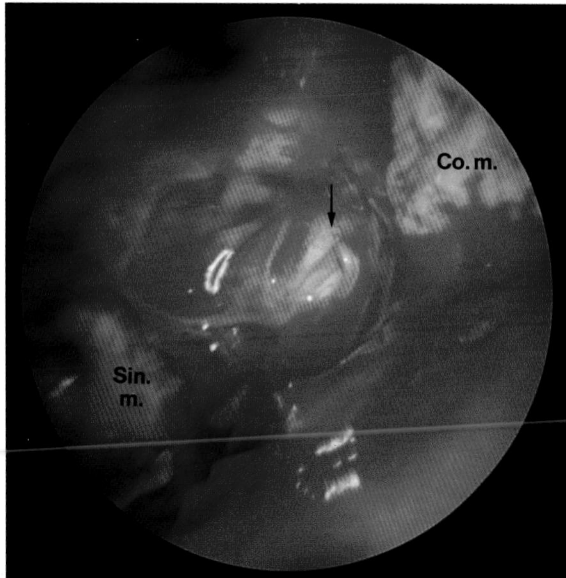

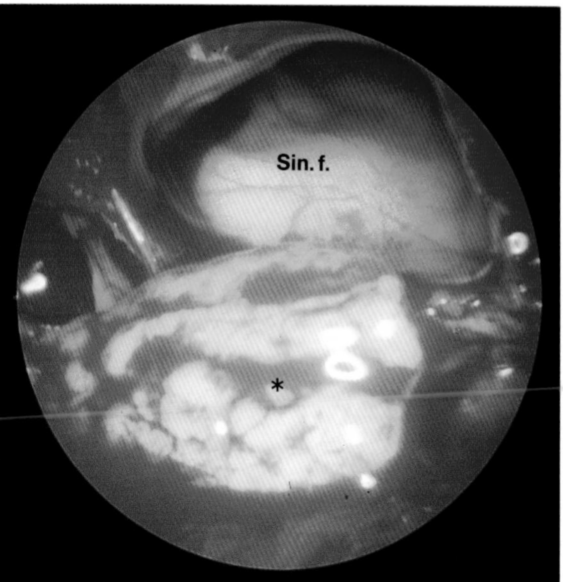

Figure 6.**61** CSF fistula after tearing of an olfactory fiber in the right nasal cavity.
a CSF fistula resulting from a tear of the olfactory mucosa at the upper attachment of the middle turbinate (marked by an arrow). The olfactory fibers are visible.

b Closure of the fistula with a glued mucosal flap from the inferior turbinate (*). The frontal sinusotomy lying anterosuperiorly is seen from below.

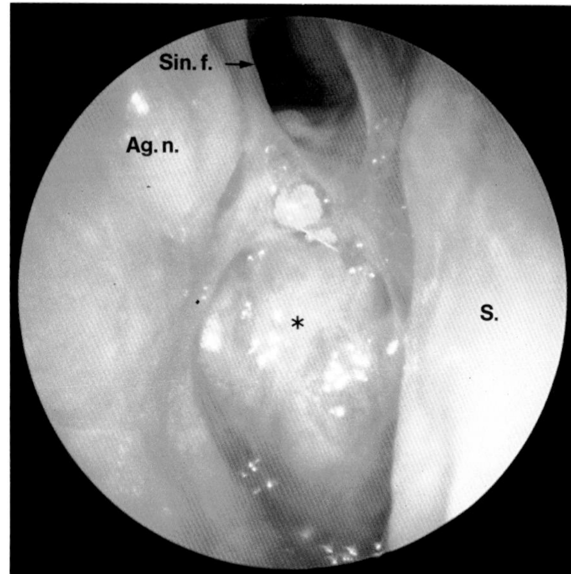

c Healed mucosal graft (*) over the CSF fistula a year later, with a view into the frontal fenestration (70° telescope).

Energetic tearing is always to be avoided as ethmoid cells and their mucosa can almost always be removed without force. A particularly dangerous dural tear may also be signalled by the oozing of dark venous blood.

A *small CSF leak* indicates tearing of an olfactory fiber (Figure 6.**61 a**). The operation should be abandoned, and the fistula closed as follows: firstly it is inspected very carefully with the endoscope, and the integrity of the neighboring bone tested by careful probing with a fine elevator. Mucosal remnants are removed from a surrounding area of 2–3 mm with a small double forceps. An oval mucosal flap is now harvested from the free edge of the inferior turbinate, carefully smoothed on its internal surface, freed of bone, but not overly thinned. This free mucosal graft is fixed over the fistula with a wide overlap using fibrin glue after hemostasis has been achieved (Figure 6.**61 b**). The procedure ends with an endoscopic check and packing, using two layers of moist gelfoam left in place for more than 2 weeks. Under this lies a layer of packing of gauze strips soaked in aureomycin exerting slight upward pressure; it too should be left in place for at least 10 days. The defect should heal within 4 weeks (Figure 6.**61 c**). Small perforations of the anterior base of the skull due to other causes can be managed in a similar manner.

Removal of the most anterior ethmoid cells under direct vision or using the endoscope requires *resection of the agger nasi.* This procedure also plays

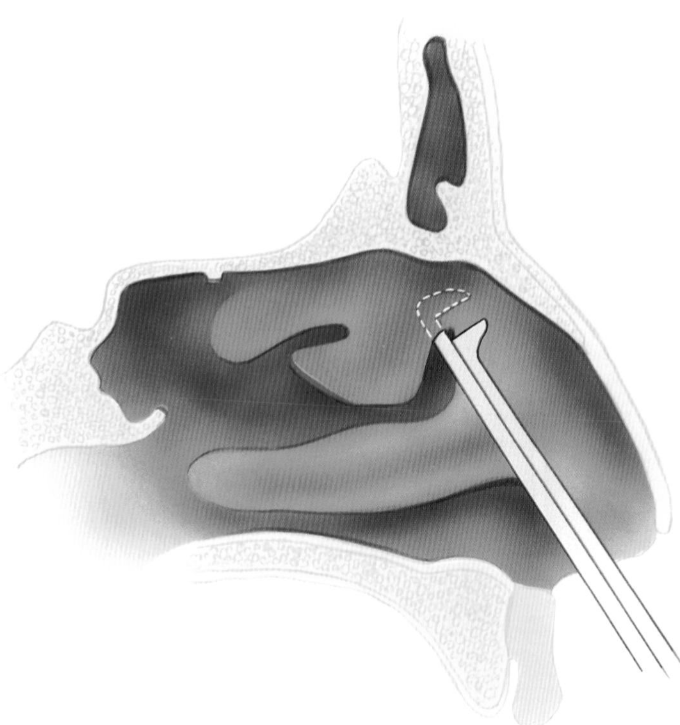

Figure 6.**62** Diagram of the exposure of the anterior ethmoid cells by resection of the agger nasi.

a key role in opening of the frontal sinus and in the prevention of recurrent polyps and cicatricial stenosis, but it destabilizes the middle turbinate whose anterior edge merges into the agger nasi. One jaw of a 90° upward-cutting punch is passed under the bony overhang uniting the most anterior part of the medial lamella and the middle turbinate with the lateral ethmoid wall (Figure 6.**62**). Under it open the agger nasi cells forming part of the most anterior ethmoid cell system, and which are usually affected by diffuse polyposis. This step can easily be done during ethmoidectomy without endoscopic control, but if it is omitted loculated sinuses remain, hindering free drainage from the frontal sinus. On the other hand too aggressive resection of the agger nasi can damage the lacrimal canal running within it.

Complete *exposure of the most anterior ethmoid cells* demands the help of the 70° telescope. The first step is control of the lateral wall of the ethmoid that is tapering both in height and breadth as it runs anteriorly. A specially designed, blunt, 45° upward-cutting ethmoidal forceps is valuable for this step: it must always be introduced parallel to the lamina papyracea. The bony septa inserting perpendicularly into the lamina papyracea can be broken down and the surface smoothed safely by closing its jaws (Figure 6.**63**).

The most anterosuperior part of the ethmoid system is often relatively acellular, and it varies widely in form. Also, a slender upper track of cells sometimes running forwards over the larger cells along the base of the skull can escape the naked eye. Endoscopic inspection is therefore necessary to pick up these small niches and clefts, and to inspect the recesses bulging laterally into the orbit.

Complete removal of mucosal polyps from the lateral anterior ethmoid cell systems is particularly important in massive polyposis, because recurrence can easily arise from remnants which are readily overlooked at this point. Small paraturbinate cells or recesses of the ethmoid are occasionally found during antrostomy even lying lateral to the insertion of the middle turbinate, and they can be the source of recurrence.

With the angular telescope it is always easy to see the transverse bar housing the ethmoid artery in the anterior part of the ethmoid roof (Figure 6.**64**). This bulge is an important landmark forming the boundary between the danger area of the ethmoid containing olfactory fibers, and the ascending part of the ethmoid roof or the posterior wall of the frontal infundibulum lying a few millimeters in front of the bar. The two are usually separated by only one cell.

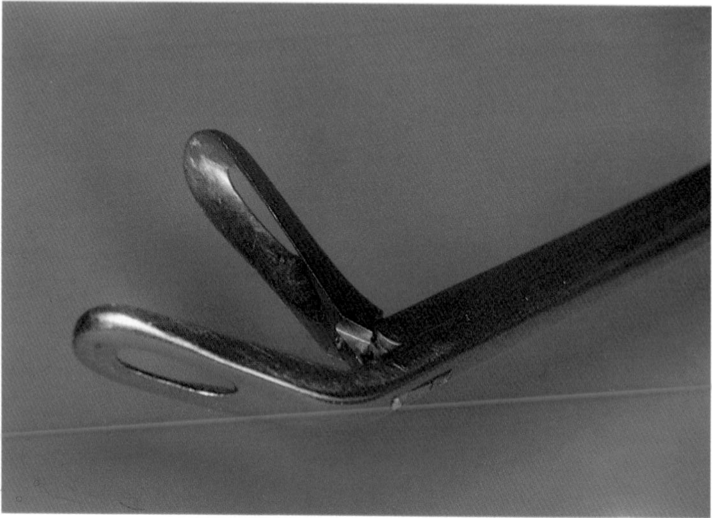

Figure 6.**63** The 45° upward-curved blunt ethmoid forceps is very suitable for the safe exenteration of the middle and anterior ethmoid cells.

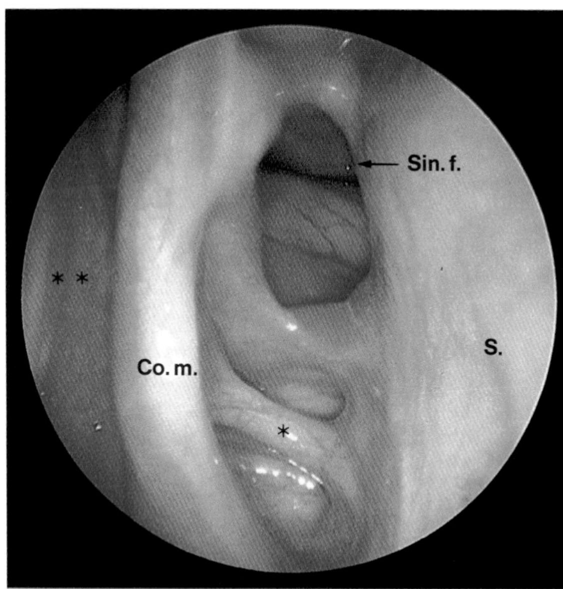

Figure 6.**64** Exenterated and healed left ethmoid sinuses with the anterior ethmoid artery running transversely in a thin bony shell (*). The frontal sinus has been widely fenestrated from below and can be seen opening anterosuperiorly. The olfactory cleft (**) and the medial lamella of the middle turbinate can be seen on the left-hand side of the picture (70° telescope).

If the artery has been damaged with the punch, the bleeding can be controlled quite easily using bipolar coagulation, but the arterial stump can retract into the orbit causing a massive extra- or subperiosteal hematoma, leading to exophthalmos or even blindness caused by compression of the optic nerve. Swelling or hematoma of the eyelids are harmless; they are treated by ice packs, but immotility of the eyeball, mydriasis or an absent light reflex demand the emergency measures already described (see page 104).

If *the orbital periosteum* is breached allowing orbital fat to enter the nasal cavity, the protruding tissue is replaced and possibly scarified using bipolar coagulation. This procedure should of course be used only for small defects. For added safety a small piece of lyophilized dura can be fixed over the defect with fibrin glue.

The above description of complete ethmoidectomy applies to polypoid pansinusitis, the most frequent indication. In consequence, it must be emphasized that *free drainage of the frontal duct* should also be secured. In most cases the ostium of the nasofrontal duct (Figure 6.**43 b**), or even a wide frontal infundibulum, opens up automatically after removal of the most anterior party walls of the ethmoids. If the duct will accept a curved size 17, or even better a size 18, suction tube, then further procedures can be omitted. The frontal sinus will heal provided that the duct is kept patent by careful aftercare. A narrow frontonasal duct may be adequate in the absence of disease. If it is inadequate to guarantee permanent aeration of the frontal sinus an intranasal frontal sinusotomy should be carried out (pages 121 ff.). In most cases widening of the narrow but visible frontal ducts by curettage directed anteriorly suffices. In other cases a wide connection to the frontal sinus is created by resection of the dividing wall between the most anterior ethmoid cells and the frontal infundibulum.

In massive polypoid pansinusitis it has proved appropriate to follow intranasal endoscopic pansinus operations by the appropriate antral procedure, once the ethmoid compartment has been attended to. Manipulation of sharp-angled instruments within the antrum via the middle meatus is considerably easier once the middle turbinate and the agger nasi have been partially resected. The severity of the disease of the maxillary mucosa does not always mirror that of the ethmoids, so that a middle meatal antrostomy, possibly even with preservation of the primary maxillary ostium, may suffice despite the need for a complete ethmoidectomy. However, in many cases the antral mucosa, too, is severely diseased with numerous polyps and thick retention cysts requiring wide resection. In this case a small window is inadequate, and the medial meatal antrostomy should be extended over the entire uncinate process, and the shape of the window must be adapted to the needs of manipulation of instruments on the floor of the antrum. Occasionally it may even be necessary to create a second, inferior, meatal antrostomy.

Anterior extension of a middle meatal antrostomy and particularly of an inferior meatal antrostomy can expose and damage the lacrimal canal, although this accident is often without sequelae.

At the end of the pansinus operation the nasal cavity and the ethmoid compartment are packed loosely for 2 days, and a breathing tube is left in place (see Figure 4.**12**).

Revision Operations on the Ethmoid

If the patient has had a previous partial or complete ethmoidectomy by either the intranasal, external or transmaxillary route, a second procedure is more difficult due to the scarring of the bony framework, and sheets of scar tissue within the cells rendering orientation and safe surgery much more difficult. Sadly, revision operations are quite often necessary but are difficult to carry out by the intranasal route if the patient has previously undergone a transfrontal procedure in which the cell tracts in the fronto-ethmoidal junction have been destroyed. Similarly a functional antro-ethmoidal procedure with mucosal preservation is often difficult and disappointing after a previous Caldwell-Luc transoral procedure because the cavities are no longer lined with mucosa capable of regeneration. There is therefore a danger of creation of lining of scar tissue arising from granulation tissue sprouting from the wound surfaces.

However, in such cases clinical examination and imaging may suggest that removal of mucosal scars or opening of loculated residual cells are indicated and an intranasal revision procedure should be tried before re-exposing the ethmoids through an external facial incision. The systematic series of steps described above is advisable: that is the examination of the posterior ethmoid and the sphenoid sinus, inspection of the ethmoid roof posteroanteriorly along the now visible base of the skull, re-exposure of the most anterior part of the ethmoid region as far as the opening of the frontal sinus, and revision of the antrostomy.

The main reasons for secondary obstruction of the frontal sinus include firstly, scar tissue obliteration of the narrow ethmoid gutter between the insertion of the middle turbinate and the lamina papyracea, and secondly prior inadequate excision of the agger nasi. The symptoms include frontal headache, a feeling of pressure in the medial canthus, and the symptoms of sinusitis and recurrent bronchitis in addition. There is no golden rule for sharp dissection and removal of the sheets of scar tissue and synechiae (Figure 6.**65**). The choice of sharp instruments such as double forceps, curettes, pointed punches, etc., must be determined by the experience of the surgeon and the local situation. It must always be borne in mind that removal of tissue creates a wound surface which will form further scar tissue, unlike the first operation which preserves at least some of the mucosa. In recent years the author has preferred the argon laser or diathermy for revision surgery, and has found that excessive granulations to reccurent scar tissue are less common, particularly after laser coagulation of cicatricial bands in the antrostomy opening. In contrast the introduction of spacers such as silicon tubes or sheet has not so far proved of value.

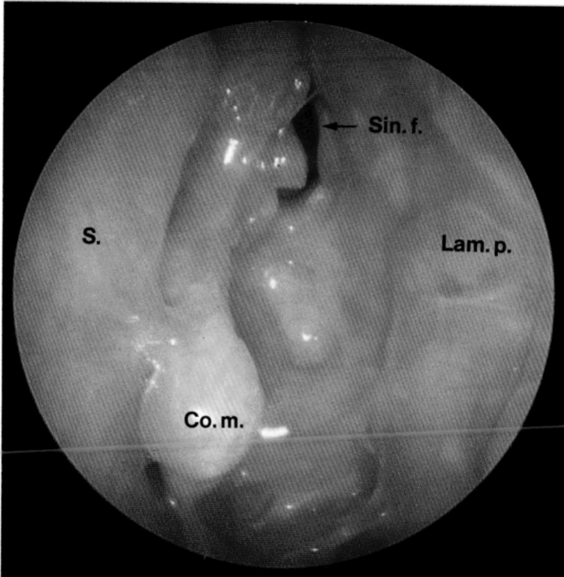

Figure 6.**65** A scarred left ethmoid after a previous operation. Wide synechiae run between the middle turbinate and the septum, and there are residual cells and polyps. In front lies the opening into the frontal sinus (70° telescope).

Ethmoidectomy in Children

Like antral operations in infancy, ethmoidectomy in children demands a conservative policy. Complete ethmoidectomy at this age is as technically possible as in the adult, and the smaller dimensions are no hindrance if fine instruments are used. The indications are limited, however, by the necessity for simultaneous mobilization of the septum which is possible but not without problems, and by intolerance to endoscopic aftercare.

If partial or complete ethmoidectomy is indicated for severe bronchial asthma, mucovicidosis, etc., good pediatric support must be ensured, and the parents must understand that the prognosis is dubious, and that one or more endoscopic examinations under general anesthesia will be required during follow-up.

The technique follows that already described for adults, but the prospect of recovery of hyperplastic polypoid or cystic lesions is better than in adults. Therefore the author would always first of all try a minor procedure limited to the middle meatus: polyps narrowing the nasal lumen or choana should be removed carefully without damaging the mucosa of the turbinates or nasal walls. The middle turbinate is displaced, the middle meatus is exposed, and an extremely careful exenteration undertaken. A hiatatotomy alone or a limited infundibulotomy, with or without middle meatal antrostomy, can suffice, or at least gain an interval of up to 3 years after which time an ethmoidectomy may be carried out. The danger of synechiae is particularly high because of the small dimensions of the ethmoids. The author is particularly opposed to the sloppy technique of indiscriminate breaking down of the ethmoidal cells.

Applications

Chronic Ethmoiditis

The decision to carry out an ethmoidal operation for chronic sinusitis must always be weighed carefully.

The indications for surgery for mucosal hyperplasia of the ethmoids demonstrated by tomography or CT scans, and particularly for endoscopically confirmed polyposis include:

- failed conservative treatment of nasal obstruction, mucosal swelling, headache, postnasal drip, dysosmia, pharyngitis and laryngitis,
- recurrent episodes of sinobronchitis complicated of bronchospasm or even established asthma; in recent years ethmoidectomy has proved to be useful for severe inflammation of the bronchial mucosa in mucoviscidosis,
- secondary ear disease such as tubal catarrh, chronic otitis media, particularly as a prelude to tympanoplasty, but also for fluctuating, progressive and otherwise unexplained sensorineural deafness,
- an inflammatory focus associated with a proved chronic ethmoiditis.

An endoscopic ethmoidectomy is contraindicated:

- if operative complications or an inadequate procedure are likely due to the surgeon's lack of experience; no operation at all is better than an unsuitable operation,
- if the patient cannot tolerate endoscopic aftercare, which is particularly true of children, oversensitive and frail patients. If the pediatrician or the internist has referred the patient for clearance of a septic focus, aftercare may require repeated general anesthesia.

The planning of the operation is determined mainly by the findings on CT scan, which may suggest partial removal of the anterior ethmoid cells or demand complete ethmoidectomy, particularly for anatomical anomalies such as aberrant cells, a low-lying ethmoid plate, etc. When talking to the patient before operation the surgeon should always keep his options open, and explain that external incision may be found to be necessary during the operation. This is particularly true of *unilateral ethmoiditis* which is unusual and which must always be suspected of concealing an inverted papilloma or even a carcinoma. In the author's material unilateral polyposis of the nasal cavity was found in 8.5% of cases whereas unilateral ethmoiditis was disclosed by radiology in only 3.3%.

The operative technique for chronic inflammation follows the guidelines already described. The view may be made worse by brisk bleeding from a highly inflamed mucosa, by arterial hypertension, by scar tissue due to a previous operation or by a septum which has been previously subjected to an inadequate operation. Repeated removal of nasal polyps is very unfavorable for the healing of the ethmoid and olfactory cleft, and damage to the septal mucosa all too often leads to adhesions between the septum and the middle turbinate. Local hemostasis using adrenalin or cocaine is very useful. Thick plates of scar tissue lying close to the dura or the orbit can occasionally indicate that the limits of operability by the intranasal route have been reached. If it is still possible to obtain a straight view into the sinus the use of an operating microscope may be helpful.

Complications of Inflammatory Disease

The categorical statement in textbooks and surgical atlases that external radical frontal and ethmoid operations are required for rhinogenic complications deserves revision.

An increasing proportion of patients with inflammatory complications of ethmoiditis requiring drainage of pus, or relief of an infective focus, can be treated by intranasal ethmoidectomy. The indications include pyoceles arising from the anterior ethmoid cells, inflammation extending to the lacrimal pathways, and subperiosteal orbital cellulitis or abscess. Osteitis of the maxilla, too, can be treated effectively by this method. The most important principle is complete endoscopic removal of the diseased ethmoid cells, wide marsupialization of a pyocele from within (Figure 6.**66**), or generous slitting of the orbital periosteum of the endoscopically visible and palpable swelling of the medial wall of the orbit. Careful drainage of the orbit with slender drains can even be achieved in this manner.

The CT scan in Figure 6.**66 a** shows expansion of the left antroethmoidal region by a large pyocele displacing the orbital contents upwards and laterally and causing double vision. It arose from mucosa entrapped at a transoral radical antrostomy with partial transmaxillary ethmoidectomy 12 years previously. The inferior meatal antrostomy had closed by scar tissue. Simple marsupialization of the mucocele into the middle meatus and exenteration of the remaining neighboring ethmoid cells led to healing of the antral lumen and the orbital contents within a few weeks. The vision returned to normal and the pain resolved immediately after release of the pressure. Figure 6.**66 b** shows a CT scan taken later, and Figure 6.**66 c** shows the noninflamed antral mucosa through the large, newly created middle meatal antrostomy.

Ethmoid inflammation spreading to the orbit is a particularly suitable indication for complete intranasal ethmoidectomy. A deep-seated orbital abscess, shown by imaging, requires a wide orbitotomy via an external facial or frontal approach, whereas an abscess in the ethmoid area can be drained intranasally. Even osteitis arising from the ethmoid and presenting externally, and meningitis in the absence of an abscess can be healed by endoscopic ethmoidectomy supplemented by antibiotics and intensive postoperative care.

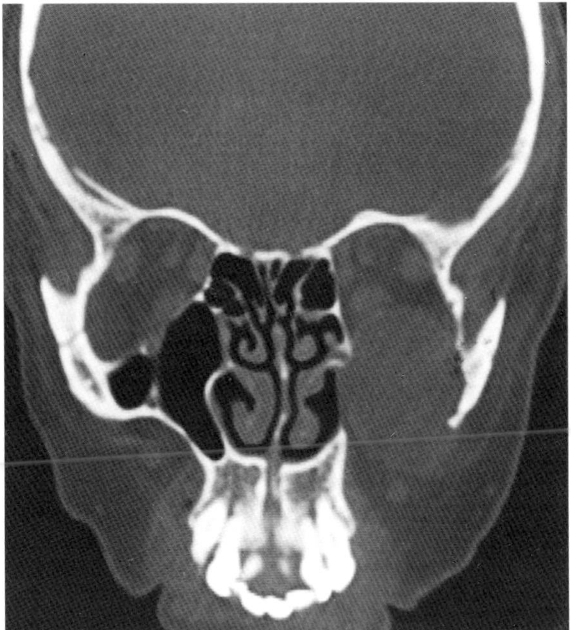

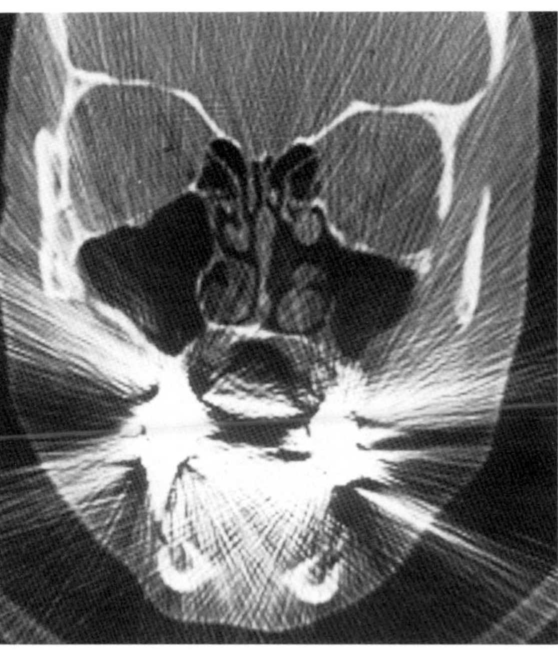

Figure 6.**66** Endoscopic management of a large left-sided antroethmoid mucopyocele. **a** CT scan showing displacement of the antral roof superiorly with the compression of the orbital contents.

b CT scan after marsupialization of the mucocele by the transethmoidal route via the middle nasal meatus.

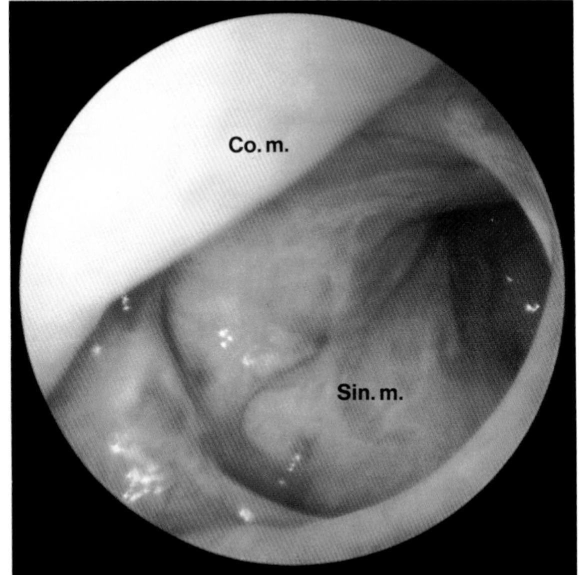

c Endoscopy of the treated mucocele via the middle meatal antrostomy (70° telescope).

Ethmoid Tumors

Benign ethmoid tumors and early localized malignant tumors can be controlled by an intranasal ethmoid procedure under endoscopic vision. An attempt at complete removal by this route is justifiable if the limits of the tumor have been defined by tomography and invasion through the roof of the ethmoids has been exluded. Specimens should be taken for histology from the wound edges to ensure complete excision of papillomas und small carcinomas. However, if the roof of the ethmoids, the septum or the orbital periosteum are invaded, an extensive external procedure must be undertaken. For large squamous carcinomas, adenoid cystic carcinomas or esthesioneuroblastomas, intranasal access may play a part in providing an inferior counter access in a combined transfrontal neurosurgical–rhinological procedure, whereas an intranasal operation alone is not to be recommended for this group.

The exposure of an *ethmoid osteoma* (Figure 6.**67 a, b**) is very simple. Since the ethmoid cells are usually not infected, only limited resection is needed, and in particular the medial wall of the middle turbinate should be completely preserved. The tumor is completely exposed by opening the ethmoid bulla, and by piecemeal removal of the overlying cells (Figure 6.**68**). If it is large or wedged by lateral processes, it can be broken up *in situ* with the diamond burr before removing it. Even an osteoma with a wide

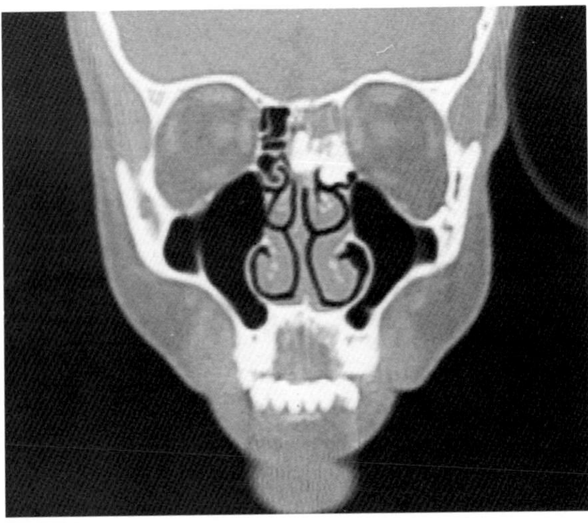

Figure 6.**67** Ethmoid osteoma. **a** CT scan before operation.

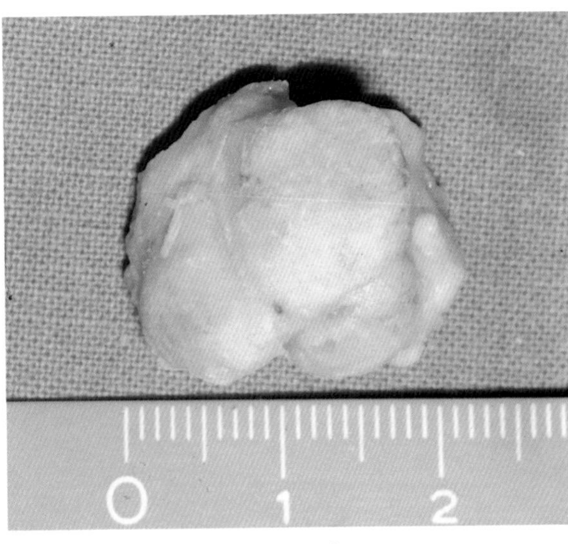

b The osteoma removed by endoscopy.

intraorbital extension can be removed in this way (Figure 6.**67 b**). The wound surface can be relied upon to re-epithelialize spontaneously because the healthy mucosa is mostly preserved.

Other benign tumors of the ethmoids are unusual, the commonest being a neurinoma. Its point of origin cannot always be defined because this tumor is often quite large before it is diagnosed due to the non-specific symptoms. If the tumor is shown by CT scan to be limited and biopsy confirms its benign nature, intranasal endoscopic removal via a limited ethmoid resection can be successful. Figure 6.**69 a–c** shows an example of a well demarcated neurinoma that was permanently controlled by subtotal resection of the middle turbinate with exenteration of the neighboring ethmoids. The differential diagnosis includes fibroma and adenoma. These must not be confused with a meningocele of the ethmoid requiring an external incision because of the accompanying defect of the base of the skull. Lymphomas are usually treated by a combination of chemotherapy and radiotherapy.

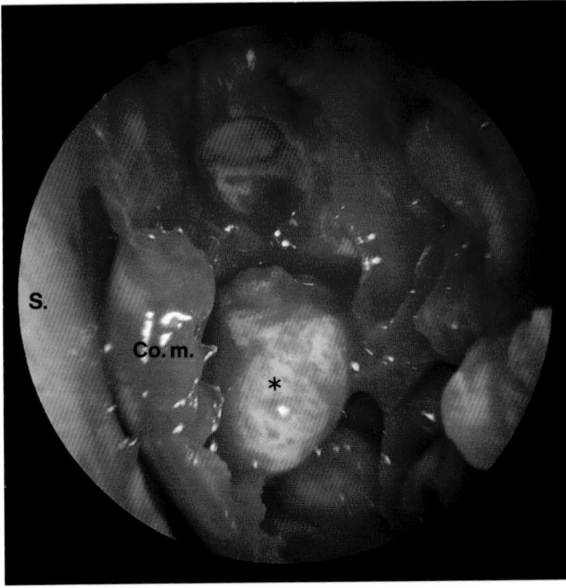

Figure 6.**68** Exposure of an ethmoid osteoma (*) by intranasal partial ethmoidectomy. The left ethmoid has been opened (70° telescope).

Inverted papillomas and small carcinomas arising from the middle meatus can be controlled by complete resection of the middle turbinate. Tissue from the neighboring cells must be submitted for histology to confirm complete excision. Ethmoid papillomas can be equally well controlled by an intranasal procedure as by the external route. Often they arise at the maxillo-ethmoidal junctional zone and extend to the antrum. Even with the endoscope it is not always possible to know whether the polypoid tissue is of a nonspecific inflammatory nature or neoplastic, so that a generous ethmoid resection should be carried out with painstaking geometrical

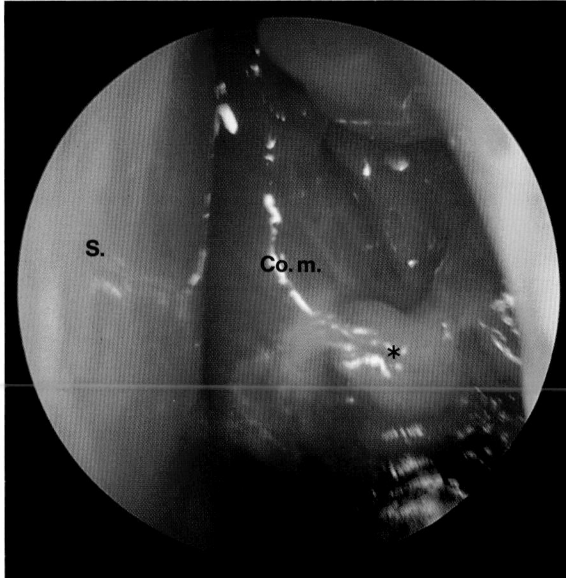

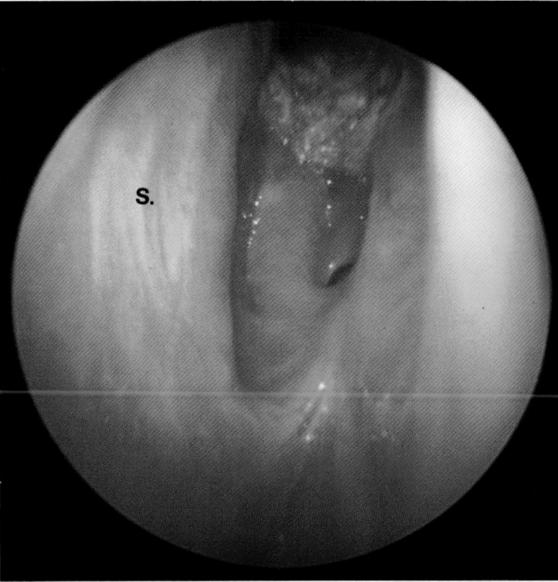

Figure 6.**69** Neurinoma of the left ethmoid. **a** Preoperative endoscopy showing a broad-based tumor (*) arising from the middle turbinate.

b Endoscopic view 2 years after intranasal removal with resection of the turbinate (70° telescope).

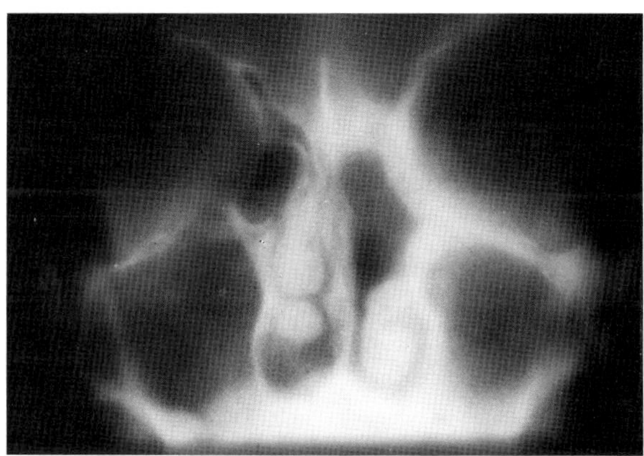

c Tomography 2 years after the operation.

removal of tissue followed by histological examination of several identified specimens. In addition to removing the mucosa completely in suspect areas, the bone should be removed with the diamond burr, using a drill with a slender shaft under endoscopic control. If the tumor extends into the antral cavity an inferior meatal antrostomy or an antrostomy through the canine fossa has proved valuable for the introduction of the drill. The drill is monitored with an endoscope introduced through the middle meatus. Cooling with physiological saline solution is difficult if the drill lacks an attached nozzle. Healing of the bone may take several months, and must be followed by endoscopy. The danger of histological misdiagnosis is very great for tumors of the nose and sinuses. Chondrosarcomas, rhabdomyosarcomas, esthesioneuroblastomas and malignant vascular tumors often demand extensive special investigation. Since they frequently extend beyond the limits of the ethmoid, they are usually not suitable for an intranasal operation.

Ethmoidectomy for Access

Intranasal endoscopic ethmoidectomy is being used with increasing frequency for access to the pituitary gland, the sphenoid sinus, the optic nerves, the lacrimal pathways and the frontal sinus. Wide experience with ethmoidectomy for chronic sinusitis is necessary before embarking upon this development in base-of-skull surgery. An experienced surgeon should be able to undertake the exposure for these specific procedures using this elegant and atraumatic technique, with the help of a microscope and an angled telescope, without reducing the efficacy of the procedure.

Internal Dacryocystorhinostomy*

M. Weidenbecher

Only a few years after Toti (1904) described external dacryocystotomy through the medial canthus, West (1911) and Polyak (1913) published a procedure for intranasal opening of the lacrimal sac. At present this operation is usually carried out by the rhinologist, with the help of an endoscope or the microscope. Compared with the external method it has two advantages: good cosmesis because there is no incision in the medial canthus, and preservation of the lacrimal apparatus. Restricted vision is a potential disadvantage, but is easily overcome with experience.

Indications for Internal Dacryocystorhinostomy

This intranasal procedure is suitable for:

- intrasaccal and postsaccal stenosis of the lacrimal ducts,
- reoperation after Toti's procedure.

Etiology of Stenosis of the Lacrimal Ducts

Narrowing of the lacrimal pathways can be caused by:

- recurrent inflammation of the ducts,
- repeated probing of the ducts,
- transmaxillary and, rarely, intranasal operations on the antrum,
- trauma to the base of the skull (impaling injuries, fractures of the lacrimal bone, Le Fort-II- and III-fractures),
- rhinoplasty,
- telecobalt irradiation causing fibrosis of the lacrimal ducts,
- tumors of the nasal cavity.

Operative technique

The operation can be carried out under either general endotracheal or local anesthesia. Visualization is improved by decongestion of the nasal turbinates and resection of a high septal deviation. A vertical mucosal incision is made with a fissure knife about 1.5 cm long over the frontàl process of the maxilla, above the anterior end of the inferior turbinate, in front of the anterior end of the middle turbinate, and about 1 cm behind the piriform aperture. A second incision is made parallel to this lying 2 cm further posteriorly (Figure 6.**70**). The mucosa is raised using an elevator and excised with a small curved conchotomy scissors. Irregular edges are straightened with the conchotome. A 15 × 20 mm mucosal defect is thus created on the lateral nasal wall (Figure 6.**71**). A septal chisel is used to create a 8 × 16 mm defect in the frontal process of the maxilla lying over the lacrimal sac (Figure 6.**72**). Since the upper edge of the lacrimal fossa is closely related to the anterior ethmoid cells, the latter may be inadvertantly opened, and must then be carefully removed. An assistant introduces a probe through the inferior lacrimal punctum, and pushes the medial wall of the lacrimal sac into the nasal lumen using the probe. Using a specially curved sickle knife as employed in ear surgery, with an irrigation-suction telescope in his left hand, the surgeon cuts the medial wall of the lacrimal sac in its entire extent. Draf (1982) has described the formation of flaps from the edges of the lacrimal sac; these flaps are then reflected and fixed with fibrin glue. However, the author regards these flaps as being unnecessary, and in any case they are usually not practicable because oft the restricted field. The excellent illumination of the surgical field provided by the endoscope allows precise surgery to be carried out so that the entire medial surface of the sac can be resected, thus largely preventing restenosis. It is advisable to intubate both canaliculae into the nasal cavity for 6 weeks to guarantee a good result. Further irrigation of the lacrimal ducts during this period is unnecessary. Loose nasal packing for 2 days reduces the risk of postoperative bleeding.

The results of this operation should not be assessed for a least a year, but personal experience and the literature show that the results are at least as good as those achieved by an external procedure, and are satisfactory in 75–80% of cases.

* Intranasal endoscopic dacryocystorhinostomy has become established as a routine in the eye and ear clinics in Erlangen. The author is particularly grateful to Prof. Dr. G.O.H. Naumann, Director of the Ophthalmological Clinic of the University of Erlangen–Nürnberg for sympathetic and fruitful cooperation.

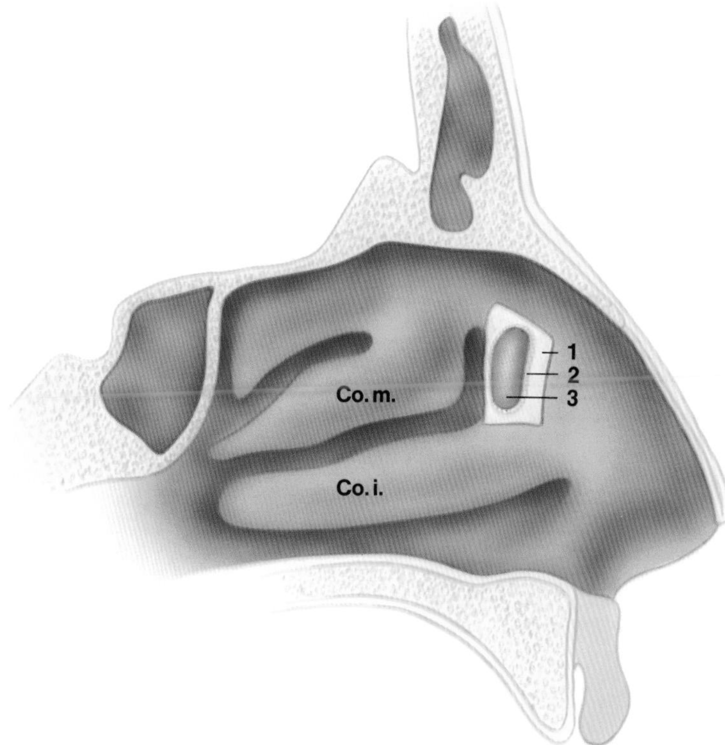

Figure 6.**70** Diagram of internal dacryocystorhinostomy: 1, mucosal defect, 2, bony window, 3, lacrimal sac.

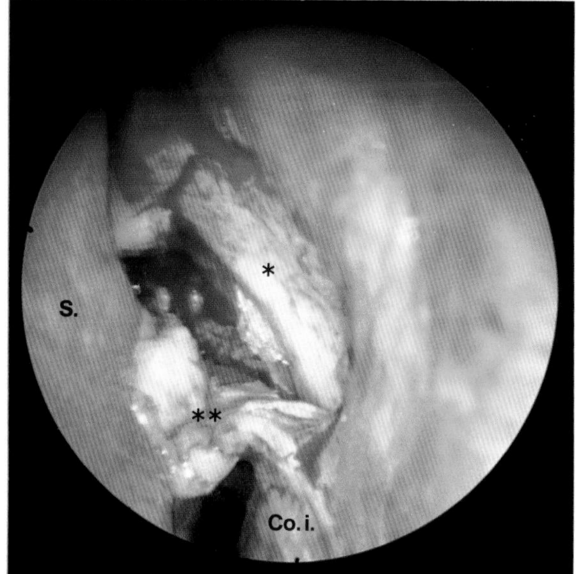

Figure 6.**71** The left lateral nasal wall (* frontal process of the maxilla) has been exposed, the mucosal flaps (**) dissected inferiorly and reflected.

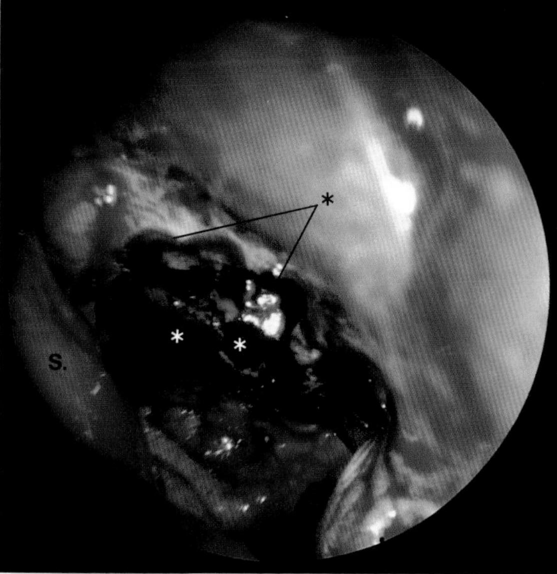

Figure 6.**72** Mucosa and bone over the left lacrimal sac have been removed (* edge of the bony window). The lacrimal sac (**) is filled with methylene blue.

Operations on the Frontal Sinus

Indications

- recurrent empyema of the frontal sinus,
- chronic frontal sinusitis,
- partial operations for diffuse hyperplastic pansinusitis,
- muco- and pyoceles,
- biopsy,
- small benign tumors,
- foreign bodies.

Principles

The goal of the operation is the removal of circumscribed pathological changes with preservation of mucosa and thus of mucociliary transport, and without extensive destruction of the bony walls of the sinus. The following are available:

- endoscopic, limited opening of the frontal sinus from below (widening of the fronto-ethmoidal junction zone),
- endoscopic monitoring of intracavity manipulations through an external bore hole,
- a limited external frontal sinus procedure using the endoscope and plastic repair of the small defect in the anterior wall of the frontal sinus, with preservation of the bony framework. If necessary a mucocele is marsupialized and tumors are reduced in size within the cavity before removal. Treatment of complications by conservative surgery is still developing, and demands intensive postoperative care.

Operative Technique

Preliminary Observations

The restricted access to the often extensive and recessed frontal sinus limits *intranasal sinus surgery*. Whereas the view into all recesses may be satisfactory for diagnostic purposes, many therapeutic manipulations are ill advised because the necessary instruments cannot be monitored endoscopically.

However, much can be achieved, contrary to what might be expected, including the generous transnasal fenestration of the floor of the frontal sinus which suffices for the treatment of most cases of sinusitis when combined with circumscribed dissection of the frontal infundibulum. Many other problems such as stenosis, foreign bodies and occasionally mucopyoceles, can be tackled if this procedure is combined with a small transfrontal portal to allow the introduction of an endoscope or instruments. When choosing between a transfacial or intranasal procedure the safety of the patient is more important than avoiding a facial scar.

Exposure of the Frontal Infundibulum

The prerequisite for endoscopic exposure of the frontal sinus from the nose is removal of the anterior part of the ethmoid area as far as the base of the skull. If the most anterior ethmoid cells have been opened intranasally during an anterior ethmoidectomy the blunt probe usually glides smoothly into the frontal infundibulum. The use of force and of pointed bougies is dangerous. An endoscope with an angled telescope should be used to expose the anterior ethmoid.

Bony overhangs, coarse mucosal tags and polyps interfering with the view into the frontal duct should be removed under vision (see Figure 6.**43 a**). These obstacles are often not present, so that removal of the most anterior cells leads directly into the frontal sinus. In those cases with a well developed cell system, the frontal duct can be easily widened to a diameter of 4–5 mm by removing small remaining septa with the punch. This step improves the prospects of healing of chronic sinusitis and prevents obstruction by scar tissue. If a curved suction tube 4 mm in diameter passes without resistance the frontal duct will usually be found to be wide enough. The resulting opening suffices for suction of thickened secretion and for the removal of polyps or cysts with the curved forceps. Further procedures are unnecessary even if the mucosa is thickened and humped because of the excellent recuperative capacity of the frontal sinus mucosa.

Care must be exercised when tearing off mucosal tags, because resulting reparative granulation tissue can lead to the formation of cicatricial stenosis. On no account must the mucosa around the entire circumference be damaged because this leads to a ring of scar tissue.

If the endoscope does *not* enter the frontal sinus and the anterior ethmoid cells apparently end blindly, or if only a narrow nasofrontal duct is visible, fenestration of the floor of the frontal sinus may be indicated, but the author usually omits this extension of the procedure if the ethmoiditis is not extensive, and radiography has shown good aeration of the frontal sinus with no mucosal swelling. On the other hand sinusotomy should be carried out for massive polyposis with an absent view into the frontal sinus indicating a disorder of drainage and aeration of the sinus. It is likewise indicated for the fenestration of frontal mucoceles.

Intranasal Frontal Sinusotomy

Two concepts are important:

1. If the nasofrontal duct has a visible diameter of only 1–2 mm, and appears incapable of ensuring satisfactory drainage for extensive polyposis of the frontal sinus, it should be widened to form a broad duct extending as far as the frontal infundibulum. This procedure corresponds to the concept of isthmus surgery. Although the surgeon is now aware of the direction of dissection, widening of the duct is often more difficult than perforation of the cells by the second method about to be described because the cells ar usually small and few in number.

Sharp forceps are usually inadequate for the often hard bone, and in this case the diamond burr should be used to resect the bone on one side in an anterior direction (but not in a circular manner) in front of the nasofrontal duct. Since ideal angled diamond burrs have not yet been developed the arch of bone hanging down from the agger nasi must be straightened, and the anterior wall of the duct itself must be drilled gradually (Figure 6.**73**). One finger of the left hand holding a long speculum should be placed on the medial canthus to detect perforation of the bone in this area immediately, and thus prevent damage to the lacrimal ducts. An assistant irrigates the drill with cool saline solution which is sucked out of the nasopharynx with a curved tube.

If a circular lesion of the mucosa has been produced, and the newly created window does not appear to be wide enough, then a spacer should be retained for from 2 to 3 weeks to prevent stenosis. The frontal duct may appear to be patent during the first weeks to be followed by cicatricial stenosis some weeks later (Figure 6.**74**).

2. Sometimes the search for the frontal duct with the endoscope proves fruitless. However, if radiographs have shown the presence of a developed frontal sinus, a careful endoscopic examination should be carried out. This maneuver is particularly delicate and demanding because inadvertent perforation of the anterior skull base is life threatening.

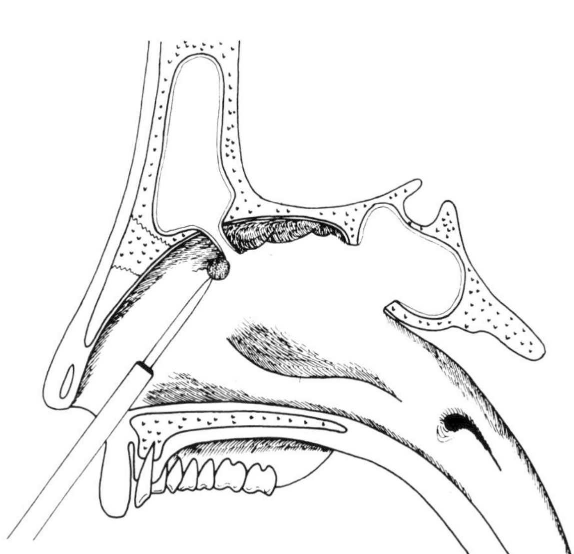

Figure 6.**73** Widening of a narrow nasofrontal duct using the diamond bur from below. The technique is explained in the text.

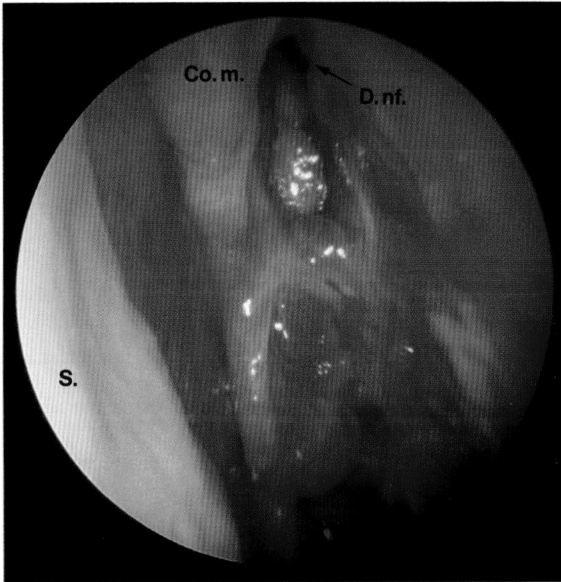

Figure 6.**74** Widened left nasofrontal duct 4 weeks after a pansinus operation (70° telescope).

The surgeon should orientate himself by the transverse bar formed by the anterior ethmoid artery, and proceed forward from there. At the same time the midpoint between the medial lamella of the middle turbinate and the surface of the already exposed lateral ethmoid wall should be estimated. Anteriorly the ethmoid may be relatively narrow. If the anterior wall of the already dissected ethmoid is now freed of its mucosa in the direction indicated, the frontal sinus can be seen shining through the most anterior ethmoid cells. Sometimes careful curettage with the curved House ear curette helps. This instrument is also particularly useful for breaking and elevating the thin bony edges to look for the pathway to the frontal infundibulum. If the point of the instrument is never directed towards the dura, damage is impossible even if the instrument has taken a false pathway behind the posterior wall of the frontal sinus. Unfortunately a highly angled diamond burr with which the bone could be removed safely has not yet been developed. After all the cell walls have been removed and the mucosa has been perforated (taking care not to confuse it with dura) the newly created passage is widened using forceps or a punch (Figure 6.**75**), but the mucosa should be removed from the anterior and lateral surfaces only.

The following are suitable landmarks for fenestration via the most anterior ethmoid cells:

- the bulge formed by the anterior ethmoid artery,
- the medial lamella of the middle turbinate at its central insertion into the ethmoid roof after removal of the agger nasi,
- the orbital wall.

Inspection with the endoscope in an anterosuperior direction towards the base of the skull reveals the prominent bar formed by the anterior ethmoid artery forming the posterior limit of the sinusotomy. One or two flat cell recesses still lie between it and the site of the nasofrontal duct anteriorly at a distance of at least 2–4 mm (see Figure 6.**64**).

The medial lamella of the middle turbinate and its insertion into the ethmoid roof form a landmark of inestimable value, because they mark the lateral limit of the cribriform plate. The surgeon must at all costs stay lateral to it when looking for the entrance to the frontal cavity and he has to stay medial to the orbital wall, which after its exposure is another guideline. The curettage may be directed anteriorly halfway between the middle turbinate and the orbital wall. The use of force inevitably leads to perforation of the base of the skull. However, it should always be possible to expose the radiologically defined frontal sinus without visualization of a nasofrontal duct by adhering to the landmarks already mentioned (Figure 6.**76 a, b**).

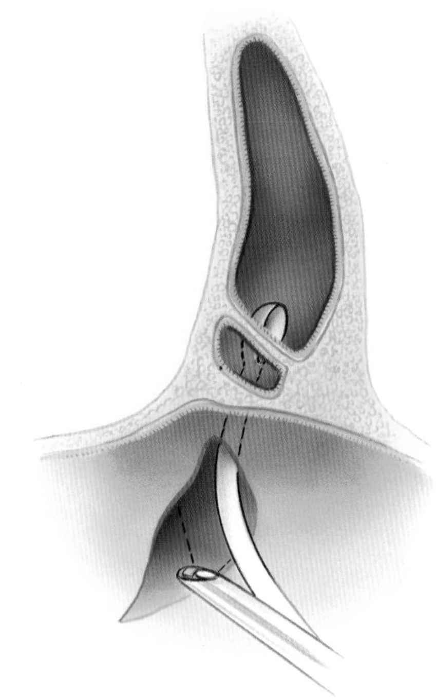

Figure 6.**75** Frontal sinusotomy using the sharp curette to break down the anterior ethmoid cells.

Endoscopic Operation on the Frontal Sinus with Two Access Ports

If the frontal sinus is affected by diffuse polyposis the first procedure should be restricted to securing the frontal duct. Only if inspection from below shows obstruction of the frontal infundibulum by polyps is it necessary, or indeed possible, to remove them. Small curved forceps which reach far into the frontal sinus are useful. If the ostium is too narrow it should be widened, usually by the procedures described above.

However, a more vigorous expansion is sometimes necessary because of hard bone or because of an obstinate tendency to stenosis. In these cases supplementary procedures such as the use of the diamond burr or laser excision of scar tissue are necessary. The *two portal* procedure has proved to be useful (Figure 6.**77 a, b**). The drill is monitored and irrigated through a transfrontal observation window immediately above the floor of the frontal sinus. The author has used this procedure several times with good results, but it is necessary to take into account inevitable scar tissue retraction of the new ostium, and to overcorrect by extending the hole by twice as much as necessary. Figure 6.**78** shows the end result from below of a frontal sinusotomy widened in this way, that led to healing of a long-stand-

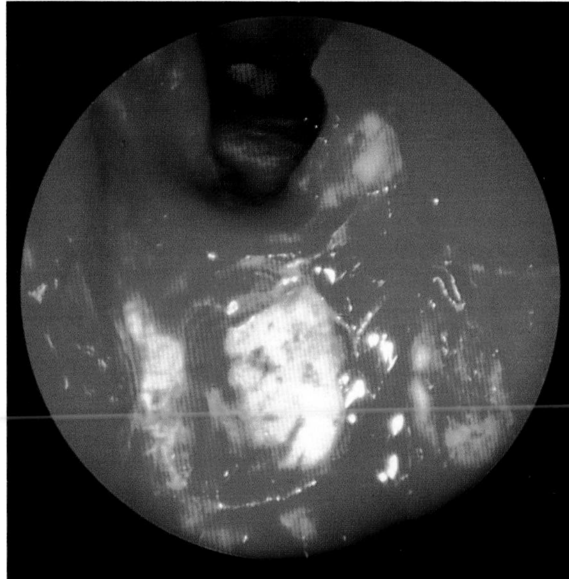

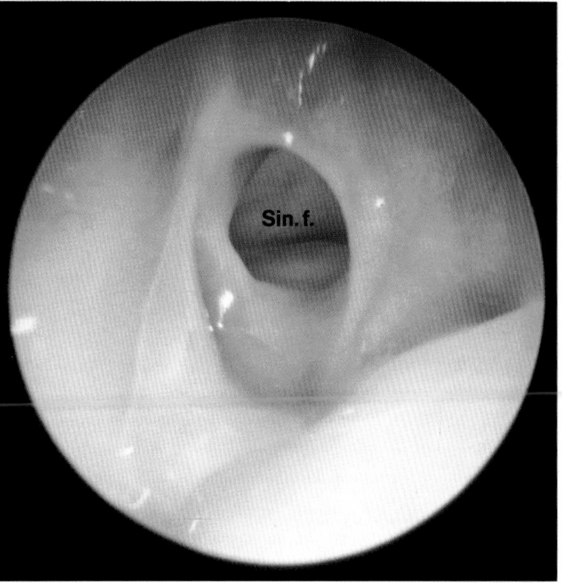

Figure 6.**76** Wide frontal sinusotomy from below using a sharp curette. **a** Operative photograph.

b Open, healed, frontal infundibulum with healthy frontal mucosa (70° telescope).

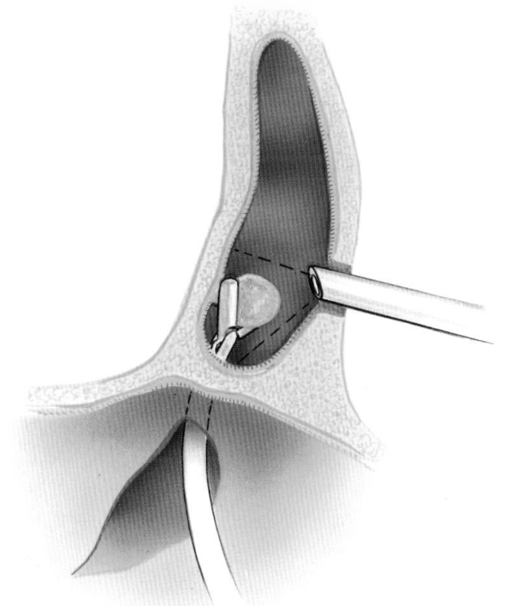

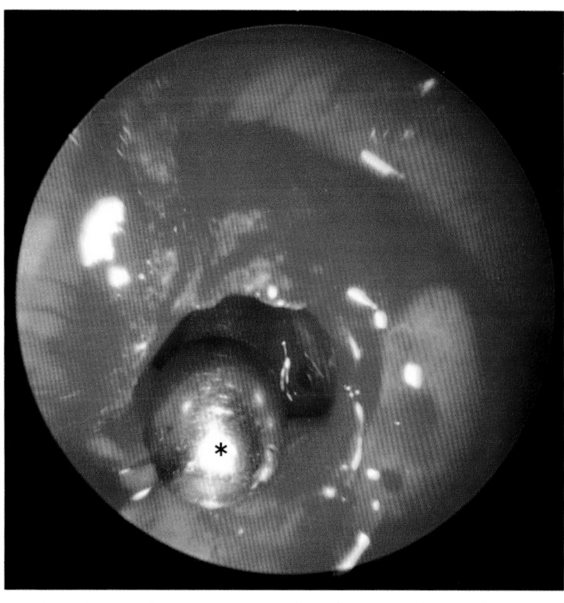

Figure 6.**77** Frontal sinus procedure through two portals. **a** Manipulation of the instruments.

b Transfrontal endoscopic view into the frontal infundibulum using the 25° microscope. An instrument has been introduced from below into the infundibulum (* = head of the forceps).

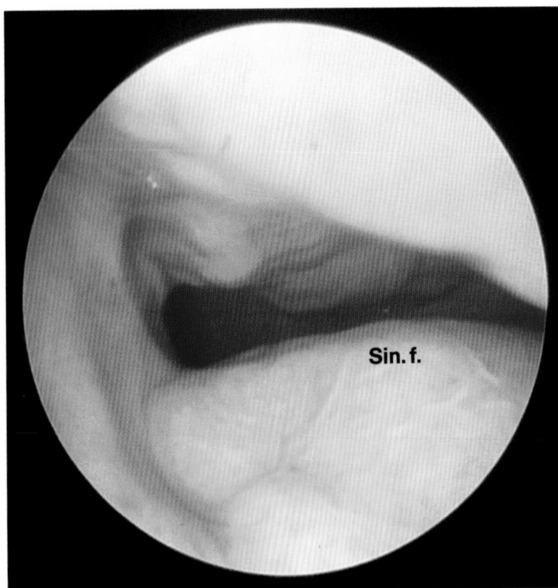

Figure 6.**78** Left frontal sinus healed aftrer a generous frontal sinusotomy from below (70° telescope).

ing frontal sinusitis after removal of polyps from within the sinus.

The histological type of a soft tissue tumor of the frontal sinus, and the best route for its removal may be determined by an endoscopic biopsy. Beck's trephine is the simplest and most direct method in most cases. If radiographic opacity of the anterior ethmoids demands that a sinusitis be distinguished from a tumor, then an anterior ethmoidectomy may be combined with endoscopic biopsy of the frontal sinus from below. In this way retention cysts, for example, can be recognized and removed at the same procedure, and a metastasis undergoing central necrosis be excluded.

Limited External Frontal Sinus Operation under Endoscopic Control

Intranasal endoscopy is not suitable for the removal of polyps, foreign bodies or benign tumors from the upper recess of the frontal sinus, because the view and scope for manipulation are unsatisfactory. Mucopyoceles and osteitis in the superior compartments are even less suitable for this procedure. However, methods are constantly being sought to achieve the goal of restitution of an aerated frontal sinus draining securely into the nose and lined with mucosa, thus avoiding an external radical procedure. A previous operation or the extent of the disease may preclude an osteoplastic procedure.

In such circumstances the frontal sinus can be opened with the usual incision in the eyebrows. Bone is removed locally, preserving bony struts, in a similar manner to preservation of the bridge in ear surgery. Endoscopić manipulations can then be carried out successfully in the angles and recesses with limited external access. The advantage is the widespread preservation of the mucosa and the bony superstructure. The access holes in the floor and anterior wall of the frontal sinus are covered with periosteum or lyophilized dura. The operation must of course include exenteration of the anterior ethmoids, and wide frontal sinusotomy into the nose. The procedure was developed to exploit the given circumstances during revision of classical frontal sinus operations, with a pre-existing often small sinusotomy.

Figure 6.**79** illustrates an endoscopic procedure for a mucocele with widening of the frontal access to the nose (Figure 6.**79 a**), and with a view through a circumscribed external window of the lower third of the frontal sinus (Figure 6.**79 b**). A small bony defect was already present at this point. The internal drainage could be secured in this manner with minimal loss of mucosa. The two small bony defects in the anterior wall of the frontal infundibulum were covered with lyophilized dura. The widened frontal duct was stented for several weeks with a polyethylene tube.

In other patients with large supraorbital mucoceles causing extensive resorption of the anterior wall of the frontal sinus (Figures 6.**80**, 6.**81**) the bony anterior wall was reconstructed with simultaneous intranasal endoscopic resection of the frontal infundibulum and the diseased ethmoids without sacrificing mucosa. This is a good example of developing functional frontal sinus surgery using endoscopic control.

The principle of minimal opening of the frontal sinus allowing preservation of its bony walls can be used to advantage for foreign bodies and tumors. The author uses the endoscope during an external operation on the frontal sinus to extract a foreign body, based on the following two concepts: (1) The patient's own bone forms a more stable support for

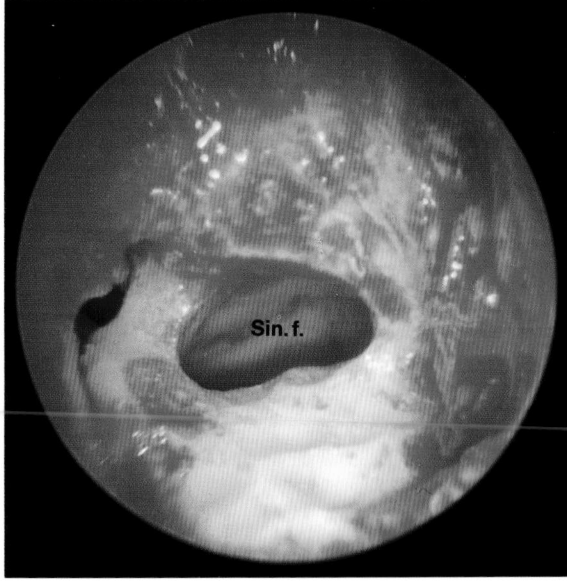

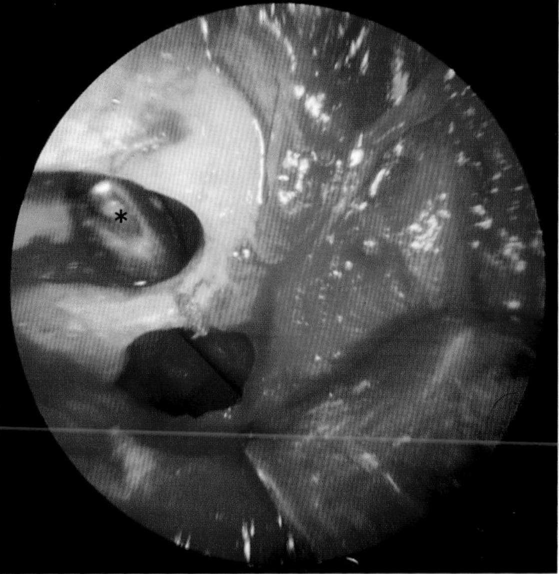

Figure 6.**79** Frontal operation through two portals allowing preservation of the bone cuff around the infundibulum of the right frontal sinus.
a Endoscopic view from within. A small spontaneous bone defect is present on the left side of the picture. The frontal sinus opens above (70° telescope).

b View from outside into the fenestrated frontal infundibulum still encased by bone. A probe has been pushed from below into the frontal infundibulum (*).

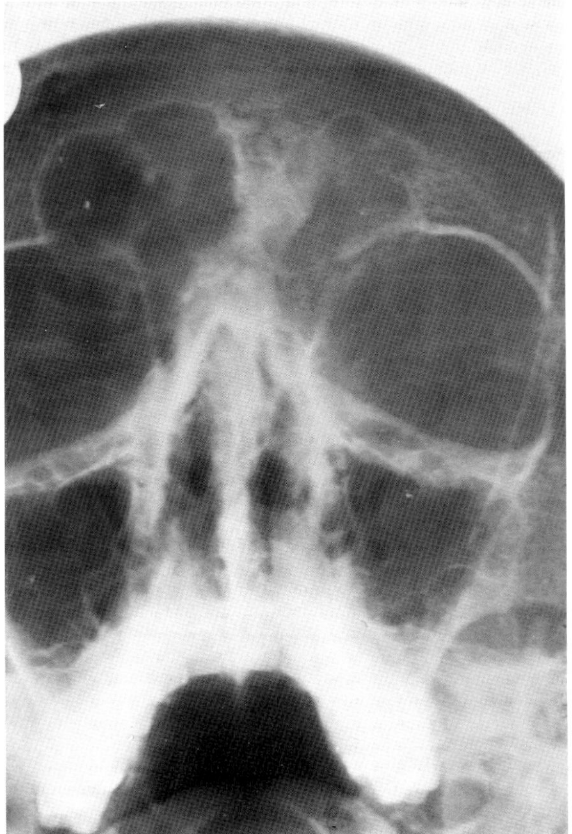

Figure 6.**80** Radiograph of a right-sided frontal mucocele before endoscopic treatment.

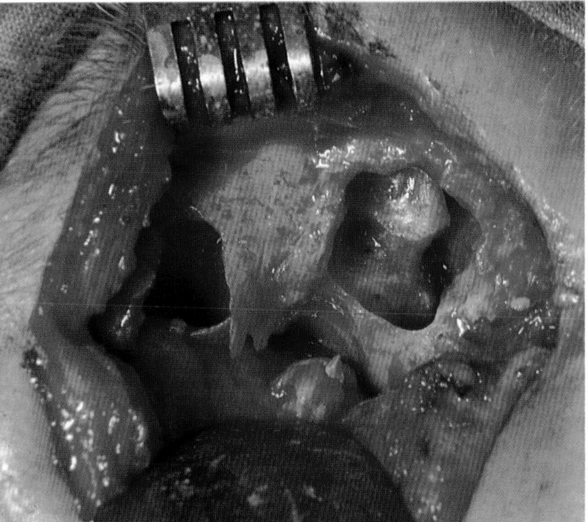

Figure 6.**81** Treatment of a right-sided frontal sinus with chronic sinusitis and a mucocele, by endoscopic monitoring of the frontal sinus operation through a limited external access with preservation of the bony frontal infundibulum (a different case from that in Figure 6.**80**).

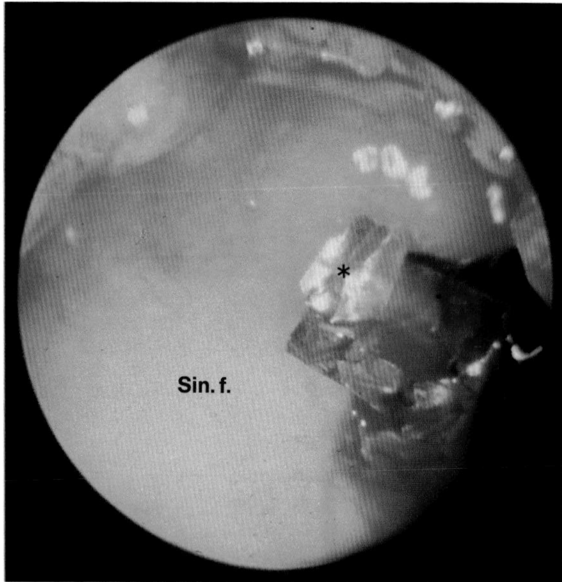

Figure 6.**82** Endoscopic removal of a foreign body from the frontal sinus via a small external access (*, splinter of safety glass).

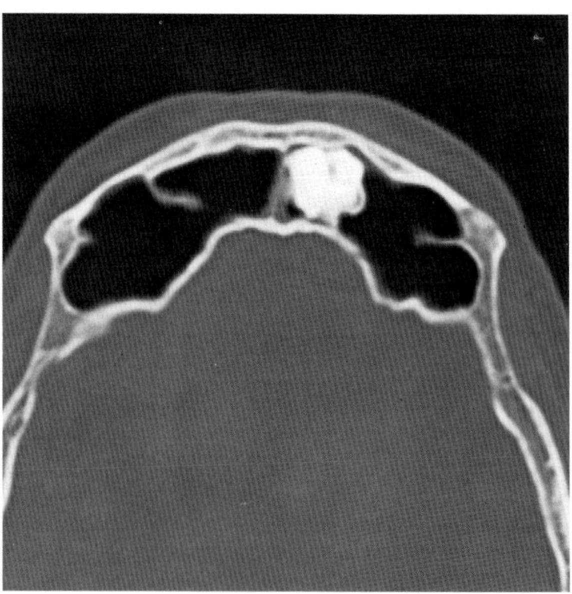

Figure 6.**83** CT scan of a frontal osteoma before removal through a small external access monitored by endoscopy.

the facial soft tissues than foreign material. (2) Several small mucosal defects are more likely to regenerate and restore the mucociliary transport necessary for the self-cleaning of the mucosa than one large defect. A small hole suffices for the observation tube, allowing the use of angled telescopes of varying degrees. One or two further holes allow the introduction of instruments for the extraction of the foreign body (Figure 6.**82**) or for drilling of a frontal osteoma to reduce it in size *in situ* (Figure 6.**83**).

Operations on the Sphenoid Sinus

Indications

- empyema,
- removal of polyps,
- removal of small benign tumors,
- removal of foreign bodies,
- biopsy,
- decompression of the optic nerve,
- resection of the vidian nerve.

Principles

The sphenoid sinus is exposed by removal of its anterior wall. Securing of the sphenopalatine artery ensures a bloodless field. The posterior edge of the nasal septum should be preserved. Manipulations on the roof and lateral wall should be carried out only under microscopic or endoscopic control. Sphenoid sinus surgery should never be carried out without previous tomography.

Operative Technique

The *exposure of the sphenoid sinus* by finding its anterior wall after removal of the posterior ethmoid cells has already been considered in detail in the section on ethmoid operations. Sphenoid sinus surgery is often regarded as being particularly dangerous and attended by severe complications. However, mistakes are usually based on inadequate preoperative investigation, lack of adequate instruments such as the endoscope and the operating microscope, and inadequate hemostasis. However, if these three prerequisites are satisfied and the surgeon is fully familiar with the endoscopic anatomy of the posterior ethmoid, then there is no particular difficulty or danger in finding the sphenoid sinus. Thus disease of the sphenoid itself can be treated by surgery, and the sphenoid sinus can be used for access to related structures.

The sphenoid sinus is often unsymmetrical, and its deep recesses can only be inspected by an angled telescope.

Applications

The *extraction of polyps* from the sphenoid sinus has already been dealt with in the section on pansinus operations. Intranasal endosopy can achieve permanently successful results in the removal of *inverted papillomas* from the antrum and ethmoids. It can be equally successful for this lesion within the sphenoid sinus. External access does not create better conditions for radical removal of papillomas, but it is the perfect exposure of the operative field with optical magnification that prevents a recurrence: intranasal access is just as good or even better for the use of the endoscope and the operating microscope. After removal of the suspect tissue with the double forceps under endoscopic control the underlying bone is drilled down with the diamond burr, again under visual control, using a long, slender handpiece. If the appropriate equipment is not available then wide exposure via the external access is of course indicated.

The transnasal removal of *benign tumors* and the *extraction of foreign bodies* from the sphenoid cavity present no difficulties using the techniques already described, but are seldom used. *Biopsy of tumors* is quite often indicated, but if the tumor proves to be malignant it usually cannot be removed surgically.

Resection of the *vidian nerve* is recommended for the treatment of nasal polyps and vasomotor rhinitis. The exposure of the nerve begins with opening of the sphenoid sinus under the operating microscope. The indications are controversial, and the author has no personal experience of Golding–Wood's technique of vidian neurectomy nor of intranasal transethmoidosphenoidal *decompression of the optic nerve.*

Strict indications are laid down in the author's clinic for decompression of the optic nerve by slitting its sheath in patients with an orbital fracture. Transorbitoethemoid access to the optic nerve has so far been preferred, but an intranasal transethmoid microdissection of the orbital apex and the canal of the optic nerve may be considered in exceptional cases with no fracture of the orbit or the ethmoids, but with loss of vision due to head injuries. A CT scan provides details about the direction of dissection with the diamond burr.

Operations on the Anterior Base of the Skull, including the Roof of the Ethmoids and the Wall of the Sphenoid Sinus

Indications

- removal of foreign bodies,
- debridement,
- closure of a small CSF leak,
- biopsy and localized removal of tissue,
- combined neurosurgical and rhinological procedures.

Principles

Ethmoidectomy provides a limited, direct endoscopic view of the lower surface of the anterior skull base. Very accurate and effective dissection and reconstruction may be carried out with slender instruments, burrs and tissue glue on the ethmoid roof and the walls of the sphenoid sinus.

Operative Technique

The anterior part of the anterior skull base is formed by the posterior wall of the frontal sinus and the roof of the orbit. In the middle lies the roof of the ethmoid, and posteriorly the sphenoid plane and the roof of the sphenoid sinus. The exposure of the ethmoid and sphenoid roof described with the intranasal endoscopic technique in the previous section, related only to dissection of the anterior skull base from below. The posterior wall of the frontal sinus is suitable for only very limited endoscopic manipulations, but the lateral and posterior walls of the sphenoid sinus are well within the reach of endoscopy.

Endoscopy of the anterior base of the skull is indicated for lesions of the anterior and middle ethmoid roof especially the cribriform plate, and for the walls of the sphenoid sinus, whereas lesions of the sphenoid plane requiring attention are unusual. For this reason anterior ethmoidectomy is the method of choice for access to the base of the skull, followed by posterior ethmoidectomy with opening of the sphenoid sinus. Individual circumstances will decide which of these is used for exposure of the base of the skull. Particular procedures do not need to be described further at this point. Ethmoidectomy in these circumstances naturally includes the radical removal of the mucosa as far as this is necessary.

For an ethmoidal-dural fistula, confirmed by CT scan, an approach via the middle meatus (preserving the middle turbinate) the ethmoid infundibulum and the ethmoid bulla is indicated. In the absence of polyposis this dissection can be very precise. If a fracture line crossing the olfactory cleft causing a CSF leak is expected, surgery should begin with a partial resection of the middle turbinate so that the base of the skull can be inspected endoscopically in the midline along the medial lamella of the middle turbinate without obstruction by the body of the middle turbinate. If an iatrogenic CSF leak after a prevois ethmoid operation requires closure, the surgery must be adapted to the prevailing situation beginning with systematic removal of scar tissue, and gradual exposure of the bony base of the skull by removal of any remaining cells.

In a case of CSF leak after a septal operation, the repair begins with separation of the two layers of the septum up to the base of the skull. Then the problem is tackled from the exposed defect with resection of olfactory mucosa followed by exenteration of the ethmoids up to this point. Most cases require complete ethmoidectomy to obtain a maximal view of the base of the skull.

There are no guidelines yet available in this still-developing endoscopic surgery of the anterior base of the skull to help in deciding whether the ethmoid should be exposed from in front or behind. Whichever is chosen, it is important always to preserve the physiological drainage of the ethmoid compartments or the sphenoid sinus which might be preserved during limited ethmoidectomy.

Procedures such as the removal of an impacted foreign body, the closure of a fistula or the removal of a tumor will not be described here in detail. The principles and the instruments are detailed on the section on sphenoid and ethmoid operations.

Applications

The anterior base of the skull is a relatively firm party wall between the paranasal sinuses and the anterior cranial fossa that resists *foreign bodies* penetrating from below, so that they often remain impacted under or in it. Foreign bodies include glass splinters and pieces of metal which become impacted during road traffic accidents, pieces of plastic and wood, and air gun pellets. These may be removed successfully by the intranasal route provided the base of the skull has not been pierced. Since the entry portal is often very small and normally requires only localized attention, an external operation is usually unnecessary. The projectile can usually be localized and the degree of injury assessed by radiography. A bullet in the wall of the sphenoid sinus (Figure 6.**84 a–c**) can often be revealed by posterior ethmoidectomy to expose the sphenoid sinus, allowing the foreign body to be removed or freed after drilling the surrounding bone. A defect in the base of the skull must be looked for, and if necessary debrided. Postoperative treatment is the same as that for secondary healing after ethmoidectomy if the dura is not injured.

The *immediate repair of a CSF fistula* caused by injury of olfactory fibers in the anterior and middle ethmoid roof has already been described under total ethmoidectomy. The technique has proved to be reliable and has therefore been developed as the standard procedure for traumatic and idiopathic dural fistulae of other types and sites. The decision between a wide external rhinological procedure, a transfrontal neurosurgical exposure of the anterior skull base or an intranasal endoscopic access for closure of a CSF fistula today should not depend on generally accepted guidelines. Traditions, a surgeon's previous training and the instruments available often carry too much weight in the decision. The advantages of intranasal debridement of a localized fracture of the base of the skull and closure of a dural defect include preservation of bony support of the floor of the frontal sinus, avoidance of division of the supraorbital nerve, and prevention of the permanent dysosmia characteristic of the neurosurgical procedure.

The technique is not difficult if the surgeon is familiar with bimanual endoscopy. After removal of as much of the middle turbinate as necessary, the ethmoid cells are cleared up to the base of the skull. Once the fistula has been found (Figure 6.**85 a** and **b**) the neighboring mucosa is removed delicately from the edge over a distance of 2–4 mm using fine curved double forceps. If the fistula reaches the nasal septum, removal of the mucosa must encompass this area. A similar procedure is followed in the roof of the sphenoid sinus (Figure 6.**86**). Here the conditions for closing the defect are considerably more favorable, as even large defects of the base of the skull in

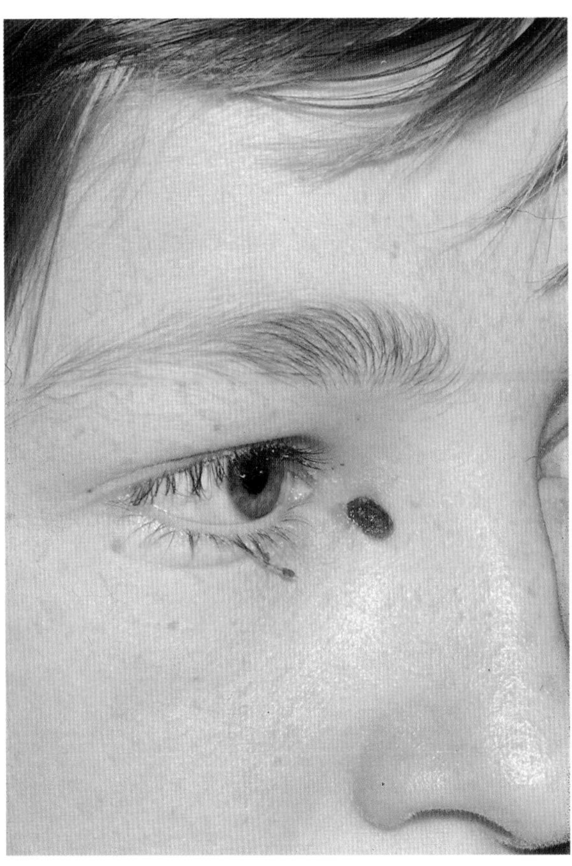

Figure 6.**84** Intranasal endoscopic removal of a bullet impacted in the wall of the sphenoid sinus.
a Entry wound in the right middle canthus.

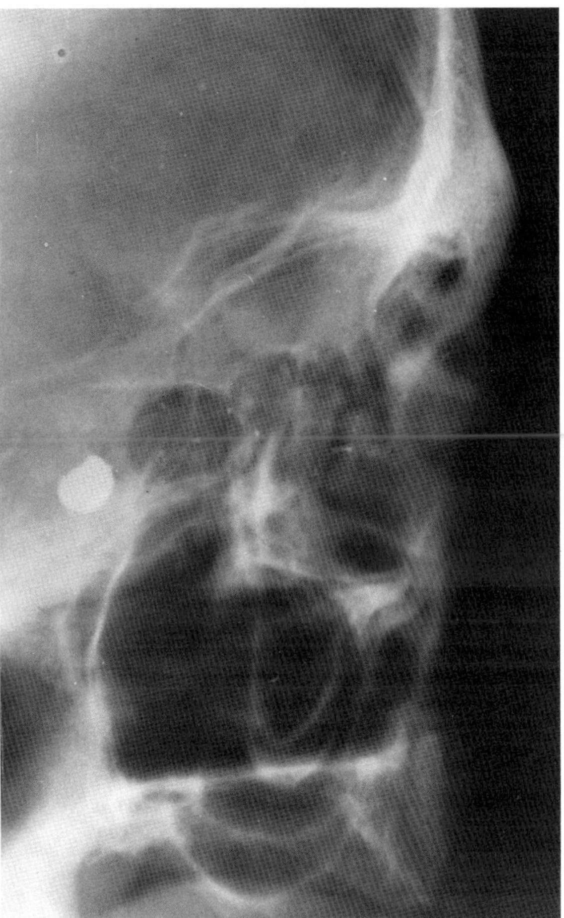

b Sagittal tomograph showing the position in the floor of the sphenoid sinus.

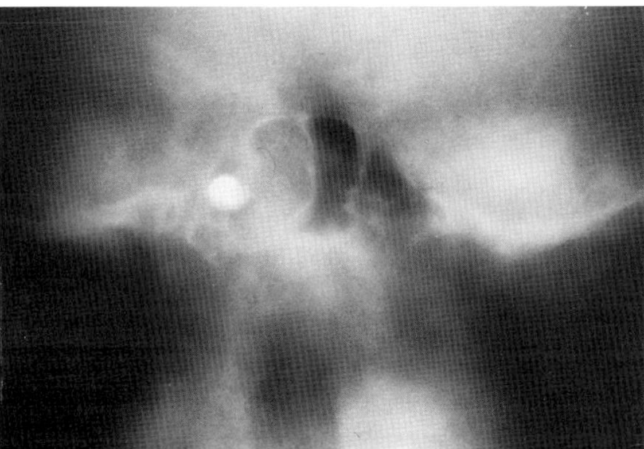

c The coronal section localizes the bullet lying in the lateral wall of the sphenoid sinus.

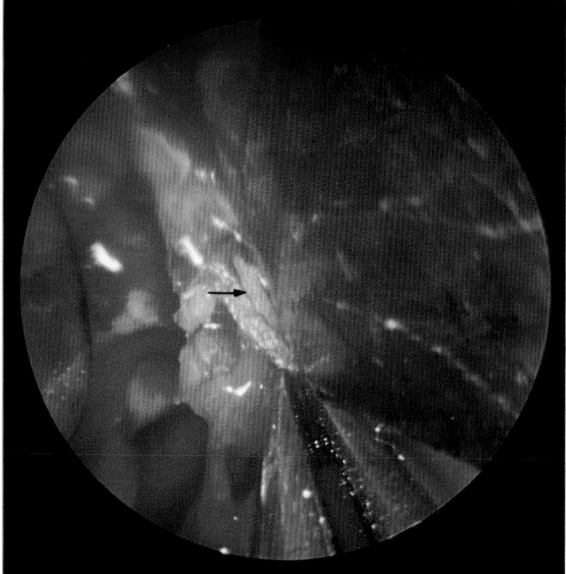

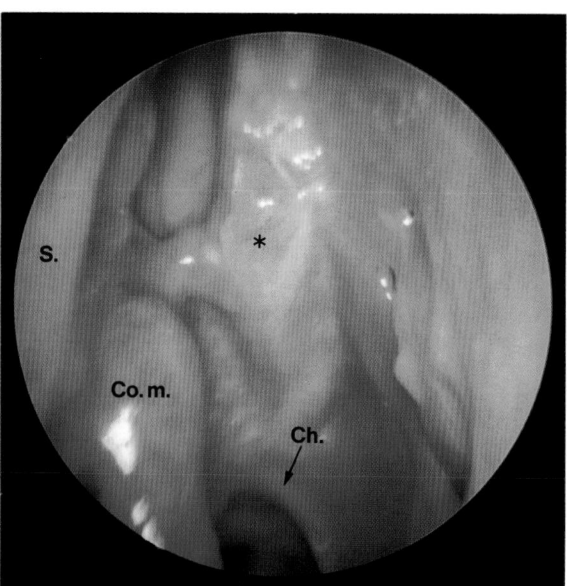

Figure 6.**85** Spontaneous dural fistula in the left anterior ethmoid.
a The greenish shiny, fistula (marked by an arrow) is shown after intranasal transethmoid exposure.

b Healed mucosal graft (*) over the fistula (70° telescope).

this area can be managed by intranasal endoscopy. The entire sphenoid sinus mucosa is removed and the cavity filled with a large piece of fascia lata, or muscle and periosteum. Additional packing with fibrin foam encourages adhesion of the connective tissue to the bone so that tissue glue is not needed.

However, tissue glue does have a place in the closure of a fistula in the roof of the ethmoid. In the absence of a counter resistance the graft must support itself by adhesion until it becomes incorporated. Thus the use of tissue glue and packing of the upper part of the nose for at least 10 days are very important. Transposition of a soft tissue flap under the denuded bony edges of a defect is very successful after wide external transfacial exposure of the posterior wall of the frontal sinus in the management of large fistulae at that point, but is scarcely practicable for small ethmoid fistulae managed by the endoscopic route.

After careful demarcation of the defect, a graft is fitted carefully over the fistula and the surrounding bone edges, and is fixed with tissue glue. A mucosal flap taken from the free edge of the inferior turbinate has proved to be very useful. Its manipulations and control with nasal forceps and an elevator is not particularly difficult but demands prior hemostasis and very careful use of the suction. The site of the graft must be checked carefully by endoscopy. The edges are then covered with a further layer of tissue glue: once this is dry the nose is packed with material such as fibrin foam which is removed at the earliest from 2 to 3 weeks later. Indeed it can be left until it is rejected spontaneously. The nasal packing of vaseline gauze introduced beneath this contact packing can be removed as soon as 10 days after the operation. Since healing of the transplanted tissue to the bone requires several weeks, reoperation should not be immediately embarked upon for a slight CSF leak in the first postoperative weeks. In this event it may be necessary to adjust the nasal packing, place the patient with the head in the upright position and drain off CSF by a lumbar drainage.

The endoscopic technique just described for closure of small CSF leaks has proved valuable for the care of spontaneous CSF rhinorrhea. The defect is usually found around the cribriform plate, particularly at its posterior edge, or in the roof of the sphenoid sinus, apparently at points of congenital weakness of the wall or of previously formed bony defects. A complete neurological work-up is indi-

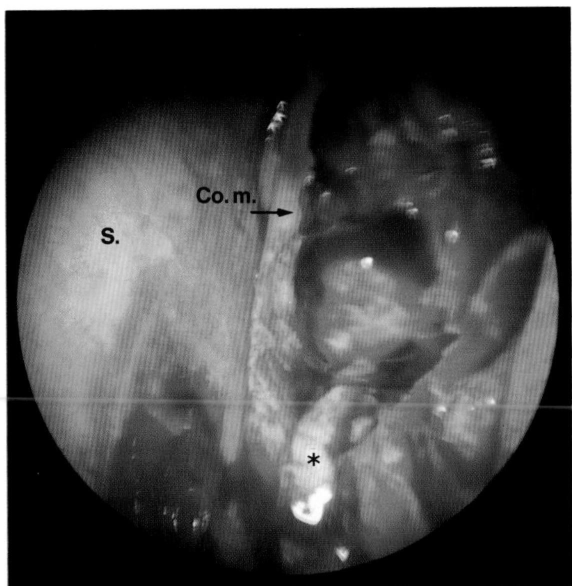

Figure 6.**86** Post-traumatic dural fistula (*) in the anterior roof of the sphenoid on the left side. Intranasal endoscopic exposure and glueing of a thick mucosal flap (70° telescope).

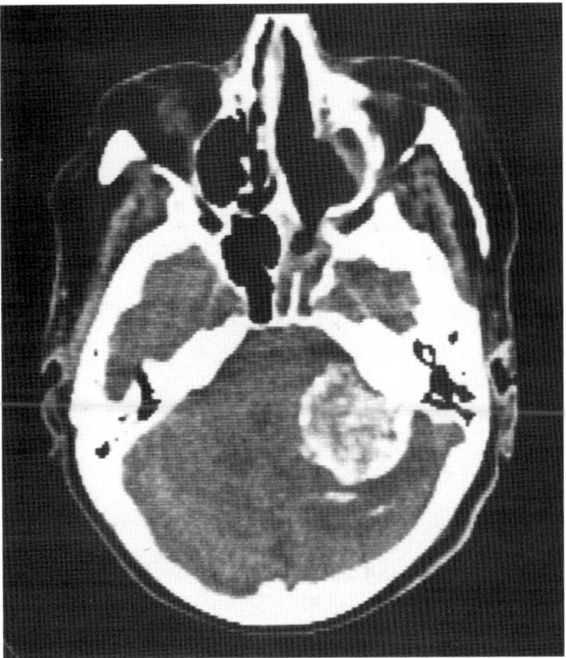

Figure 6.**87** Large acoustic neuroma in a 78-year-old lady causing a spontaneous CSF fistula through the right ethmoid roof. The fistula was exposed by the intranasal endoscopic route, and the tumor was debulked by translabyrinthine partial resection.

cated. In one case of spontaneous recurrent CSF rhinorrhea, we found a large acoustic neuroma (Figure 6.**87**) with no other lesions of the anterior skull base.

Intranasal endoscopic exposure of the anterior skull base using a similar technique to that for closure of small CSF fistulae is suitable for *debridement.* Limited endoscopic exposure of the ethmoid and skull base is the procedure of choice for destruction of structural support, cell septa and lamellae found during a procedure for a fracture of the middle third of the face and of the anterior skull base, where the differential diagnosis of an opacity shown by precise imaging includes sinusitis, an organized hematoma or a meningocele.

The advantages of *endoscopic biopsy, localized removal of tumor* and nontraumatic, very precise *aftercare* have already been mentioned. Invasion of the skull base by a tumor mandates the inclusion of endoscopy in the diagnosis, treatment and follow-up. Tissue diagnosis, marginal biopsies, removal of residual tumor, and the palliation of inoperable disease need only be mentioned at this point. However, the curative procedure for inverting papillomas which has been developed in the Erlangen Clinic needs emphasis. This intranasal, endoscopic technique embraces ethmoidectomy and sphenoid sinusotomy for tumors invading the walls of the sphenoid and skull base. Endoscopic follow-up and biopsy (Figure 6.**88**) has on several occasions indicated the necessity for a revision operation or retreatment with irradiation (Figure 6.**89**).

The example of an ossifying nasopharyngeal fibroma (Figure 6.**90 a** and **b**) shows that occasionally even a large benign tumor can be controlled by intranasal endoscopy. An initally explorative procedure could be extended to a completely successful removal because the tumor was well demarcated and was avascular.

Thanks to increasing cooperation in the search for the optimal solutions for patients with difficult problems* we have recently carried out several *neurosurgical-rhinosurgical combined operations* in-

* The author wishes to express his particular thanks to the founders of the International Skull Base Study Group and to Prof. Dr. R. Fahlbusch, Director of the Neurosurgical Clinic at Friedrich-Alexander University.

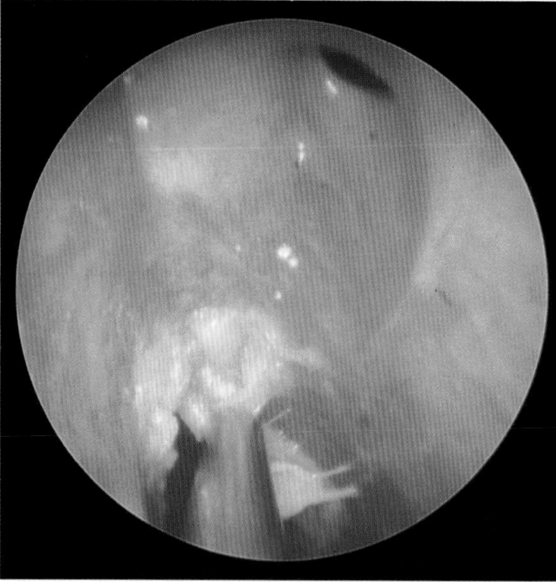

Figure 6.**88** Endoscopic follow-up after removal of a tumor from the roof of the left ethmoid. A biopsy taken from a persistent ulcer, with crusting, showed no recurrence (70° telescope).

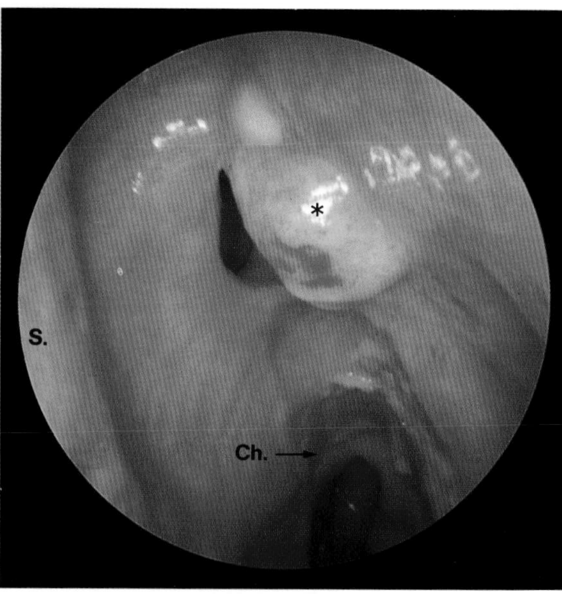

Figure 6.**89** Endoscopic follow-up after removal of a tumor from the base of the skull showing recurrence (*) of a carcinoma on the lateral ethmoid wall. Left side of the nasal cavity (70° telescope).

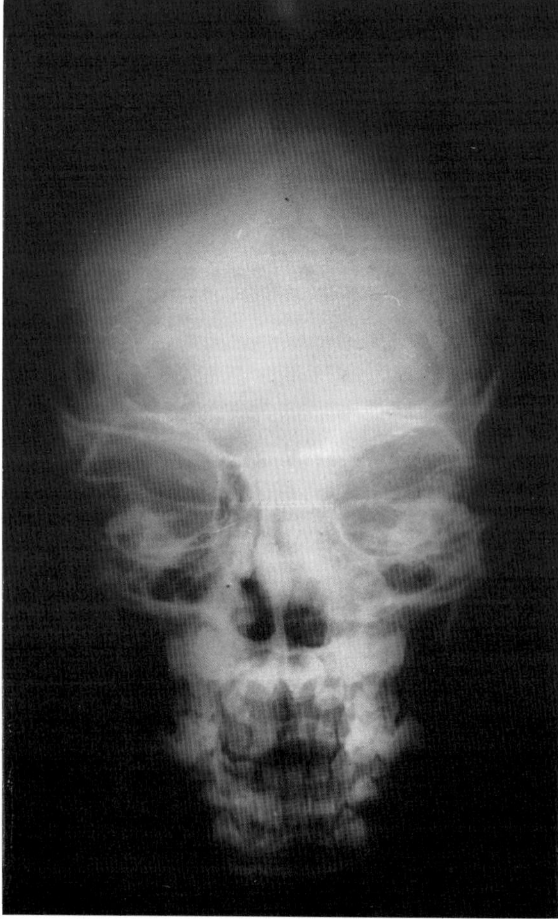

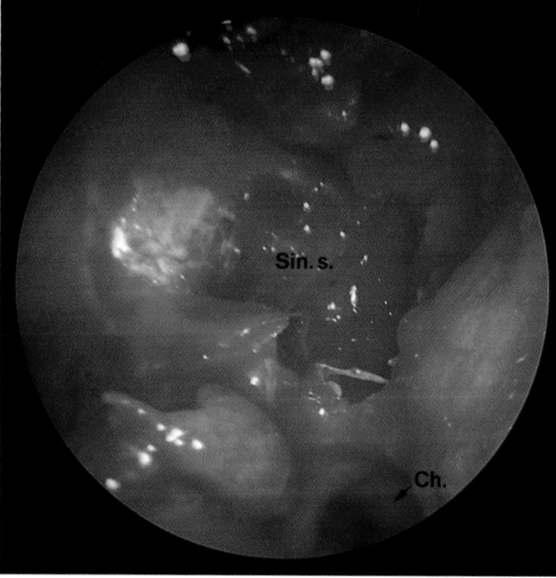

Figure 6.**90** Ossifying nasopharyngeal fibroma. **a** Skull view showing opacity of the right ethmoid region. **b** Intra-operative view into the sphenoid after intranasal removal of the moderately vascular fibroma. The open sphenoid cavity is shown on the right and above, and the choana on the right and below.

corporating intranasal endoscopic techniques. The contributions to this developing field include the following:

- Histological specimens have been obtained on several occasions by localized exploration of the base of the skull for supra and intrasphenoid tumors and orbital tumors infiltrating into the skull base.
- In some cases the nasal procedure was carried out from below at a different sitting either before or after a neurosurgical procedure to resect and reconstruct a large part of the base of the skull. Occasionally a combined procedure is carried out at the same time (Figure 6.**91**).
- Combined neurosurgical-intranasal resection of large tumors of the anterior skull base using the operating microscope, via a unilateral or bifrontal approach offers greater advantages because of the very wide exposure of the anterior cranial fossa so that a good margin can be obtained round an invasive ethmoid carcinoma or esthesioneuroblastoma. In this procedure the rhinologist excises the ethmoid block, the sphenoid sinus and the nasal septum. The use of the microscope with an angled telescope can be very useful for inspection of all the concealed recesses such as the edges of the maxillary sinus.
- Intranasal endoscopic closure of CSF leaks has also proved very useful in these combined procedures allowing late defects in the dural closure to be repaired. It has also been used successfully for a few cases of CSF rhinorrhea after transethmoidal operations on the pituitary gland.

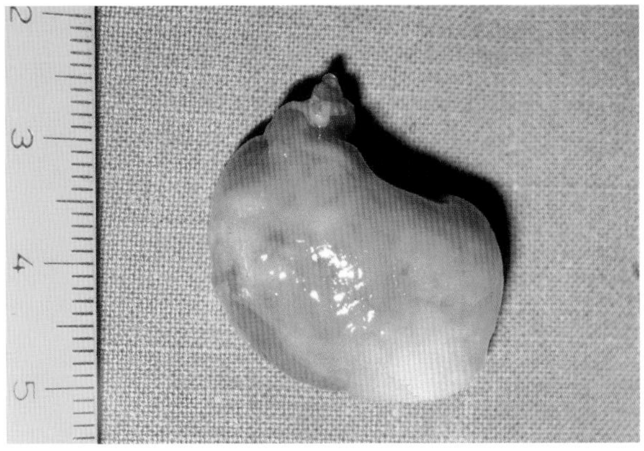

Figure 6.**91** Compact esthesioneuroblastoma arising on a pedicle from the middle turbinate, after intranasal endoscopic removal.

7. Results of Endoscopic Sinus Surgery

Overall Assessment and Evaluation Criteria

If several means of treatment of a group of diseases are available a comparison of the results with respect to several parameters helps the responsible doctor to come to a decision about the chances of healing, the complication rates and the application to the individual patient. These data will be of particular interest to a specialist contemplating adopting a new operative technique, to allow him to assess whether it is worthwhile, and to provide a comparison with his own results. Furthermore, standard values must be available for family practitioners and other referring colleagues who must answer medicolegal questions, and provide a detailed explanation to the patient.

The data given in the literature are difficult to interpret because of the large number of variable factors which influence the results, such as referral patterns, indications for surgery, equipment and variations in surgical skill. Furthermore, the results may improve over the course of time, even for the same surgeon. Even more influential factors are the criteria of success and failure, and these are seldom the same in different reports. What is "very good, good and moderate" in the assessment of treatment of sinusitis? Does it refer to the satisfaction of the patient or to the endoscopist? How liberally were the results classified and for how long were the patients followed-up? Was like compared with like? Were the patients similar with respect to other diseases and risk factors? Were related lesions such as septal deviation, defects of bone or mucosa after previous antral operations or scarring after previous ethmoid operations taken into account? All these parameters can have a marked effect on the results of a later intervention so that the choice of a homogenous group for comparison is not always possible, even in a large series of patients. As a clinician the author cannot agree with the statisticians' viewpoint that a large series of cases from several centers compensates for any bias.

Endoscopic antral operations, the most frequent intranasal sinus procedure, will serve as an example. The outcome is determined by the precision of the technique, but it depends much more on the indication: was the lesion truly an isolated antral cyst, or was it an occult ethmoiditis or a paradental granuloma? How often is the patient's dental state investigated accurately before an antral operation, or ethmoiditis looked for by a CT scan? How often is an abnormal nasal septum corrected, or a supplementary turbinectomy performed? Can allergic cofactors be excluded with certainty?

The list of unknown factors can be prolonged almost indefinitely and be extended to the other nasal sinuses. Confounding factors of this type plague the comparison of almost all statistics of surgery of the sinuses. The inevitably imprecise presentation of the data means that the results must be regarded with suspicion. Criteria for evaluation must be as objective as possible, conclusive, representative, easy to compare, should include a subjective assessment by the patient, and should not be too demanding in documentation. The follow-up of small, well defined, complete and clearly defined groups of cases is more conclusive than observation of a large heterogeneous series, and a retrospective study of this kind is as informative as a prospective controlled trial.

Material

Intranasal endoscopic sinus surgery was introduced at the Erlangen ENT Clinic in 1975, initially as an inferior meatal antrostomy. Intranasal ethmoid operations were introduced in 1976, and middle meatal antrostomy in 1981; during the same period ethmoid operations have been developed into partial resections or complete ethmoidectomy. Intranasal procedures on the anterior base of the skull were begun in 1976; since 1981 other indications have been developed such as the treatment of mucoceles and periorbital inflammation, and since 1986 intranasal dacryocystorhinostomy has been undertaken.

The intranasal operative technique is now part of the training program for all assistants. The number of operations by the classical transoral (Caldwell-Luc) or external (Ritter-Jansen) access to the sinuses has decreased markedly, and these operations are not performed at all for chronic sinusitis. In a teaching clinic the proportion of successes and failures is of necessity different from that in a highly specialized personal series. Although the results from an academic hospital may be interesting, it is doubtful whether they are worth publishing because of the difficulty of comparison with other series. For this reason only the author's data will be given below. The postoperative care and follow-up have usually been carried out by the ENT surgeon who referred the patient initially.

Table 7.**1** shows the number of endoscopic intranasal procedures carried out by the author. It can be seen that most patients had a bilateral procedure: unilateral operations are seldom indicated except for recurrent antral empyema or simple antral cysts.

Some of the analyses of the data have already been published, some are more recent and are awaiting publication. The relevant publications from the Erlangen Clinic are given in the reference list.

The review is arranged in the following main categories:

1. *Subjective assessment* by the patient himself.
2. *Objective evaluation* of the following parameters:
   - change in the previous medication,
   - endoscopic follow-up of the mucosa,
   - radiographic follow-up of aeration of the sinuses,
   - olfactometry.
3. *Complications:*
   - during or immediately after the operation,
   - late complications due either to the operative technique or to inadequate healing.

Table 7.**1** Author's series of intranasal endoscopic procedures (1975–1986).

Procedure	Number
Inferior meatal antrostomy	921 (644 patients)
Middle meatal antrostomy	567 (338 patients)
Inferior plus middle meatal antral operations	218 (126 patients)
Partial ethmoidectomy	91 (60 patients)
Complete ethmoidectomy including frontal or sphenoid sinusotomy	1015 (511 patients)
Operations on the anterior skull base	21 (18 patients)
Operations for patients presenting with complications of sinusitis	8 (8 patients)

Antral Operations for Chronic Maxillary Sinusitis

The intranasal endoscopic antral procedures available for evaluation were carried out for the following indications:

- isolated or oligotopic antral cysts,
- recurrent antral empyema,
- isolated polyposis of one antral cavity,
- polypoid hyperplastic pansinusitis.

Table 7.**2** presents the results of verbal and written answers to a simple questionnaire. The high proportion reporting favorable results contrasted with only 9% of patients whose symptoms were unchanged or worse, emphasizes the value of the technique.

Facial pain was relieved in 84%, nasal discharge reduced in 75%, and nasal obstruction resolved in 86% of cases, as might have been expected after intranasal antral procedures combined with restitution of the normal nasal airway by septoplasty. However, it is of interest that pharyngitis improved in 74% of cases and bronchitis in 62%, and furthermore a similar proportion of patients with an allergic rhinitis reported an improvement. Dysosmia was less likely to improve.

Endoscopic follow-up can only be carried out on a proportion of patients for more than 1 year, and patients reporting back after this time usually had a recurrence of their symptoms.

Table 7.**2** Subjective assessment of isolated antral operations (n = 234).

Very good, symptom-free	58%
Clearly improved	33%
No change or worse	9%

Endoscopy of the operated antral cavity often showed mild anomalies such as localized swelling of the mucosa or retention cysts, despite the absence of symptoms (Table 7.**3**). These are of no importance because they are also found in healthy subjects. However, small polyps or cysts could cause continuing drainage of secretions and intermittent pain. Localized lesions in the antral cavity can often not be discovered and thus cannot be included in a classification of results.

Of 234 patients, 21 (9%) were submitted to repeat endoscopy for continuing symptoms. In 34% the inferior meatal antrostomy was found to be restenosed or closed, but in 24% no pathological abnormality was found. Table 7.**4** shows that a middle meatal antrostomy is more likely to remain open than an inferior meatal antrostomy. In some patients the antrostomy narrows or closes within weeks or months, particularly in children, more than 25% of whom suffer this fate, but closure of the antrostomy does not necessarily lead to recurrence of symptoms.

Table 7.**3** Endoscopic follow-up of the nasal mucosa using a rigid 70° telescope after intranasal antral operations via a middle and/or inferior meatal antrostomy.

Antral mucosa	Antrostomy Inferior (n = 30) meatal	Middle (n = 24) meatal	Middle plus inferior meatal (n = 8)
Intact and free of inflammation	40%	63%	50%
Hyperplasia	17%	13%	38%
Cysts	7%	–	–
Scars	10%	4%	–
Not assessable	26%	20%	12%

Table 7.**4** Patency of nasoantrostomies after simultaneous maxilloethmoid operations.

Antrostomy:	Inferior meatal	Middle meatal	
Wide window	71%	86.8%	
Stenosis	19%	9 %	
Reclosure	10%	4.2%	
Total	117	142	3-year observation period

The transport function cannot be deduced from the size and shape of the window. Hosemann (1985) has produced photographic evidence showing that transport function is better after middle than after inferior meatal antrostomy.

Cysts, synechiae, or secreting hyperplastic antral mucosa were found in 24% of patients with persistent symptoms, that is about 2% of the whole series.

Radiographic check-up was only carried out for recurrent symptoms of sinusitis. Where radiography was carried out coincidentally in the absence of symptoms, 43% were normal, 38% much improved and only 19% the same or worse.

The only data available about healing of *sinusitis in children* after an endoscopic antral procedure is that of Panis et al. (1979) (Table 7.**5**). Unfortunately, children cannot be subjected to routine endoscopic follow-up, and the indications are stricter: at the present time antral and ethmoid operations in infants are rare.

Table 7.**5** Results of antral operations for sinusitis in children after failed conservative treatment including dental attention and adenoidectomy.

Free of symptoms	90%
Unremarkable endoscopic findings	75%
Clear sinuses on X-ray	80%

Revision operations are particularly difficult to evaluate. In the author's experience second operations can be compared within limits with a previous purely intranasal first operation. However, if the former procedure was a Caldwell-Luc radical antrostomy, the massive scarring of the cavity and the absence of mucosa does not permit comparison with isthmus surgery. In these cases the prospect of mucosal healing is considerably worse.

In the author's own series of failures, particularly after ethmoid procedures, the proportion of patients who had undergone a previous Caldwell-Luc procedure was much higher than that in the whole series. A detailed study of intranasal revision procedures after a Caldwell-Luc antrostomy has not yet been reported.

The *complications* after intranasal antral procedures in the author's own series were negligible. In the early years there were difficulties with the lacrimal ducts after inferior meatal antrostomy, and one patient later needed a Toti dacryocystorhinostomy. However, this problem and postoperative pain no longer occur.

Ethmoid Operations for Chronic Ethmoiditis

The separation of intranasal endoscopic ethmoidectomy from the other sinus operations is justified only by the relative newness of the procedure and its subdivisions. From the point of view of treatment of the disease, such separate assessment is questionable since isolated long-standing ethmoiditis without extension to the sphenoid or antral cavities is unusual. The grouping is therefore rather arbitrary and provisional. It includes partial ethmoidectomies for localized ethmoiditis and those cases where ethmoidectomy for serious diffuse polyposis of the ethmoid sinus was the main point of interest. In the latter cases the less severely affected frontal antral and sphenoid cavities underwent sinusotomy at least.

The number of *partial ethmoidectomies* is still too few to allow final evaluation based on long-term follow-up. The frequency and the progress of localized mucosal thickenings in the semilunar hiatus and the middle ethmoid outflow tract have only been elucidated by the wider use of polycyclic tomography and CT scans since 1980. In addition, the author's series contains a higher proportion of advanced or previously treated cases of sinusitis, so that the number of partial ethmoidectomies is low. Experience with this procedure has been extremely favorable: chronic inflammation of the ethmoid and antral sinuses healed after minor procedures in the middle meatus, although the results were occasionally disappointing. Sometimes the ethmoiditis extended to other previously healthy regions, so that a supplementary operation with complete ethmoidectomy became necessary. Therefore the indications cannot yet be fully evaluated.

In the author's series of intranasal endoscopic ethmoid operations *complete ethmoidectomy* for severe diffuse polyposis was the commonest procedure. The *subjective assessment* is based on 220 answers returned to 310 questionnaires. The outcome for the symptoms of sinusitis is summarized in Table 7.**6**.

Table 7.**6** Influence of intranasal ethmoid operations on preoperative symptoms in 220 patients.

Symptom	Healing/improvement	No change	Worse
Pain in the head and face	93.4%	5.0%	1.7%
Nasal obstruction	93.3%	4.8%	1.9%
Nasal discharge	85.5%	9.5%	5.0%
Olfactory disorders	84.9%	8.3%	6.9%
Throat discomfort	84.7%	11.2%	4.1%
Disorders of taste*	79.3%	17.2%	3.4%
Epiphora	78.9%	15.8%	5.3%
Proneness to infection	78.7%	14.8%	6.5%
Ear symptoms	71.7%	22.6%	5.7%

* Not quantifiable for sweet, salty, bitter and sour.

Table 7.**7** Subjective judgment of particular groups of patients undergoing intranasal ethmoid operations.

	Patients without asthma and no analgesic sensitivity	Asthmatics without analgesic sensitivity	No asthma but analgesic sensitivity	Asthma-polyposis-analgesic sensitivity triad
Healing from sinusitis	51.0%	52.7%	–	38.5%
Improvement	34.1%	26.2%	50.0%	30.8%
No change	9.9%	15.8%	37.5%	15.3%
Worse	5.0%	5.3%	12.5%	15.4%

Of the patients who were asked to summarize the results of intranasal complete ethmoidectomy, 82% rated the disease as healed or improved. It is now possible to define subgroups of patients with an increased risk of a poorer subjective result. These include ones with bronchial asthma or asthmatic bronchitis, and particularly those with a known sensitivity to nonsteroidal anti-inflammatory agents such as aspirin. The results for this prognostically important group of patients are shown separately in Table 7.**7**.

The proportion of the author's patients with diffuse chronic polypoid sinusitis suffering clinically manifest asthma was 23%. Their assessment of the results of the operation relative to the nasal symptoms is reported in Table 7.**7**; 57% of these patients reported a varying improvement of their asthma.

Previous operations may also affect the subjective assessment of the results: patients who had undergone a previous transmaxillary ethmoidectomy were much less satisfied with a revision operation than those who had previously undergone an intranasal procedure.

Endoscopic follow-up can only be achieved in a proportion of cases. The offer of a free follow-up

Table 7.**8** Endoscopic findings after complete ethmoidectomy for severe diffuse ethmoid polyposis (90 patients, 168 sides).

	Sphenoid sinus	Ethmoid sinus	Maxillary antrum
Normal findings	95%	52%	72%
Homogenous mucosal thickening	–	5%	14%
Slight hyperplasia	5%	25%	13%
Polyps	–	18%	1%

Table 7.**9** Sense of smell before and after complete ethmoidectomy for diffuse ethmoid polyposis. Consecutive series of 35 cases.

Preoperative function		Postoperative function Normosmia	Hyposmia	Anosmia
Normosmia	21	21	–	–
Hyposmia	3	3	–	–
Anosmia	11	9	1	1
Total	35	33	1	1

examination was only accepted by 41% of the patients, and they do not represent a random sample. Controlled studies run into difficulties for several reasons, for example many patients do not turn up for the follow-up investigation, and readmission is discouraged because it increases costs. Therefore, follow-up endoscopic findings (Table 7.**8**) are not fully representative: patients with persistent symptoms are more likely to report for follow-up than those who are symptom-free, so that the true results are probably more favorable.

The recurrent polyps shown in Table 7.**8** were sometimes amenable to conservative treatment. There was often a remarkable discrepancy between the subjective assessment of the symptoms by the patient and the findings on endoscopy. Thus the subjective assessment of a sub-group of patients with bilateral unsatisfactory healing of the mucosa was just a good as that of a further small group with completely healed non-inflamed mucosa on both sides.

The *sense of smell* before and after ethmoidectomy is a yardstick of the severity of the disease, the efficacy of treatment, and also the precision of the mucosa-sparing technique. The patients themselves often regard the recovery of a long-absent olfactory function as being more important than the improved nasal respiration and relief from headache. Table 7.**9** presents the author's experience with a relatively small series: the sense of smell was regained in a large proportion of cases, whereas olfactory deterioration was exceptional.

An illuminating example of the pathological mechanism of dysosmia in nasal and ethmoid polyps may be of interest. After a septal correction done elsewhere, a 45-year-old patient complained of loss of the sense of smell due to mechanical occlusion of the olfactory cleft by mucosal swelling and polyps. At the first investigation he was found to have hyposmia (Figure 7.**1a**). When he presented for operation a few months later he had become anosmic. The entrance to both olfactory clefts was found to be narrowed by scar tissue at follow-up several months after ethmoidectomy (Figure 7.**1b**). At this time the sense of smell was relatively poor, but improved greatly after division of synechiae. A follow-up osmogram (Figure 7.**1c**) indicated a return to normal on one side and improvement on the opposite side.

Finally the *early and late complications* of intranasal ethmoidectomy are of great interest. Fifty years ago it was the high proportion of visual defects, blindness, CSF fistulae and meningitis that brought intranasal ethmoidectomy into disrepute, rather than the poor results. The complication rate will determine whether the reborn intranasal sinus surgery, now supplemented by endoscopes, can gain a permanent place in rhinological surgery.

The complications in the author's second series were relatively minor, with no permanent injury (Table 7.**10**). However, a series of similar size of operations carried out by more than thirty full-time academic staff and assistants in training in the au-

Table 7.**10** Complications after complete ethmoidectomy for diffuse ethmoid polyposis (n = 220).

Asthma attack immediately after operation*	4 (1.8%)
Neuralgia of face and head	4 (1.8%)
Postoperative anosmia	2 (0.9%)
Intraoperative CSF leak, tearing of olfacactory fibers	2 (0.9%)
Orbital hematoma	1 (0.5%)
Ethmoid mucocele	1 (0.5%)
Death	0
Blindness	0
Paresis, double vision	0
Meningitis	0
Ozena	0

* After pain medication in patients with undiagnosed sensitivity to analgesics.

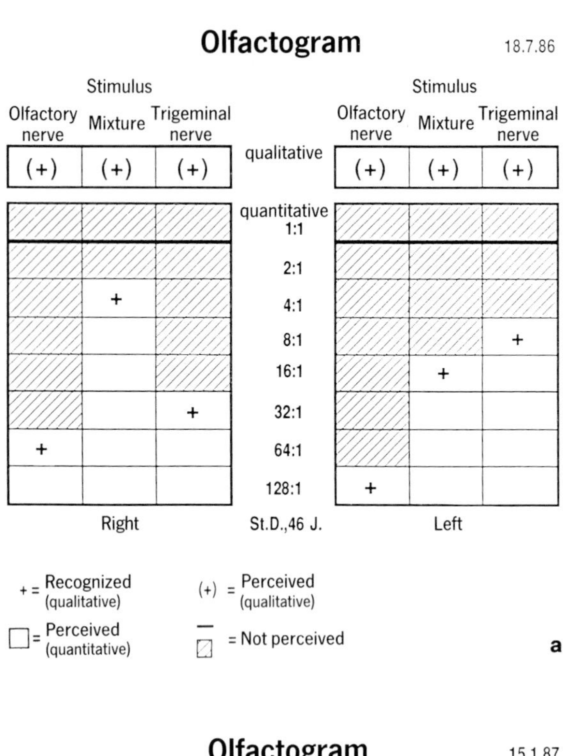

a

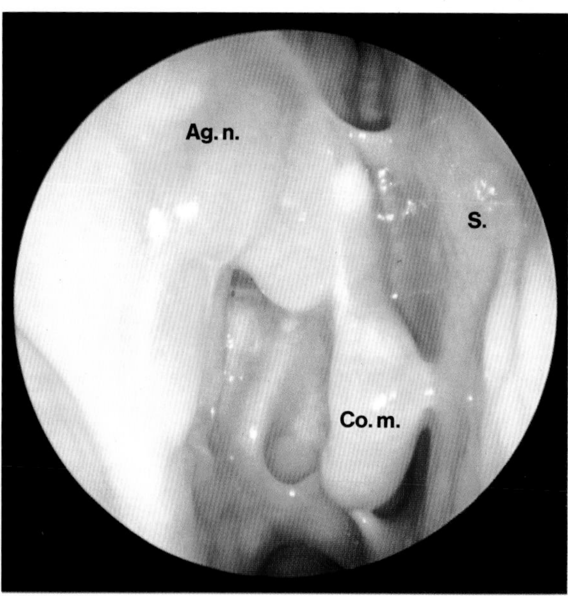

b

Olfactogram

15.1.87

Right: Olfactory nerve	Right: Mixture	Right: Trigeminal nerve	Stimulus	Left: Olfactory nerve	Left: Mixture	Left: Trigeminal nerve
(+)	(+)	(+)	qualitative	+	+	(+)
	+		quantitative 1:1	+	+	+
			2:1			
			4:1			
+		+	8:1			
			16:1			
			32:1			
			64:1			
			128:1			

Right St.D.,46 J. Left

+ = Recognized (qualitative) (+) = Perceived (qualitative)

□ = Perceived (quantitative) = Not perceived

c

Figure 7.1 Mechanical obstruction of the right olfactory cleft by bridges of scar tissue. **a** Olfactogram of hyposmia in chronic polypoid pansinusitis. **b** Five months after ethmoidectomy the olfactory cleft is again partially closed by synechiae and the patient again complains of severe hyposmia (70° telescope). **c** The sense of smell returned almost completely to normal after endoscopic division of the scar tissue.

thor's clinic, included one meningitis and brain abscess with a fatal outcome, and one case of blindness due to postoperative intraorbital bleeding. However, the brain abscess presented 2 weeks after the operation, and it is not clear whether it was already present before the operation or was caused by the operation itself.

In 1988 one fatal case due indirectly to a sphenoid operation was recorded: probing of the sphenoid cavity with a blunt suction tube before any tissue was removed led to brisk arterial bleeding causing a critical fall of blood pressure despite packing of the posterior ethmoid area. The patient died 5 days later of generalized bilateral cerebral edema despite immediate anesthesiological support and rapid transfusion. The autopsy showed that the internal carotid artery was protruding into the lumen of the sphenoid sinus, and had almost no protective bony covering. This 46-year-old patient had presented cerebral symptoms before the operation. He did not suffer intracranial bleeding, but died as a result of a chain of complications set in motion by a relatively minor injury to the wall of the sinus by the suction tube.

It is often stated that an ethmoid procedure for chronic polypoid sinusitis in asthmatics is complicated by a major asthmatic attack, so that internists sometimes advise against the operation. The author's experience with many long-standing asthmatics is quite to the contrary: practically all were almost entirely symptom-free in the first postoperative phase provided that they had prophylactic antibiotic cover but without administration of corticosteroids. Status asthmaticus only occurred in four of 220 (1.8%) ethmoid operations within the first few hours, probably because analgesics had been given to sensitive patients.

The symptoms of asthma may recur a few days later, rarely a few weeks later, and more commonly a few months later. They are probably caused by recurrent inflammation due to walling off of mucosal surfaces by scar tissue. This view is strengthened by the further resolution of the symptoms of asthma after a revision operation.

Intraoperative CSF leak due to injury to the olfactory mucosa was seen only eight times. It was not due to a perforation of the base of the skull by instruments, but rather to radical removal of polyps from the olfactory cleft with tearing of the olfactory fibers. It was permanently controlled in every case by a free mucosal graft. A late fistula was as uncommon as a late intracranial complication. The author has encountered only one mucocele of the ethmoids after intranasal ethmoidectomy, and he has never seen postoperative ozena. It was noted that 13% of patients complained of crusting, often prolonged, and 5.3% found it troublesome. However, in all cases a hyperexudative and usually purulent mucositis was found under the crusts, and never a dry atrophic mucous membrane.

8. Historical Overview

Current endoscopic surgery of the nasal sinuses derives its stimulus from two sources: intranasal surgery extending back to the nineteenth century and sinoscopy which was originally used only for diagnosis. A historical review must therefore encompass the early stages of both components. Furthermore it must not only chronicle the past but should also point the way to future developments.

Not every reference can be analyzed, because of lack of time and space, and it has therefore not always been possible to establish the priority of reporting of a technique. Moreover new ideas and practical innovations are often not published at all, or are only reported long after they have been presented at meetings and operative courses and taken up by other surgeons. It seems more important to name the paramount contributions to anatomy, pathophysiology, diagnosis and treatment that have influenced the author's concepts.

Beginnings of Intranasal Sinus Surgery

The first intranasal antral operation is usually ascribed to *von Mikulicz,* who reported *opening of the antral cavity through the middle meatus* in 1886. In 1886 *Ziem* stated that *Schaeffer* had also used this method often to simplify irrigation for the treatment of a chronic antral infection. *Claoué* used antrostomy for the same indication, and published a 10-year-personal experience in 1912.

Dahmer (1909) created a large inferior meatal antrostomy by resecting the anterior end of the inferior turbinate. He curetted the mucosa from the floor of the antrum itself, and claimed that the resulting ease of irrigation was the actual purpose of his operation. Indeed the patient could carry out the regular irrigations himself.

Other European rhinologists such as *Boenninghaus* and *Hajek* who had adopted the method of wide inferior meatal antrostomy, sometimes with resection of the head of the inferior turbinate, had declared themselves satisfied with the rapid decrease of purulent secretion after the operation (cited by *Claoué* 1912). In America in 1897, *Lothrop* carried out a wide inferior meatal antrostomy leading to resolution of suppuration due to various causes, but the antrostomy was regarded merely as a means of irrigation to control the suppuration.

Middle meatus antrostomy described by *Siebenmann* in 1899 and 1900 had the same purpose, that is the creation of an easily accessible nasoantral opening for long-term irrigation of the antral cavity by the patient himself. He proposed resection of the head of the middle turbinate, and breaking down the fontanelle with the little finger. *Zuckerkandl's* (1882) statement that this window generally remained fully patent deserves mention: it was already known at that time that the inferior meatal antrostomy easily closed again (*Lothrop* 1897). *Kubo* in 1912 expressed a preference for a middle meatal antrostomy and *Onodi* designed a perforator for this purpose in 1902. *Gerber* (1905), like Onodi, favored middle meatal antrostomy; he created the window in the middle meatus after transoral antral procedures.

Others had different preferences: for example *McBride* (1900) stated that an antrostomy lying as deeply as possible in the inferior meatus was more correct on surgical principles (for example *Halle* 1906). *King* (1935) stated that even hyperplastic sinusitis could heal after a simple antrostomy in the inferior meatus, although the radiographic contrast medium was mainly transported to the natural ostium. Thus *Lavelle* and *Harrison* in 1971 compared two series and found a higher rate of healing of chronic maxillary sinusitis with fewer complications after a middle meatal antrostomy. A list of advantages of this procedure was presented by *Bryant* in 1960. *Halle* in 1906 thought that this route of access was impractical because it lay close to the orbit.

Those who prefer middle meatal antrostomy emphasize that the physiological transport pathways of the antral cavity lead to the maxillary ostium. The credit for the photographic recording of their corkscrew course should be given to *Hilding* (1931, 1932) who also showed that carbon particles bypassed an inferior meatal antrostomy, and could leave the antral cavity and re-enter it again before finally leaving through the natural ostium. Accurate descriptions were given by *Proetz* (1941). *Messerklinger* and *Stammberger* have provided an impressive film demonstrating this process.

Hilding (1941) recommended making the antrostomy as far as possible from the ostium. Every time that he created an antral window at the maxillary ostium in the healthy antral cavity of the rabbit a persistant inflammation arose which resolved if a new ostium was created at a distance from it. He warned of the caution necessary when transferring the results of animal experiments to the surgical treatment of human disease.

The combination of two antrostomies was described by *McKenzie* (1921, 1927) and the removal of the entire medial antral wall by *Sluder* (1927) who preserved only the inferior turbinate. In 1903 *Réthi* recommended a large bimeatal perforation and removed the anterior two-thirds of the inferior turbinate.

Straatman and *Buiter* (1981) recently resurrected the old principle of fontanellotomy which had been in disuse for many decades. They have developed a precise operative technique using the endoscope, and fenestrate the posterior fontanelle under vision using a special instrument.

It is difficult to establish who was the first to surpass simple intranasal antrostomy, and who was the first to carry out *transnasal manipulations within the antral cavity* without an angled telescope.

In 1900 *Dahmer* removed chronic hyperplastic mucosa partially or sub-totally based on the concept of radical surgery. He resected the anterior third of the middle turbinate and created a wide opening from the floor of the nose up to the middle meatus, and turned a mucosal flap from the nasal wall into the opening. *Réthi* (1903) excised all the suspect tissue from the antral cavity using a sharp curette after removing the anterior two-thirds of the inferior turbinate and creating a large bimeatal window. The intracavity manipulations described by *Sturmann* (1910) are not included under this heading, although his was an intranasal procedure. He used an approach through the piriform aperture, and also resected the anterior wall of the antrum.

It can be assumed that gross lesions of the antral mucosa were removed intranasally by other surgeons through a wide antrostomy created with a punch, as *Unterberger* emphasized in 1932. However, *Schicketanz* in 1959 was the first to mention that isolated mucosal cysts could be removed via the inferior meatus. *Davison* (1969) removed polyps from the antrum using forceps and curettes, but he used the Caldwell-Luc procedure for long-standing disease. All intranasal procedures without endoscopic monitoring should be regarded as modified antrostomy, but they do not meet the criteria of mucosal microsurgery.

Intranasal ethmoid surgery with the unaided eye is also subject to the same limitations, and it is uncertain how complete, precise and safe it has been. This is doubtless the reason that the method, indications, results and operative dangers of intranasal ethmoidectomy remain controversial.

Killian described his technique of resection of the uncinate process with widening of the neighboring ostium in 1900 (Figure 8.**1**). *Halle* was probably the first surgeon with extensive personal experience of intranasal ethmoidectomy and frontal and sphenoidal sinusotomy. The important points, such as uniting all individual cells into a common cavity, difficulties with the most anterior cells, indications for chronic empyema, prevention of blind dissection, the topical use of adrenalin and the use of special curved instruments were all described in his work which appeared in 1906. In the English-speaking world, *Mosher* (1912) initiated intranasal ethmoidectomy for chronic ethmoiditis, centered upon the fine structure of the ethmoid labyrinth. He resected the

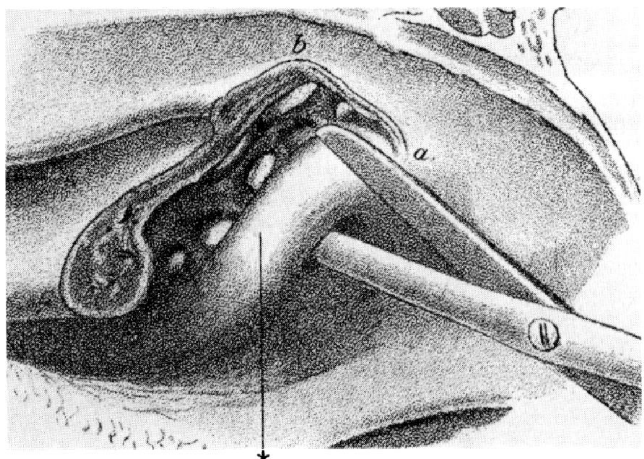

Figure 8.**1** Resection of the uncinate process (*) with the scissors to expose the ethmoid infundibulum (from *Killian*, 1900).

middle turbinate widely, thus improving the view of the sphenoid and posterior ethmoid sinuses and making the operation safer. Numerous authors adopted the same view including *Lederer* (1953), *Weille* (1959), *Yankauer* (1921), *Kidder* et al. (1974) and *Friedman* et al. (1982). It is interesting that *Gruenwald* had recommended radical amputation in 1896 and warned against a faint-hearted approach. Others such as *Pratt* (1925), *Davison* (1969), *Eichel* (1972), *Guggenheim* (1972), *Freedman* and *Kern* (1979) and *Dixon* (1983) emphasized the value of preservation of the middle turbinate to prevent the symptoms of dryness because the nasal cavity would otherwise become too large.

A similar divergence of opinions and results appears in the statements about completeness of ethmoidectomy. *Eichel* (1972) confirmed that many rhinologists term a limited opening of a few middle ethmoid cells an ethmoidectomy. Many understand the term total ethmoidectomy to include opening of the sphenoid sinus (*Dixon* 1983, *Wigand* 1981, *Eichel* 1972, *Friedman* et al. 1982) and an antrostomy as well (*Davison* 1969, *Ashikawa* et al. 1982, *Wigand* 1981). Others usually leave the sphenoid sinus unopened. *Messerklinger* (1984) and *Stammberger* (1985) open the antral cavity if indicated by the individual radiological findings. Many of these aspects can only be discussed if intranasal sinus surgery is raised to the status of precise endoscopic sinus surgery.

Early Stages of Endoscopic Sinus Surgery

The start of endoscopic sinus surgery cannot be ascribed to one date or one person. It began with endoscopic diagnosis which could be combined with the removal of tissue for histology. From this step endoscopic surgical treatment of sinus disease slowly emerged.

Draf in his monograph of 1978 reviewed the literature on endoscopic diagnosis. *Hirschmann* (1903) was the first to use a reflector, a speculum and the true endoscope for the inspection of the nose and sinuses. His endoscope was made by the firm of Reiniger, Gebbert and Schall in Berlin, based on the cystoscope designed by *Nitze* in 1897. Other pioneers of this new method refined it for endoscopic diagnosis of the nasal passages, the antrum and the nasopharynx. However, *Reichert, Valentin* and *Sargnon* rapidly extended its use to minor procedures such as cautery, opening of cysts, irrigation (*Reichert* 1902), measurement of tubal opening (*Valentin* 1903) and removal of foreign bodies (*Sargnon* 1908, *Imhofer* 1910). Until that time the endoscope had only been introduced into the antral cavity through an open dental socket or via the anterior antral wall *(Sargnon)*, but it is suspected that *Spielberg* (1922) in the USA was the first to use the intranasal route through the inferior meatus. He used the nasopharyngoscope described by *Holmes* for inspection of the antral cavity. He named the procedure antroscopy, and used it for work-up before a radical antrostomy or conservative treatment with irrigation. In 1925, *Maltz* described the sinuscope made for him by the firm of Wolf in Berlin. He also used an approach through the inferior meatus or through the anterior antral wall. In the succeeding years these and other almost exclusively rigid telescopes with proximal illumination by a very small bulb were used, almost always for diagnosis, including the removal of specimens for biopsy (*Portmann* 1925, *Watson-Williams* 1930, *Slobodnik* 1930, *Luedecke* 1932, *Christensen* 1946, *Hahn* 1955, *von Riccabona* 1955 and *Bauer* and *Wodak* 1958). The details were summarized by *Draf* in 1978.

Endoscopy of the nose and sinuses received a further stimulus by the development of better illuminated endoscopes, such as the telescopes made by *Storz* with a Hopkins rod, by Wolf with a Lumina telescope with varying angles of vision, and flexible glassfiber bundles for illumination. The intensity of light was increased sixfold, and the size of the field was expanded threefold. The recognition of disease, minor manipulations and photographic documentation were thus considerably facilitated (*Timm* 1964, *Messerklinger* 1972, *Gruenberg* 1971, *Hellmich* and *Herberhold* 1971, *Draf* 1973, 1978).

Reports of techniques allowing excision of biopsy specimens and more precise removal of tissue such as cysts followed rapidly: small grasping forceps were integrated into the endoscope (*Draf* 1973), and a two-channel instrumentation, the bimeatal antral endoscopy was described by *Hellmich* and *Herberhold.*

The improved diagnostic capability of nasal and sinus endoscopy was also taken up in other European countries: *Illum* and *Jeppesen* (1972) and *Draf* (1978), compared the reliability of radiography with sinuscopy. *Buiter* (1976) and *Terrier* (1973, 1975) demonstrated its value in recording mucosal lesions.

Reynolds and Brandow in 1975 reported intranasal antrostomy for chronic sinusitis: they drilled a small opening into the antral cavity in front of the head of the inferior turbinate under an operating microscope. They introduced a sinuscope through the anteromedial antral window, and were able to inspect the antrum, to carry out irrigation and biopsy, and to insert a Teflon button.

Terrier and *Baumann* (1976) assessed the validity of endoscopic assessment of mucosal lesions using histomorphology, and established a classification of sinusitis. The value of this diagnostic procedure is also recognized by maxillofacial surgeons (*Schmidseder* and *Lambrecht* 1977). *Draf* has extended endoscopy to the frontal and sphenoid sinuses.

Flexible fiberoptic endoscopes have been developed for the investigation of the nose and the nasal sinuses. They include the ENF-P2 rhinolaryngoscope made by Olympus Company with an external diameter of only 3.4 mm, an 85° angle of vision and a 230° arc of the visual field. It can be used for pain-free endoscopy in children and adults, but has not yet replaced the widespread use of the rigid sinus endoscope because of the poorer light output and the necessary bimanual manipulation. Its place is in diagnostic nasopharyngolaryngoscopy (*Yamashita* et al. 1984, *Lancer and Jones* 1986).

Endoscopic surgery of the nasal sinuses is defined as a range of procedures based on the use of endoscopes with an angled telescope or the microscope. The history of its development is relatively short, and coincides with the renaissance of older intranasal operative techniques that it has influenced continuously in recent times.

The beginning can be dated from 1958 when *H. Heermann* reported intranasal surgery with the use of a binocular microscope, designed especially for more precise clearance of the middle and posterior ethmoid cells and the sphenoid cavity; it also facilitated the removal of polyps from the olfactory cleft (*J. Heermann* 1982). The microscopic view into the antral cavity through the inferior meatus for removal of antral mucosa had previously been mentioned by *J. Heermann* in 1974. *Bagatella and Mazzoni* (1980) reported the advantages of the microscope using a lens of 250 or 300 mm focal length for ethmoidectomy for polyposis of the middle and posterior ethmoid cells. *Draf* (1982) also used the microscope but combined it with an angled telescope. In 1983 *Dixon* emphasized the increased safety achieved by the microscope for ethmosphenoidectomy, but had to admit that not all regions were visible with this technique.

Trans-septal trans-sphenoidal microsurgery under optical control can be regarded as intranasal sinus surgery, and is the standard procedure for pituitary adenomas.

The rigid endoscope with an angular optical axis offers clear advantages in viewing the sinuses and their recesses compared with the straight field of vision provided by the operating microscope, but it has disadvantages including the tendency to misting and soiling by the warm and bleeding operative field. A much needed technical improvement was the suction-irrigation surgical endoscope with a rotary and interchangeable angled telescope that could remain *in situ* for a long time (*Wigand* 1981). With its help, the intranasal technique of antral surgery could be extended to all forms of chronic maxillary sinusitis (*Wigand and Steiner* 1977) and to the intranasal surgery of all nasal sinuses (*Wigand* 1981).

About the same time other authors began to monitor intranasal procedures in the middle meatus using the rigid-angled telescope: for example *Buiter and Straatman* (1981) used it for fontanellotomy, and *Messerklinger* (1980, 1984) and *Stammberger* (1985, 1986) used it for both partial and total ethmoidectomy. However, both used a straight telescope without suction-irrigation. In the meantime other surgeons have described their experiences (*Dixon* 1983, *Fenner* 1984, *Friedrich* 1985, *Kennedy* 1985). Whereas flexible endoscopes have a certain value in pre- and postoperative diagnosis *Yamashita, Mertens and Rudert* 1984), they have not established themselves for intraoperative use.

The passage of fine instruments alongside the endoscope is preferable to transendoscopic instrumentation. The working channels which need to be integrated in the endoscope are too small, whereas the options for instruments introduced alongside the observation tube are much wider. Thus, the surgical laser has so far only been used by the paraendoscopic method (*Wigand* 1981, *Buiter* 1984) although specially designed flexible endoscopes may become available if the type of laser, for example Nd:Yag or argon, allows them to be used.

The abundance of new proposals appearing every year illustrates a fascinating chapter of nasal surgery in which technical developments and biological knowledge supplement each other in the perfection of medical treatment.

References

Ackermann, W.: Diagnostik und Indikation zur Revision der voroperierten Nasennebenhöhle unter besonderer Berücksichtigung von Stirnhöhlen und Siebbein. Diss., Erlangen 1984

Ashikawa, R., H. Ohkushi, T. Ohmae, T. Matsuda: Clinical Effects of the Nasal Cavity (Takahshi's Method). Auris-Nasus-Larynx (Tokyo) 9 (1982) 91–98

Ashikawa, R., Y. Kasahara, T. Matsuda, K. Katsume, S. Yoshimura: Surgical anatomy of the nasal cavity and paranasal sinuses. Auris-Nasus-Larynx (Tokyo) 9 (1982) 75–79

Baenkler, H. W., W. Schaubschläger, H. Behnsen: Antigen induced histamine release from mucosa in nasal polyposis. Clin. Otolaryngol. 8 (1983) 227–230

Baenkler, H. W., F. Dechant, W. Hosemann: In vitro histamine release from nasal mucosa upon bacterial antigens. Rhinology 25 (1987) 17–22

Bagatella, F., A. Mazzoni: Transnasal microsurgical ethmoidectomy in nasal polyposis. Rhinology 18 (1980) 25–29

Bagatella, F., C. R. Guirado: The ethmoid labyrinth: an anatomical and radiological study. Acta Otolaryngol. Suppl 403 (1983) 1–19

Bauer, E., E. Wodak: Neuerungen in der Diagnostik und Therapie der Nasennebenhöhlen. Arch. Ohr.-, Nas.- u. Kehlk.-Heilk. 171 (1958) 325–329

Berger, E.: La chirurgie du sinus sphènoidale. Octave Doin, Paris 1890

Boenninghaus, G.: Die Operationen an den Nebenhöhlen der Nase. In Katz, L., F. Blumenfeld: Handbuch der speziellen Chirurgie des Ohres und der oberen Luftwege. Kabitzsch, Leipzig 1923

Bryant, F. L.: Management of chronic maxillary sinusitis in children. J. La Med. Soc. 112 (1960) 390–393

Buiter, C. T.: Endoscopy of the upper airways. Excerpta Med. Amsterdam. American Elsevier, New York 1976

Buiter, C. T.: Endoscopic ND-Yag laser therapy in the upper airways. In P. A. R. Clement: Recent Advances in E.N.T.-Endoscopy. Sci. Soc. Med. Inform. Gent 1985

Buiter, C. T., N. J. A. Straatman: Endoscopic antrostomy in the nasal fontanelle. Rhinology 19 (1981) 17–24

Christensen, H.: Endoscopy of the maxillary sinus. Acta otolaryngol. (Stockh.) 34 (1946) 404

Claoué, R.: Empyème du sinus maxillaire gauche – infection aigue secondaire des sinus sus-nasaux gauches – accidents méningitiques – mort. Rev. Hebdom. Laryngol. 16 (1895) 805–810

Claoué, R.: Dix ans de pratique de "l'opération de Claoué" pour le traitement de la sinusite maxillaire chronique. Arch. Int. Laryngol. 33 (1912) 355–361

Conley, J. J.: The use of plastic tubing in the treatment of chronic maxillary sinusitis. Ann. Otol. 56 (1947) 678–683

Dahmer, R.: Die breite Eröffnung der Oberkieferhöhle vor der Nase mit Schleimhautplastik und persistierender Öffnung. Arch. Laryngol. Rhinol. 21 (1909) 325–333

Davison, F. W.: Intranasal surgery. Laryngoscope 79 (1969) 502–511

Dixon, F. W.: Clinical results in patients treated by intranasal ethmoidectomy. Arch. Otolaryngol. 43 (1946) 59–62

Dixon, H. S.: Microscopic sinus surgery, transnasal ethmoidectomy and sphenoidectomy. Laryngoscope 93 (1983) 440–444

Draf, W.: Wert der Sinuskopie für Klinik und Praxis. Z. Laryngol. Rhinol. 52 (1973) 890–896

Draf, W.: Die Endoskopie der Nasennebenhöhlen. Diagnostische und therapeutische Möglichkeiten. Z. Laryngol. Rhinol. 54 (1975) 209–215

Draf, W.: Endoskopie der Nasennebenhöhlen. Technik – Typische Befunde – Therapeutische Möglichkeiten. Springer, Berlin 1978

Draf, W.: Die chirurgische Behandlung entzündlicher Erkrankungen der Nasennebenhöhlen. Arch. Otorhinolaryngol. 235 (1982) 133–305; 367–377

Eckert-Möbius, A.: Endonasale Kieferhöhlenoperation. Zbl. Hals.-, Nas.- u. Ohrenheilk. 30 (1938) 642–643

Eggert, J.: Ergebnisse endonasaler Siebbeinoperationen. Diss., Erlangen 1979

Eichel, B. S.: The intranasal ethmoidectomy procedure: historical, technical and clinical considerations. Laryngoscope 82 (1972) 1806–1821

Eichel, B. S.: Revision sphenoidethmoidectomy. Laryngoscope 95 (1985) 300–304

Fehle, R.: Ergebnisse endonasaler Siebbeinoperationen unter endoskopischer Kontrolle. Diss., Erlangen 1988

Fenner, T.: Technik der endonasalen, endoskopisch kontrollierten Ethmoidektomie. ORL (Bern) 7 (1984) 190–197

Flock, H.: Sinusitis maxillaris im Kindesalter und ihre Behandlung. H.N.O. 6 (1957) 165–167

Freedman, H. M., E. B. Kern: Complications of intranasal ethmoidectomy: a review of 1000 consecutive operations (Mayo Clinic Rochester, Minn.). Laryngoscope 89 (1979) 421–432

Friedman, W. H., G. P. Katsantonis, R. G. Slavin, P. Kannel, P. Linford: Sphenoidectomy: its role in the asthmatic patient. Otolaryngol. Head Neck Surg. 90 (1982) 171–177

Friedrich, J.-P.: Sinus surgery by endoscopic guidance. In P. A. R. Clement: Recent Advances in E.N.T.-Endoscopy. Sci. Soc. Med. Inform. Brüssel 1985

Gerber: Prinzipien der Kieferhöhlenbehandlung. Arch. Laryngol. Rhinol. 17 (1905) 56–63

Golding-Wood, P. G.: Observations on petrosal and Vidion neurectomy in chronic vasomotor rhinitis. J. Laryngol. 75 (1961) 232

Grünberg, H.: Die primär chronische Sinusitis maxillaris im endoskopischen Bild. Z. Laryngol. Rhinol. 50 (1971) 813–817

Grünwald, L.: Die Lehre von den Naseneiterungen. Lehmann, München 1896

Guggenheim, P.: Present status of surgery for chronic sinusitis. Rhinology 10 (1972) 17–25

Hahn, W.: Die Anwendung des Antroskops in der Kieferheilkunde. Zahnärztl. Rdsch. 64 (1955) 175

Hajek, M.: Indikation der verschiedenen Behandlungs- und Operations-Methoden bei den entzündlichen Erkrankungen der Nebenhöhlen der Nase. Z. Hals.-, Nas.- u. Ohrenheilk. 4 (1923) 511–522

Halle, M.: Externe oder interne Operation der Nebenhöhleneiterungen. Berl. Klin. Wschr. 43 (1906) 1369–1372; 1404–1407

Halle, M.: Die intranasalen Operationen bei eitrigen Erkrankungen der Nebenhöhlen der Nase. Arch. Laryngol. Rhinol. 29 (1915) 73–112

Halle, M.: Über Therapie der Stirnhöhlenerkrankungen. Arch. Laryngol. Rhinol. 29 (1915) 466–475

Halle, M.: Nebenhöhlenoperationen. Z. Hals.-, Nas.- u. Ohrenheilk. 4 (1923) 489–510

Halle, M.: Schädigung der Zähne nach Radikaloperationen der Oberkieferhöhle. Arch. Ohr.-, Nas.- u. Kehlkopfheilk. 126 (1930) 251–259

Hartmann, A.: Atlas der Anatomie der Stirnhöhle, der vorderen Siebbeinzellen und des Ductus nasofrontalis. Bergmann, Wiesbaden 1900

Heermann, H.: Über endonasale Chirurgie unter Verwendung des binoculären Mikroskopes. Arch. Ohr.-, Nas.- u. Kehlkopfheilk. 171 (1958) 295–297

Heermann, J.: Endonasale mikrochirurgische Resektion der Mukosa des Sinus maxillaris. Laryngol. Rhinol. Otol. 53 (1974) 938–942

Heermann, J.: Endonasale mikrochirurgische Siebbeinausräumung bei Blutdrucksenkung am halbsitzenden Patienten. H.N.O. 30 (1982) 180–185

Hellmich, S., C. Herberhold: Technische Verbesserungen der Kieferhöhlen-Endoskopie. Arch. Ohr.-, Nas.- u. Kehlkopfheilk. 199 (1971) 678–683

Hilding, A.: Physiology of drainage of nasal mucous: experimental work on accessory sinuses. Amer. J. Physiol. 100 (1932) 664

Hilding, A. C.: Experimental sinus surgery: effects of operation windows on normal sinuses. Ann. Otol. Rhinol. Laryngol. 50 (1941) 379–392

Hilding, A. C.: The role of ciliary action in production of pulmonary atelectasis, vacuum in the paranasal sinuses, and in otitis media. Ann. Otol. 52 (1944) 816–833

Hilding, A. C.: Physiologic basis of nasal operations. Calif. Med. 72 (1950) 103–107

Hirschmann, A.: Über Endoskopie der Nase und deren Nebenhöhlen. Eine neue Untersuchungsmethode. Arch. Laryngol. Rhinol. 14 (1903) 195–202

Hosemann, W.: Mukoziliärer Transport der Nasennebenhöhlenschleimhaut nach Kieferhöhlenfensterung. Arch. Otorhinolaryngol. Suppl. II 245–246 (1985)

Hosemann, W., M. E. Wigand: Örtliche Unterschiede im Gewebebild der chronisch-hyperplastischen Nasennebenhöhlenschleimhaut. H.N.O. 33 (1985) 311–315

Hosemann, W., M. E. Wigand, R. Fehle, J. Sebastian, D. L. Diepgen: Ergebnisse endonasaler Siebbein-Operationen bei chronisch-diffuser Sinusitis paranasalis. H.N.O. 36 (1988) 54–59

Hosemann, W., M. E. Wigand, J. Nikol: Klinische und funktionelle Aspekte der endonasalen Kieferhöhlen-Operation. HNO (in press)

Illum, P., F. Jeppesen: Sinoscopy: endoscopy of the maxillary sinus. Technique, common and rare findings. Acta Otolaryngol. (Stockh.) 73 (1972) 506–512

Imhofer, R.: Entfernung eines Fremdkörpers aus der Kieferhöhle mit Hilfe der Endoskopie. Z. Laryngol. Rhinol. 2 (1910) 429–437

Jahnke, V.: Ultrastruktur der normalen und allergischen Nasenschleimhaut. Fortschr. Med. 89 (1971) 691

Kennedy, D.: Functional endoscopic sinus surgery. Arch. Otolaryngol. 111 (1985) 643–649

Kidder, T. M., R. J. Toohill, J. D. Unger, R. H. Lehmann: Ethmoid sinus surgery. Laryngoscope 84 (1974) 1525–1534

Killian, G.: Die Krankheiten der Kieferhöhle. In P. Heymann: Handbuch der Laryngologie und Rhinologie, III. Band, 2. Hälfte. Hölder, Wien 1900 (S. 1004–1096)

Killian, G.: Die Nebenhöhlen der Nase in ihren Lagebeziehungen zu den Nachbarorganen. Fischer, Jena 1903

King, E.: A clinical study of the functioning of the maxillary sinus mucosa. Ann. Otol. 44 (1935) 480–482

Kubo, J.: Über die supraturbinale Eröffnung bei der Sinusitis maxillaris chronica. Arch. Laryngol. Rhinol. 26 (1912) 351–356

Lancer, J. M., A. S. Jones: The flexible fiberoptic rhinolaryngoscope. Brit. Med. J. 293 (1986) 712–713

Lang, J.: Klinische Anatomie der Nase, Nasenhöhle und Nebenhöhlen. Thieme, Stuttgart 1988.

Lavelle, R. J., M. S. Harrison: Infection of the maxillary sinus: the case for the middle meatal antrostomy. Laryngoscope 81 (1971) 90–106

Lederer, F. L.: Diseases of the Ear, Nose and Throat, 6th ed. Davis, Philadelphia 1953

Legler, U.: Die Lateroposition der unteren Muschel – ein einfacher Eingriff zur Verbesserung der Luftdurchlässigkeit der Nase. Z. Laryngol. Rhinol. Otol. 49 (1970) 386–391

Lenz, H., H. Preußler: Histologische Veränderungen des respiratorischen Schleimhautepithels der unteren Nasenmuscheln nach Argon-Laserstrichkarbonisation (Laser-Muschel-Kaustik) bei Rhinopathia vasomotorica. Laryngol. Rhinol. Otol. 65 (1986) 438–444

Lothrop, H. A.: Empyema of the antrum of Highmore: a new operation for the care of obstinate cases. Boston Med. Surg. J. 136 (1897) 455–462

Lüdecke, E.: Die verbesserte Antroskopie. Z. Hals.-, Nas.- u. Ohrenheilk. 31 (1932) 507–513

Maltz, M.: New instruments: the sinuscope. Laryngoscope 35 (1925) 805–811

McBride, P.: The indications for the intranasal treatment in diseases of the ear. Brit. Med. J. (1900) 636–638

Messerklinger, W.: Über die Drainage der menschlichen Nasennebenhöhlen unter normalen und pathologischen Bedingungen. 1. Mitteilung. Mschr. Ohrenheilk. 100 (1966) 56–68

Messerklinger, W.: Technik und Möglichkeiten der Nasenendoskopie. H.N.O. 20 (1972) 133–135

Messerklinger, W.: Endoscopy of the nose. Urban & Schwarzenberg, München 1978

Messerklinger, W.: Das Infundibulum ethmoidale und seine entzündlichen Erkrankungen. Arch. Otolaryngol. 222 (1979) 11–22

Messerklinger, W.: Diagnostische und therapeutische Möglichkeiten des niedergelassenen HNO-Arztes bei der Sinusitis. In H. Ganz: HNO-Praxis Heute 1. Springer, Berlin 1980

Messerklinger, W.: Rezidivierende Rhinosinusitis. Endoskopische Diagnose und Chirurgie. Film 1984

Messerklinger, W.: Die Rolle der lateralen Nasenwand in der Pathogenese, Diagnose und Therapie der rezidivierenden und chronischen Rhinosinusitis. Laryngol. Rhinol. Otol. 66 (1987) 293–299

Mikulicz, J.: Zur operativen Behandlung des Emphyems der Highmorshöhle. Arch. Klin. Chir. 34 (1887) 626–634

Morgenstein, K. M., M. K. Krieger: Experiences in middle turbinectomy. Laryngoscope 90 (1980) 1596–1603

Mosher, H. P.: The applied anatomy and the intra-nasal surgery of the ethmoidal labyrinth. Trans. Amer. Laryngol. Ass. 34 (1912) 25–39

Mosher, H. P.: The surgical anatomy of the ethmoidal labyrinth. Amer. Acad. Ophthalmol. Otolaryngol. (1929) 376–410

Naumann, H. H.: Die Mikrozirkulation in der Nasenschleimhaut. Thieme, Stuttgart 1961

Naumann, H. H.: Gedanken zum gegenwärtigen Stand der Stirnhöhlenchirurgie. Z. Laryngol. Rhinol. 40 (1961) 733–749

Naumann, H. H.: Neue Trends in der Nebenhöhlen-Chirurgie? Laryngol. Rhinol. Otol. 66 (1987) 57–59

Naumann, H. H., W. H. Naumann: Kurze Pathophysiologie der Nase und ihrer Nebenhöhlen. In J. Berendes, R. Link, F. Zöllner: Hals-Nasen-Ohrenheilkunde in Praxis und Klinik, Bd. I. Thieme, Stuttgart 1977 (S. 10.1–10.55)

Nitze, M.: Erste Mitteilung eines Cystoskops. Wien. Med. Wschr. 29 (1879) 649–652; 896–910

Onodi, A.: Die Eröffnung der Kieferhöhle im mittleren Nasengang. Arch. Laryngol. Rhinol. 14 (1903) 154–160

Panis, R., W. Thumfart, M. E. Wigand: Die endonasale Kieferhöhlenoperation mit endoskopischer Kontrolle als Therapie der chronisch rezidivierenden Sinusitis im Kindesalter. H.N.O. 27 (1979) 256–259

Polyak: Über die Technik der intranasalen Dacryocystostomie. Verh. Ver. dtsch. Laryngol., Würzburg 1913, XX, 194–202

Portmann, G.: Le sinuso-pharyngoscope. Rev. Laryngol. (Bordeaux) 46 (1925) 387

Pratt, J. A.: The present status of the intranasal ethmoid operation. Arch. Otolaryngol. 1 (1925) 42–50

Proetz, A. W.: Essays on the Applied Physiology of the Nose. Annals Publ. St. Louis 1941

Reichert, M.: Über eine neue Untersuchungsmethode der Oberkieferhöhle mittels des Antroskops. Berl. Klin. Wschr. 39 (1902) 401–404; 478

Réthi; L.: Zur Radikaloperation hartnäckiger Kieferhöhlenempyeme von der Nase her. Wien. Med. Wschr. 53 (1903) 545–548

Reynolds, W. V., E. C. Brandow Jr.: Recent advances in microsurgery of the maxillary antrum. Acta Otolaryngol. 80 (1975) 161–166

Sargnon: De l'endoscopie directe du sinus maxillaire par les fistules. Arch. Int. Laryngol. (1908) 705–710

Scheler, F.: Diagnostik der Sinusitis maxillaris und Resultate der endonasalen Kieferhöhlen-Operation. Diss., Erlangen 1980

Schickedanz, H. W.: Indikationen zur Kieferhöhlenfensterung im unteren Nasengang und deren Ergebnisse. Z. Laryngol. Rhinol. 38 (1959) 240–249

Schmidseder, R., T. Lambrecht: Anwendungsmöglichkeiten und Indikationen der Sinuskopie aus zahnärztlicher und kieferchirurgischer Sicht. Österr. Zahnärztetagung, Villach 1977

Sebastian, J.: Endoskopische Nachuntersuchung nach endonasalen Siebbein-Operationen bei chronisch-diffuser Sinusitis paranasalis. Diss., Erlangen (in preparation)

Siebenmann, F.: Beitrag zur Lehre von der Entstehung und Heilung kombinierter Nebenhöhleneiterungen der Nase. Mschr. Ohrenheilk. 46 (1912) 656–661

Siebenmann, G.: Die Behandlung der chronischen Eiterung der

Highmorshöhle durch Resektion der oberen Hälfte (Pars supraturbinalis) ihrer nasalen Wand. Münch. Med. Wschr. 47 (1900) 31–33

Slobodnik, M.: Die direkte Untersuchung der Kieferhöhle durch Endoskopie. Z. Laryngol. Rhinol. 19 (1930) 437–443

Sluder, G.: Nasal Neurology: Headache and Eye Disorders. Kimpton, London 1927

Spielberg, W.: Antroscopy of the maxillary sinus. Laryngoscope 32 (1922) 441–443

Stammberger, H.: Unsere endoskopische Operationstechnik der lateralen Nasenwand – Ein endoskopisch-chirurgisches Konzept zur Behandlung entzündlicher Nasennebenhöhlenerkrankungen. Laryngol. Rhinol. Otol. 64 (1985) 559–566

Stammberger, H.: Endoscopic surgery for mycotic and chronic recurring sinusitis. Ann. Otol. Rhinol. Laryngol. Suppl. 11 (1985) 94

Stammberger, H.: Endoscopic endonasal surgery: concepts in treatment of recurring rhinosinusitis, part I: anatomic and pathophysiologic considerations; part II: technique. Otolaryngol. Head Neck Surg. 94 (1986) 143–156

Stammberger, H., S. J. Zinreich, W. Kopp, D. W. Kennedy, M. E. Johns, A. E. Rosenbaum: Zur operativen Behandlung der chronisch-rezidivierenden Sinusitis – Caldwell Luc versus funktionelle endoskopische Technik. H.N.O. 35 (1987) 93–105

Straatman, N. J. A., C. T. Buiter: Endoscopic surgery of the nasal fontanel. Arch. Otolaryngol. 107 (1981) 290–293

Sturmann, D.: Erfahrungen mit meiner intranasalen Freilegung der Oberkieferhöhle. Arch. Laryngol. Rhinol. 23 (1910) 143–152

Teatini, G.: Personal communication, in "Corso Chirurgia dei Seni Paranasali". Ferrara 1980

Teatini, G., G. Simonetti, U. Salvolini, W. Masala, F. Meloni, F. Rovasio, G. L. Dedola: Computed tomography of the ethmoid labyrinth and adjacent structures. Ann. Otol. Rhinol. Laryngol. 96 (1987) 239–250

Terrahe, K., P. Drücke, K. P. Backwinkel: Die terminale Strombahn der Nasenschleimhaut bei hyperergischer Sofortreaktion. Arch. Ohr.-, Nas.- u. Kehlkopfheilk. 197 (1970) 265–277

Terrahe, K., K. Mündnich: Gefahren und Komplikationen bei der transmaxillären Siebbein-Keilbeinhöhlenoperation. Laryng. Rhinol. Otol. 53 (1974) 313–320

Terrier, F., G. Terrier, D. Rüfenacht, J.-P. Friedrich, W. Weber: Die Anatomie der Siebbeinregion: topographische, radiologische und endoskopische Leitstrukturen. Ther. Umsch. 44 (1987) 75–85

Terrier, G.: L'endoscopie rhino-sinusale. Rev. Méd. Suisse Rom. 93 (1973) 231

Terrier, G.: L'endoscopie du sinus maxillare en pathologie traumatique et infectieuse. Ther. Umsch. 32 (1975) 628

Terrier, G., R. P. Baumann, J. M. Pidoux: Endoscopic and histopathological observations of chronic maxillary sinusitis. Rhinology 14 (1976) 129–132

Timm, C.: Die Modifikation der Nebenhöhlendiagnostik und -therapie durch Anwendung der Sinuskopie. Arch. Ohr.-, Nas.- u. Kehlkopfheilk. 185 (1965) 776–783

Tos, M., C. Mogensen, Z. Novotny: Quantitative histology of the normal ethmoidal sinus. ORL 40 (1978) 172–180

Toti, E.: Dacryocystorhinostomia. Clin. Med. Firenze 33 (1904)

Unterberger, S.: Konservative Kieferhöhlenoperation und Zähne. Z. Laryngol. Rhinol. 22 (1932) 467–474

Valentin, A.: Die cystoskopische Untersuchung des Nasenrachens oder Salpingoskopie. Arch. Laryngol. Rhinol. 13 (1903) 409–420

von Riccabona, A.: Erfahrungen mit der Kieferhöhlenendoskopie. Arch. Ohr.-, Nas.- u. Kehlkopfheilk. 167 (1955) 359–365

Waller, G., M. Weidenbecher, H.-J. Pesch, H. Baenkler: Vergleichende klinische, histomorphologische und immunologische Untersuchungen zur Ätiologie der Polyposis nasi et sinuum. Laryngol. Rhinol. Otol. 55 (1976) 174–178

Watson-Williams, P.: A new endo-rhinoscope or salpingoscope. Zbl. HNO 14 (1930) 855

Weigand, I. G.: Beeinflussung des Asthma bronchiale durch die chirurgische Sanierung von Infektionen der oberen Luftwege. Diss., Erlangen 1983

Weille, F. L.: A practical technique for intranasal ethmoidectomy and an evaluation of its usefulness. Laryngoscope 69 (1959) 449–462

West, J. M.: Eine Fensterresektion des Ductus naso-lacrimalis in Fällen von Stenose. Arch. Laryng. Rhinol. 24 (1911) 62–64

Wigand, M. E.: Eine einfache, knorpelerhaltende Methode der Septumkorrektur. Wien. Med. Wschr. 128 (1978) 376–377

Wigand, M. E.: Ein Saug-Spül-Endoskop für die transnasale Chirurgie der Nasennebenhöhlen und der Schädelbasis. H.N.O. 29 (1981) 102–103

Wigand, M. E.: Transnasale, endoskopische Chirurgie der Nasennebenhöhlen bei chronischer Sinusitis. I. Ein biomechanisches Konzept der Schleimhautchirurgie. H.N.O. 29 (1981) 215–221

Wigand, M. E.: Transnasale, endoskopische Chirurgie der Nasennebenhöhlen bei chronischer Sinusitis. II. Die endonasale Kieferhöhlen-Operation. H.N.O. 29 (1981) 263–269

Wigand, M. E.: Transnasale, endoskopische Chirurgie der Nasennebenhöhlen bei chronischer Sinusitis. III. Die endonasale Siebbeinausräumung. H.N.O. 29 (1981) 287–293

Wigand, M. E.: Transnasal endoscopical surgery of the anterior skull base. Proc. XIIth ORL World Congr., Budapest, Hungary, 1981, Publ. House Hung. Acad. Sci. (1981) 137–140

Wigand, M. E.: Transnasal ethmoidectomy under endoscopical control. Rhinology 19 (1981) 7–15

Wigand, M. E.: Renaissance des opérations transnasales des sinus par léndoscopie chirurgicale. J. Franc. d'Oto-rhino-laryngol. 5 (1982) 319–322

Wigand, M. E.: Aktuelles in der Otorhinolaryngologie 1982: Transnasale Chirurgie der Nasennebenhöhlen und der vorderen Schädelbasis. Österr. HNO-Kongreß, Bad Kleinkirchheim 1982. Thieme, Stuttgart 1983

Wigand, M. E., W. Hosemann: Endoscopic Ethmoidectomy for Chronic Sinubronchitis. In: E. Myers: New Dimensions in Otorhinolaryngology – Head and Neck Surgery, Vol. 1. Elsevier, Amsterdam (1985) 549–552

Wigand, M. E., W. Steiner: Endonasale Kieferhöhlenoperation mit endoskopischer Kontrolle. Laryngol. Rhinol. Otol. 56 (1977) 421–425

Wigand, M. E., W. Steiner, M. P. Jaumann: Endonasal sinus surgery with endoscopical control: from radical operation to rehabilitation of the mucosa. Endoscopy 10 (1978) 255–260

Wittmaack, K.: Über die normale und die pathologische Pneumatisation des Schläfenbeines einschließlich ihrer Beziehungen zu den Mittelohrerkrankungen. Fischer, Jena 1918

Yamashita, K., J. Mertens, H. Rudert: Die flexible Fiberendoskopie in der HNO-Heilkunde. H.N.O. 32 (1984) 378–384

Yankauer, S.: The complete sphenoethmoid operation. Laryngoscope 31 (1921) 831–842

Ziem: Über Bedeutung und Behandlung der Naseneiterungen. Mschr. Ohrenheilk. 20 (1886) 33–43; 79–84; 137–147

Zuckerkandl, E.: Normale und pathologische Anatomie der Nasenhöhle und ihrer pneumatischen Anhänge. W. Braumüller, Wien, Leipzig, Bd. I. 1882, B

Index

VANDERBILT UNIVERSITY
3 0081 027 803 885